BRITISH MEDICAL BULLETIN
VOLUME 63   2002

New developments in hearing and balance

Scientific Editors

Brian C J Moore

Jonathan Ashmore

Mark Haggard

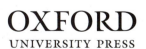

OXFORD

UNIVERSITY PRESS

PUBLISHED FOR THE BRITISH COUNCIL BY
OXFORD UNIVERSITY PRESS

OXFORD UNIVERSITY PRESS
Great Clarendon Street, Oxford OX2 6DP, UK

British Library Cataloguing in Publication Data
A catalogue record for this book is available from the British Library
ISBN 0–19–851625–8
ISSN 0007–1420

Subscription information *British Medical Bulletin* is published quarterly on behalf of The British Council. Subscription rates for 2002 are £170/$290 for four volumes, each of one issue. Prices include distribution; the British Medical Bulletin is distributed by surface mail within Europe, by air freight and second class post within the USA*, and by various methods of air-speeded delivery to all other countries. Subscription orders, single issue orders and enquiries regarding volumes from 2001 onwards should be sent to:

Oxford University Press, Great Clarendon Street, Oxford OX2 6DP, UK
(Tel +44 (0)1865 353907; Fax +44(0)1865 353485; E-mail: jnl.orders@oup.co.uk

*Periodicals postage paid at Rahway, NJ. US Postmaster: Send address changes to *British Medical Bulletin*, c/o Mercury Airfreight International Ltd, 365 Blair Road, Avenel, NJ 07001, USA.

Back numbers of titles published 1996–2000 (see inside back cover) are available from The Royal Society of Medicine Press Limited, 1 Wimpole St, London W1G 0AE, UK. (Tel. +44 (0)20 7290 2921; Fax +44 (0)20 7290 2929); www.rsm.ac.uk/pub/bmb/htm).

Pre-1996 back numbers: Contact Jill Kettley, Subscriptions Manager, Harcourt Brace, Foots Cray, Sidcup, Kent DA14 5HP (Tel +44 (0)20 8308 5700; Fax +44 (0)20 8309 0807).

This journal is indexed, abstracted and/or published online in the following media: Adonis, Biosis, BRS Colleague (full text), Chemical Abstracts, Colleague (Online), Current Contents/ Clinical Medicine, Current Contents/Life Sciences, Elsevier BIOBASE/Current Awareness in Biological Sciences, EMBASE/Excerpta Medica, Index Medicus/Medline, Medical Documentation Service, Reference Update, Research Alert, Science Citation Index, Scisearch, SIIC-Database Argentina, UMI (Microfilms)

Editorial services and typesetting by BA & GM Haddock, Ford, Midlothian EH37 5RE
Printed in Great Britain by Bell & Bain Ltd, Glasgow, Scotland.

BRITISH MEDICAL BULLETIN Volume 63 2002

New developments in hearing and balance

Scientific Editors: Brian C J Moore, Jonathan Ashmore, Mark Haggard

http://www.bmb.oupjournals.org

Acknowledgements

The planning committee for this issue of the British Medical Bulletin was chaired by **Mark Haggard** and also included **Jonathan Ashmore, David Baguley, Andrew Forge, Guy Richardson** and **Matthew Holley.**

The British Council and Oxford University Press are most grateful to the Scientific Editors **Brian CJ Moore, Jonathan Ashmore** and **Mark Haggard** for their expert assistance in the completion of this volume.

Material Disclaimer

Drug Disclaimer

Preface

It is now 15 years since the last review on hearing was published in the *British Medical Bulletin*. The previous review had been published over 30 years earlier. The shortening interval reflects the pace of scientific communication, but it also reflects the spectacular growth in what we know about hearing mechanisms and the prospects for treating deafness. That the *British Medical Bulletin* has chosen to devote this issue to hearing is a signal of the recognition that hearing – or rather the consequences of a lack of hearing – is one of the biomedical areas where UK research has made major contributions. In countries with ageing populations and lower mortality from disease, we should like to think that the fruits of current hearing research are already making a really significant contribution to improving the quality of life of their people.

In this issue we have tried to bring together a balance of chapters that reflect the startling progress in understanding hearing. As anticipated in the preface to the 1987 *British Medical Bulletin* issue on hearing, there has been further movement in the field away from the strict diagnosis of hearing loss towards the basic understanding of both peripheral and perceptual mechanisms. This is not to imply that diagnosis and management will be removed from the centre stage of audiology, for (as shown in several chapters) these remain the core skills in the clinic. There is, however, a growing appreciation that studying the basic mechanisms of hearing and hearing loss can form the only rational basis for treatment. Progress in the field has depended on both the application of new technologies and on new treatment methods. To carry this programme forward requires, as it has done over the past three decades in the UK, groupings of researchers, clinicians and healthcare workers interacting and exchanging their particular expertise.

The new element is molecular biology. No one could have failed to notice the explosive development of molecular biological technologies over the past decade. These have provided techniques that are particularly well matched to understanding hearing mechanisms where the amount of tissue is very small. The tools of molecular genetics have been particularly successful in finding the causes of hereditary hearing losses (see the chapter by Bitner-Glindzicz). One of the more surprising consequences is that the intricacies of the cochlea are now known to a much wider scientific community. The identification in 1994 of the gene mutation responsible for a hereditary hearing loss (Usher type 1B) and recognition of the gene product as an unexpected motor molecule (myosin 7a) introduced the inner ear as an important system to cell biologists. This work, the outcome of a collaborative project by UK hearing researchers, may have been instrumental in bringing a new generation of researchers into the studying hearing. It also means that the inner ear, as a topic for study, has moved into the student textbooks from where it had been banished for a very long time.

Although some of the methods of molecular biology were forecast in the 1987 review, it was hard to anticipate how all-pervasive the molecular technologies would become. We have moved from what was then called a biochemistry of hearing, where the techniques were poorly adapted to the very small amounts of tissue available in the auditory system, to a molecular biology and even a nanotechnology of hearing where single molecules, the natural units of the inner ear, can be investigated. It is difficult sometimes to appreciate the scale of this change in viewpoint. The way in which mouse and animal models of hearing and balance loss have informed human hearing loss has been a major theme of the past decade. These topics are taken up in the chapters by Forge and Wright, Ashmore and Richardson. With the detailed maps of human and mouse genomes reaching completion we are now in a 'post-genomic' era where the interactions between proteins, and not just the gene sequence, becomes the goal. A major current that has run through the past 15 years has been how to restore hearing using biological rather than surgical repair. Despite a number of inflated claims and false starts, there are now cautious signs of progress. These are described in the chapters of Raphael and of Holley.

As well as concentrating on the very small, hearing research has taken advantage of the emerging whole brain imaging technologies. It has been clear that new diagnostic techniques in neuro-otology would open up major new avenues of investigation. The use of fMRI and PET are now almost taken for granted in studies of brain function, but for obvious reasons (MRI scanners produce sound levels in excess of 110 dB) the study of auditory function has lagged behind the understanding of vision and of other senses. Largely due to the efforts of workers in the UK at Nottingham the situation has now been improved and, as described by Palmer in this volume, we are now engaged in understanding the neural basis of auditory cognitive tasks. Bronstein and a pioneer user of imaging the UK, Griffiths, describe the clinical opportunities in the relatively under-explored areas of neuro-otological symptoms and of central pathologies. Development of the central auditory system is a recurrent theme in hearing research. How experience affects the central connections and how central auditory processing affects the development of language are taken up in the chapters by Moore and by Bailey and Snowling. Long-standing questions about auditory development have their roots in the study of the plasticity and form of brain connections that are problems in neuroscience. In contrast, tinnitus research, reviewed by Baguley, contains so many novel and competing proposals about the basic mechanisms that it is hard to avoid the conclusion that this is a field set for an explosive growth over the next few years.

This volume of the *British Medical Bulletin* is necessarily selective of topics for reasons of space. We have tried to choose several areas where there have been significant changes and improvements in audiological technology. Ramsden surveys the recent developments in cochlear implants and the future possibilities of placing the implant stimulus more centrally. Despite these newer developments, there has been some radical rethinking of how traditional hearing aids work and how best to optimise their use. These topics are described by Moore and by Gatehouse. The discussion seems appropriate as we have now reached a time where digital hearing aids, in view of the size of the market, should be cheap enough to be classified as consumer electronics, on a par with many other 'hi tech' items we take for granted. The year 2003 is the 25th anniversary of the original description of oto-acoustic emissions by Kemp and his chapter develops the current thinking behind their use for early screening of deafness.

Standing back from research carried out in the UK, it seems clear that, by any international standards, the UK hearing research community has made a major contribution. This is no reason to be complacent. We must recognise that the resources devoted to hearing research in this country are very modest. For those of us who have sat on funding committees, the position of hearing research needs continuous defence against claims that it is a very small and specialist field and therefore cannot be sustained. The Medical Research Council has however maintained strong support for the Institute of Hearing Research at Nottingham. The MRC and the Wellcome Trust also retain a fellowship programme that supports clinically qualified individuals who wish to build bridges to the basic biomedical research communities. The major change over the past 15 years has been the growth of funding for hearing research projects from charities. These include the major player, the Wellcome Trust, as well as the critically important but more modest charities such as Defeating Deafness, the Royal National Institute for Deaf People and the British Tinnitus Association. The support for focused hearing research on a major scale has so far been indirect, with the Wellcome Trust, whose annual spend surpasses the MRC, funding a new Centre for Auditory Research at UCL as part of the joint infrastructure fund (JIF) designed to maintain UK university research.

As every science funding cycle reveals, communities of research workers are fragile. Movement of just a few key research teams nationally and internationally can make or break a research speciality. These are interesting times. After 25 years as Director, Mark Haggard has stepped down at the MRC's Institute of Hearing Research at Nottingham and David Moore has become its new director. UK research may thus be at a watershed where new directions may soon be established. A further driver for mobility has been the recent three UK University Research Assessment

Exercises, where universities have recruited aggressively to build up research expertise. On the whole this has not redistributed hearing research significantly although there has been some movement to the south-east over the past 5 years. Whatever national movements are apparent, there are now extensive collaborations and exchanges of expertise and researchers between the UK and centres in Europe and in the US. If there is one lesson to be learnt from the past decade it is that hearing research depends on national and international free collaboration between its scientists.

This volume tries to give an overall picture of activity in what has been a dynamic period in the field. The aim has been to convey some of the scientific excitement in a way which provides pointers to the past literature and to future developments. We hope this issue of the *British Medical Bulletin* can be used as a resource that points not only to what is already known but as a signpost to the key hearing laboratories, developments and opportunities of the next decade.

Jonathan Ashmore

The molecular architecture of the inner ear

Andrew Forge and **Tony Wright**

UCL Centre for Auditory Research and Institute of Laryngology & Otology, University College London, London, UK

The inner ear is structurally complex. A molecular description of its architecture is now emerging from the use of contemporary methods of cell and molecular biology, and from studies of ontogenetic development. With the application of clinical and molecular genetics, it has now become possible to identify genes associated with inherited, non-syndromic deafness and balance dysfunction in humans and in mice. This work is providing new insights into how the tissues of the inner ear are built to perform their tasks, and into the pathogenesis of a range of inner ear disorders.

The inner ear provides sensory information relating to hearing (from the cochlea) and balance (from the vestibular system). It comprises a series of interconnected fluid-filled membranous canals (the membranous labyrinth) inside bony channels at the base of the skull (Fig. 1). In

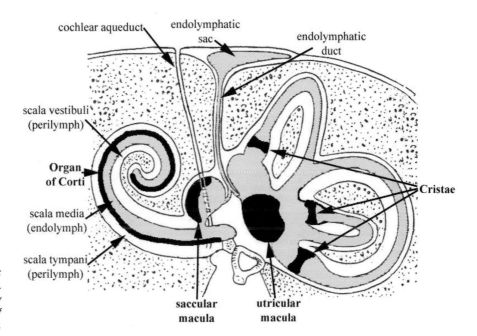

Fig. 1 Diagram of the inner ear in cross-section of the human temporal bone.

Correspondence to:
Prof. Andrew Forge, UCL Centre for Auditory Research, Institute of Laryngology & Otology, 330–332 Gray's Inn Road, London WC1X 8EE, UK

humans and higher primates, the bony labyrinthine channels are in the temporal bone, the hardest bone in the body, which is fused with the skull. In other mammals, the inner ear is contained within an auditory bulla that can be isolated quite easily. The fluid inside the lumen of the membranous channels is endolymph. This has an unusual composition for an extracellular fluid. It has a high potassium ion (K^+) concentration (~140 mM) but is low in sodium ions (Na^+)[1]. In the cochlea, but not the vestibular system, endolymph also has a high positive electrical potential, the endocochlear potential (EP), of around +80 mV. The fluid that fills the bony channels is perilymph. Perilymph is close to normal extracellular fluid and has a high Na^+/low K^+ composition. The border between the two fluids lies at the level of the junctions between the epithelial cells that surround the endolymphatic spaces. Maintenance of this permeability barrier is essential for function of the inner ear.

Three types of epithelium surround the endolymphatic compartment: sensory epithelia, ion transporting epithelia, and relatively unspecialised epithelia. The sensory epithelium of the cochlea is the organ of Corti, a narrow spiral of cells. The vestibular system of mammals contains five sensory epithelial sheets: the maculae of the utricle and saccule, and the three cristae, one in each of the semi-circular canals. Sensory epithelia are composed of sensory hair cells and accessory supporting cells (Fig. 2A). Each hair cell is surrounded and separated from its neighbours by supporting cells so that no two hair cells contact each other. The sensory epithelium is covered by an acellular extracellular matrix structure: the tectorial membrane in the cochlea, the otolithic membranes of macular organs, and the cupulae of the cristae. The hair cells derive their name from the organised bundle of rigid projections at their apical surface (Fig. 2B,C). Deflection of the hair bundle caused by either sound waves or changes in head position modulates the flow of K^+ ions from endolymph through the hair cells, altering the hair cell's resting electrical potentials and exciting hair cell activity. Hair cells are thus mechanotranducers converting a mechanical stimulus (movement) into an electrical signal. The ion transporting epithelia, the stria vascularis of the cochlea (Fig. 3A,D) and the dark cell regions of the vestibular system, are involved in active (energy consuming) ion transport necessary to maintain the unusual endolymph composition. The less specialised epithelia, Reissner's membrane in the cochlea (Fig. 3A) and the epithelium of the roof of the saccule, utricle, ampullae of the semi-circular canals and the semi-circular canals, form permeability barriers separating the fluid spaces. Rupture of these membranes would be expected to result in fluid mixing and physiological dysfunction. It is thought this event may occur to Reissner's membrane in Menière's syndrome. These simple epithelia will not be discussed further. What follows is a selective account of some details of sensory epithelia generally and then of the organ of Corti and stria vascularis of the mammalian cochlea more specifically.

Hair cells

The hair bundle and cuticular plate

The hair bundle is formed of rows of stereocilia that increase in height in one particular direction across the bundle, and a single kinocilium located behind the row of longest stereocilia (Fig. 2B,C). Stereocilia are

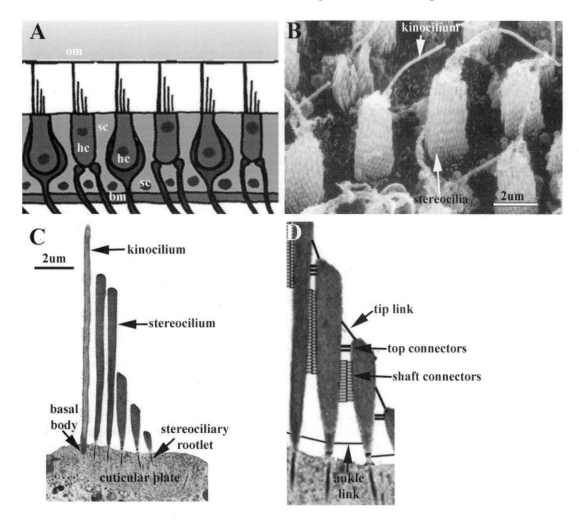

Fig. 2 General features of hair cell containing sensory epithelia. (**A**) Diagram to illustrate the general organisation of a mechanotransducing epithelium of the inner ear (in this case a mammalian macula). hc, hair cell; sc, supporting cell; bm, basement membrane; om, overlying extracellular matrix (otoconial membrane in the maculae). (**B**) The apical surface of a sensory epithelium (mammalian utricular macula) as viewed by scanning electron microscopy, showing organised hair bundles on the hair cells. Each hair cell is separated from its neighbour by intervening supporting cells the surfaces of which are covered with microvilli. (**C**) The apical structures of a hair cell in the mammalian utricle. The thin section in a composite montage image illustrates the general features and organisation. (**D**) Interstereociliary cross-links in diagrammatic representation. The thicknesses of the various links are not drawn to scale.

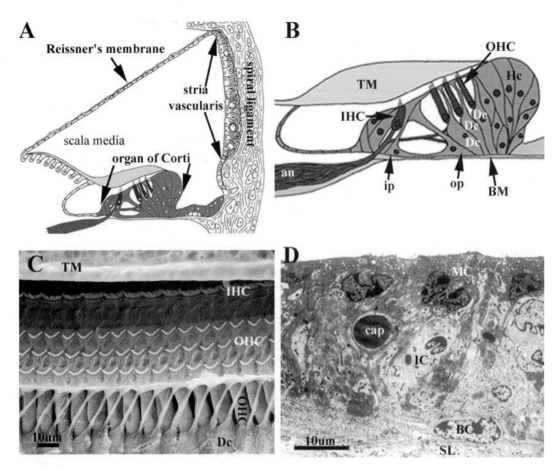

Fig. 3 The mammalian cochlea. (**A**) Diagram of a cross-section through a single turn of the cochlear spiral. (**B**) The organ of Corti in cross section. IHC, inner hair cell; OHC, outer hair cell; Dc, Deiters' cell; ip, inner pillar cell; op, outer pillar cell; Hc, Hensen's cells; TM, tectorial membrane; BM, basilar membrane. (**C**) SEM of the organ of Corti (gerbil) to show the arrangement of hair cells (IHC, OHC) and supporting cells at the apical surface. The Hensen's cells have been removed to expose the bodies of the outermost row of outer hair cells (OHC) and the bodies and phalangeal processes of the outermost row of Deiters' cells (Dc). (**D**) Thin section through the stria vascularis (mouse) (endolymph at the top). MC, marginal cell; IC, intermediate cell; BC, basal cell; cap, capillary; SL, spiral ligament.

plasma membrane bound projections enclosing filaments of the cytoskeletal protein, actin, while the kinocilium is a true cilium, similar to motile cilia. In the hair cells of the organ of Corti, the kinocilium is present only during development, becoming reduced as the cochlea matures to remain only as the basal body in the apical cytoplasm at one side of the stereociliary bundle. The position of the kinocilium (or the basal body) and the longest row of stereocilia define the polarity of the asymmetric hair bundle (Fig. 2B,C). Deflection of the stereocilia towards the longest opens ion channels (the transducer channels), K+ enters and the hair cell becomes depolarised. Deflection in the opposite direction closes the transducer channels and the hair cell becomes hyperpolarised. The transducer channels are located towards the tops of the stereocilia[2].

The parallel actin filaments in the stereocilia are closely packed in a semi-crystalline array[3] and are cross-linked by fimbrin[4] and espin[5]. The high density of actin filaments and the extensive cross-linking between them imposes rigidity on the shaft of the stereocilium, which tapers at its proximal end (at the apical surface of the hair cell; Fig. 2C) such that, when deflected, the stereocilium pivots at the taper like a stiff rod. The espin gene is mutated in one mouse strain; these 'Jerker' mice are deaf and show a vestibular disorder, recognised from their erratic, circling behaviour[5]. This reveals the importance of actin bundling and the maintenance of stereociliary rigidity to hair cell function. The stereocilia are supported on the cuticular plate (Fig. 2C), a rigid platform formed of a meshwork of actin filaments in the apical cytoplasm of the hair cell at the level of the junction between the hair and supporting cells[6]. Actin filaments descend from the stereocilium into the cuticular plate as a rootlet (Fig. 2C) which is cross-linked into the actin meshwork. In addition to actin, the cuticular plate contains spectrin[7], a protein which cross-links between actin filaments and has elastic, deformation-resisting properties, and tropomyosin[6], a protein that binds round actin and stiffens it. Around its lateral margin, the cuticular plate is linked to the lateral plasma membrane at the level of the intercellular junction[8] with which on the supporting cell side, actin and other cytoskeletal proteins are also associated. This may provide a means of support for the cuticular plate so that the stereocilia themselves are supported on a rigid platform enhancing their ability to respond to small displacement forces.

Various members of the myosin family of motor proteins, types 1c, 6, 7a and 15 – all unconventional (non-muscle) isotypes, are also localised in the cuticular plate region and the stereocilia. As shown in Table 1, mice with mutations in the genes for myosins 6, 7a or 15 all show deafness and balance disorders and abnormalities in their stereociliary bundles[9]. In the mouse mutant where myosin 6 is defective (Snell's waltzer), stereocilia are fused and greatly lengthened[10]. Interestingly, a similar anomaly is seen in the human organ of Corti from elderly people and may be related to hearing loss with age[11]. It has been suggested that myosin 6 may be involved in holding the apical plasma membrane of the hair cell on to the cuticular plate in the regions between the stereociliary bases so that individual stereocilia can be maintained and when it is defective that membrane region becomes detached. In mice where myosin 15 is mutated (Shaker 2) stereocilia are greatly reduced in height[12] indicating that this myosin isotype may have some role in stereociliary maintenance, but its precise function is not yet clear. Mutations in the myosin 7a gene are responsible for Usher's syndrome type 1B[13]. The mutant mouse strain carrying this mutation (Shaker 1)

Table 1 Mouse strains and mutations referred to in the text. For further information see also Steel and Kros[9] or *Hereditary Hearing Impairment in Mice* <http://www.jax.org/research/hhim>

Mouse strain[a]	Affected molecule	Site of defect	Human disorder/ locus name[b]	Gene name
Jerker	Espin	Hair cells	Not yet identified	–
Shaker 1	Myosin 7a	Hair cells	**Usher 1B (DFNA11/DFNB2)**	MYO7a
Shaker 2	Myosin 15	Hair cells	DFNB3	MYO15
Snell's Waltzer	Myosin 6	Hair cells	DFNA22	MYO6
Ames Waltzer	Protocadherin 15	Hair cells	**Usher 1F**	PCDH15
Waltzer	Cadherin 23	Hair cells	**Usher 1D (DFNB12)**	CDH23
–	Collagen 4A5	Basilar membrane	**Alport syndrome**	COL4A5
transgenic	Collagen 4A3	Basilar membrane	**Alport syndrome**	COL4A3
	Usherin	Basilar membrane	**Usher 2A**	
Twister	Otogelin	Tectorial/otolithic membranes	Not yet identified	
transgenic	Tectorin	Tectorial/otolithic membrane	DFNA8/12	TECTA
	Connexin 26	Gap junctions: supporting cells, cochlear lateral wall	DFNA3/DFNB1	GJB2
	Connexin 30	Gap junctions: supporting cells, cochlear lateral wall	DFNA3/DFNB1	GJB6
	Connexin 31	Gap junctions: cochlear lateral wall	DFNA2	
transgenic	IsK potassium channel	Marginal cells of stria vascularis	**Jervell and Lange-Neilsen syndrome**	KCNE1
dominant spotting (pigmentation anomaly)	Tyrosine kinase receptor (c-kit)	intermediate cells of stria vascularis	**Piebald trait**	KIT

[a]The capitalised names refer to naturally occurring mouse strains. No entry means that there is no mouse model. Transgenic is used to mean engineered (knockout) mouse strains with the targeted gene disrupted.
[b]Locus names are used as descriptors for the condition. DFNA are autosomal dominant; DFNB are autosomal recessive.

shows hair bundles in which groups of stereocilia are separated from each other at the hair cell apex and the kinocilium is misplaced suggesting an effect on maintenance of orientation and interstereociliary stabilisation[14]. Myosin 7a may have a role in the various cross-links that are present between stereocilia.

The stereocilia in an individual hair bundle are connected by a variety of fibrillar extracellular cross-links (Fig. 2D)[15]. Lateral links connect the shaft of one stereocilium to its neighbours. A 'tip-link' runs from the top of a stereocilium to the shaft of an adjacent longer stereocilium along the line of morphological and functional polarity[16]. The tip-link is thought to be a gating element that controls the opening of the transduction channel[17]. As the bundle moves in the excitatory direction, tension on the link opens the channel; when the bundle moves in the opposite direction, tension is relieved and the channel closes. High resolution imaging has suggested that the tip-link is formed of coiled filaments[18,19]. Currently, the molecular identity of the tip-link, or that of the transduction channel, is unknown. The transduction channel was initially assumed to be at the lower end of the tip-link, *i.e.* on the top of the shorter stereocilium, but more recent evidence has shown that transduction channels can be present at the top end, *i.e.* on the side of the taller stereocilium[20]. Myosin 1c localises to the region near the upper insertion point of the tip-link (on the shaft of the longer stereocilium)[21] and is thought to be involved in an adaptation motor that closes the transduction channel when the stereocilium is exposed to a sustained excitatory deflection, thereby restoring sensitivity to further stimulation. Elegant experiments involving genetic manipulations of the structure of the myosin 1c molecule have recently shown that this molecule is indeed involved in adaptation in vestibular hair cells[22]. Myosin 7a may also play a role in controlling tip-link tension. In the cochlea, defects in myosin 7a cause a large decrease in the sensitivity of transduction channel opening to stereociliary deflection suggesting that in the absence of functional myosin 7a the channels are generally closed and that tension on the gating spring is significantly reduced[23].

There are thought to be at least three different types of lateral links between stereocilia (Fig. 2D)[24,25]. Ankle links (which are absent from the hair cells of the organ of Corti, but present in the hair bundles of mammalian vestibular organs and the auditory and vestibular hair cells of non-mammalian vertebrates) connect stereocilia at their proximal ends. Shaft connectors are present along the mid-region of the stereociliary shaft. Top-connectors link stereocilia laterally just below the level of the tip-links. These subpopulations of lateral links have been identified through the use of antibodies that specifically label each sub-population separately. This indicates differences in composition between the links and their distinction from the tip-link. The lateral links may have a role in holding the bundle together to stabilise it and to couple mechanically deflections of the stereocilia so that the stereocilia in a single bundle all move as a unit. Mutations in the genes for two different members of the cadherin family, proteins involved in adhesion between the plasma membranes of adjacent cells, have been shown to cause deafness and balance disorders: (i) protocadherin (Pcdh15) which is defective in the 'Ames waltzer' mouse mutant[26] and is the protein defective in Usher's syndrome type 1F;[27] and (ii) cadherin 23 (Cdh23) which is defective in the 'waltzer' mouse strain and is the underlying cause of Usher's syndrome type 1D in humans[28]. These proteins localise to the stereocilia and, in the mutant mouse strains where they are defective, the stereocilia are splayed out. Pcdh15 and Cdh23 are, therefore, good candidates for proteins of which lateral links may be composed. Myosin 7a may be associated with some of the lateral links. It localises to this region of the stereocilia and the molecule contains a domain that can complex with a protein called vezatin that has been localised to the basal region of the stereocilia and that in turn can complex with cadherins[29]. Myosin 7a, vezatin and cadherins may form complexes that maintain lateral tension between stereocilia keeping them both separate but functionally co-ordinated and consequently mutations in the myosin 7a gene lead to a break up of the bundle.

The lateral plasma membrane

The lateral membrane of a hair cell is characterised by the presence of a variety of ion channels (see Ashmore, this volume)[30]. Outwardly rectifying K[+] channels open when the hair cell is depolarised following stereociliary deflection and permit the outward flow of K[+] to re-polarise the hair cell. Depolarisation also leads to the opening of voltage-gated Ca^{2+} channels allowing influx of Ca^{2+} that stimulates the release of neurotransmitter at the synapses on to the primary afferent nerve endings. In this way, stereociliary deflection opening transduction channels and producing depolarisation is coupled to neural discharge. Hair cells in some rodent species also possess inwardly rectifying K[+] channels, that open when the cell is hyperpolarised to restore hair cell resting potentials. Channels with these general properties can have different physiological characteristics in terms of their voltage-dependence, the speed with which they respond (fast or delayed) and the size of the current that flows through them. A number of different types of hair cell are recognised depending of their location (auditory or vestibular), innervation pattern (afferent or efferent) and species; there are differences between hair cell types in the numbers of ion-channels and which members of the various physiological types of ion-channel, each the product of different genes, they possess[30].

In addition to ion-channels, hair cells in the organ of Corti show other specialisations of their lateral plasma membrane that are associated with particular unique functions that these cells perform (see below).

Supporting cells

The supporting cells provide mechanical support to the epithelium and the hair cells. Their cell bodies contact each other and rest on the extracellular matrix that underlies the sensory epithelium (Fig. 2A), but the nature of the adhesion molecules involved in the cell–matrix interaction are not yet known. Phalangeal processes run from the cell body between the hair cell bodies to the lumenal surface where they expand to fill the spaces between hair cells (Figs 2A & 3B). Supporting cells posses a fairly extensive cytoskeletal system that is particularly well developed in the supporting cells of the organ of Corti (see below). In the apical cytoplasm, there are cytoskeletal assemblies containing the β-form of actin in filamentous bundles that run parallel to the lumenal surface of the cell anchoring to the adherens-like region of the intercellular junction of the adjacent hair cell. They also contain intermediate filaments, cytoskeletal proteins, mainly several different isotypes of cytokeratins[31], an intermediate filament type usually associated with epidermal cells, but vimentin also is present in supporting cells[31,32]. Vimentin is usually associated with mesenchymal cells, especially muscle cells. Its presence in the epidermal supporting cells is unusual but, since vimentin provides rigidity, its presence in supporting cells may be a reflection of the role in providing a rigid structural support to hair cells that these cells play.

Supporting cells are coupled to each other by large numbers of large gap junctions[33,34]. Gap junctions are sites of direct communication between adjacent cells where clusters of channels in the membrane of one cell are in direct register with clusters of channels in the membrane of its neighbour to form continuous aqueous pores connecting the cytoplasms of the adjacent cells. The protein sub-units that form gap junction channels are members of the connexin protein family. At least 20 different types, or isoforms, of connexin have been identified. Six connexins form a hemi-channel called a connexon, and the connexons of two adjacent cells align symmetrically to form the communication pathway between the cells. Each gap junction can contain up to several thousand connexons (channels). The channels allow the passage of small metabolites (up to 1.2 kDa in size), ions, and second messengers, coupling the cells both electrically and chemically. Numerous gap junctions are present at points of contact adjacent supporting cell bodies and between the head regions of adjacent cells, but there are no gap junctions associated with hair cells. The large size and number of gap junction plaques between all supporting cells mean that the supporting cell population can be regarded as a functional syncitium, but hair cells are functionally isolated from the surrounding supporting cells. Some of these gap junction plaques in inner ear sensory tissues are enormous, amongst the largest in the whole body, several square micrometres (μm^2) in area and containing several thousand channels. One role for supporting cells is thought to be to remove K^+ ions from the intercellular spaces of the sensory epithelium as they flow through hair cells and thereby maintain the low K^+ environment around the body of the hair cell necessary for transduction and sensitivity to stimulation. It has been proposed that the gap junctions provide a means to ferry the K^+ away preventing local accumulation. The gap junctions on the organ of Corti and in vestibular sensory epithelia in mammals contain two connexin isoforms, cx26 and cx30. Mutations in the genes for at least three different connexins, connexin 26 (Cx26), Cx30 and Cx31, have been identified as causes of hereditary sensorineural hearing loss. Mutations in the Cx26 gene are the most common cause of non-syndromic hereditary deafness. However, connexin mutations do not appear to cause balance dysfunction. The effects on hearing maybe related, in addition, to the presence of gap junctions in the lateral wall of the cochlea (see below).

The organ of Corti

The mature organ of Corti (Fig. 3A–C) is a ridge of cells resting on the basilar membrane, the underlying extracellular matrix. The basilar membrane and attendant organ of Corti coil in a spiral the length of which varies with species; in humans it is about 35 mm long (range, 28–40 mm)[35] but around 20 mm in guinea pigs and 40 mm in whales. The width increases systematically from the base, where high frequency sounds are detected, to the apex which is most sensitive to low frequencies. The two hair cell types, inner and outer hair cells (IHC, OHC), are regularly arranged in most mammals with a single row of IHC on the inner side of the spiral and three, sometimes four, rows of OHC (Fig. 3C). The human organ of Corti, however, appears less well ordered with sometimes two ranks of IHC and the rows of OHC being less clearly definable and less evenly spaced than in the cochleae of lower mammals[35]. Within the body of the organ of Corti are large extracellular spaces around the OHC – the spaces of Nuel – and between the outer hair cell region and the inner hair cells – the tunnel of Corti (Fig. 3B). These spaces are created by morphological specialisations of the supporting cells in which the phalangeal processes between the cell body region and expanded head at the apical (lumenal) end become reduced in width. The spaces are filled with perilymph as the basilar membrane is freely permeable to ions. The border between perilymph and endolymph thus lies at the level of the junctions at the lumenal side of the organ of Corti.

Hair cells

IHC are approximately flask shaped and their hair bundles are in an approximately straight line or wide 'U'-shape so that their hair bundles appear to form an almost continuous fence along the inner aspect of the organ of Corti (Fig. 3C). The hair bundles of the IHC do not appear to contact the overlying tectorial membrane. OHC are cylindrical, with a basally positioned nucleus. Their hair bundles form a characteristic 'W'-shape (Fig. 3C) and contact the underside of the overlying tectorial membrane in which impressions of the longest stereocilia from the OHC can be seen. The two hair cell types show very different innervation patterns[36]. IHC are innervated exclusively by afferent nerves and

90–95% of all the afferent nerves from the cochlea to the brain arise from IHCs with several different afferents synapsing with each IHC. Efferent endings to the IHC region arise ipsilaterally from the lateral superior olive in the mid-brain and contact the afferent nerves below the level of the hair cell, not the hair cells themselves. These efferent nerves constitute only about 20% of the efferent innervation to the organ of Corti. OHC, in contrast, are directly innervated by several large bouton-like efferent endings. About 80% of the efferent cochlear innervation terminates on OHCs. These OHC efferent nerves arise mainly contralaterally in the medial portion of the superior olive. Afferent nerves to the OHC region, which constitute only 5–10% of the total cochlear afferent innervation, branch considerably within the organ of Corti so that an individual neurone synapses with several OHC. These innervation patterns alone indicate that IHC are the primary receptor cells, while OHCs would appear to have some modulatory role.

OHCs increase in length systematically from the base of the cochlear spiral to the apex. They are longer in the apical cochlear coils than in basal coils. In the guinea pig, for example, OHC length varies from ~20 μm at the basal end to ~65 μm in apical coils[37]. The length of the longest stereocilia on OHC also increase in height systematically along the organ of Corti, in humans from ~2.5 μm in the basal coils to ~7.0 μm at the apex[38]. At any one position of the organ of Corti, OHC length and stereocilia height also increase from the innermost row to the outermost. These systematic changes mean that the length of the cell body and height of the stereocilia for a particular OHC are precisely defined for its position on the basilar membrane. In contrast, the length of IHC and the height of their stereocilia do not vary greatly.

The loss of OHCs in the continued presence of functioning IHCs results in hearing threshold shifts of ~60–80 dB and in loss of fine tuning in auditory nerves and thus of the exquisite frequency discrimination of which the cochlea is normally capable. These findings suggested the OHCs as sites of a 'cochlear amplifier'. Isolated OHCs maintained in short-term culture undergo fast reversible length changes at up to auditory frequencies (at least 20 kHz) when stimulated electrically. It is thought that *in vivo* changes in OHC potential deriving from the normal transduction mechanism drives the length changes[39], and these changes feed into the basilar membrane motion to enhance it in a frequency specific manner. The end result is to fine tune and amplify the signal that reaches the IHC[40].

The motor protein that drives the fast motile response is located in the lateral plasma membrane of the OHC. Freeze-fracture, a technique which exposes membranes in face view, shows the plasma membrane of OHC to contain an unusually high density of closely packed, large intramembrane particles (~6000 per mm^2)[41]. These particles represent intramembrane proteins and no other hair cell type shows similarly high intramembrane protein densities. During organ of Corti maturation, the acquisition and increase in number of these particles on OHC membranes coincides with the time course and onset of motile properties[42]. The particles are, therefore, thought to represent the motor protein. In recent elegant studies, identification of mRNAs unique to OHCs in comparison with IHCs enabled the cloning of the complementary DNA of the OHC motor protein which has been christened 'prestin'[5]. This protein is unique to OHCs. Immunolocalisation studies show prestin to be present in the lateral plasma membrane exclusively in OHC, that its appearance during development coincides with the onset of motile responses, and its forced expression in unspecialised epithelial cells in cultures results in those cells acquiring electrical characteristics and motile responses similar to OHCs[43]. It is thought prestin interacts with intracellular anions, principally chloride, which cause a reversible conformational change in the prestin molecules that results in enlargement of membrane surface area[43].

Immediately underlying the lateral plasma membrane of the OHC is an organised cytoskeletal complex, the cortical lattice[44], composed of actin filaments running helically around the cell cross-linked by spectrin, a protein with elastic properties. Regularly arranged short pillar-like structures appear to link the lattice to the inner side of the plasma membrane[41,45]. It has been suggested that the lattice gives rigid support to the plasma membrane preventing deformation, but also acts like a spring providing a restoring force after length increase, with the pillar-like structures, so far of unidentified composition, coupling plasma membrane shape change to the lattice. Inside the lattice and parallel to the lateral plasma membrane is one to several (depending on species and location along the organ of Corti) layers of membrane-bound sacs, the lateral cisternae, which appear to form a continuous network-like system within the entire lateral wall of the OHC[46]. Ca^{2+}-ATPase (an enzyme that actively transports Ca^{2+} against a concentration gradient) localises to the membranes of the cisternae[47] and many mitochondria are located along the inner aspect of the innermost cisternal layer. The function of this specialised smooth endoplasmic reticulum system has not been fully identified, but the presence of the Ca^{2+}-ATPase and the association of mitochondria suggest the cisternae sequester Ca^{2+}.

Supporting cells

Several different morphologically recognisable types of supporting cell are present in the mature organ of Corti (Fig. 3B)[6]. The Deiters' cells between OHCs have cell bodies in contact with each other and rest on the basilar membrane. Each one forms a cup-shaped enclosure around the very base of an OHC and its nerve endings. The thin phalangeal processes extend through the space of Nuel so that the entire lateral side of each OHC is free of contact with supporting cells; contact between the OHC and its surrounding supporting cells is only at the apical junctional complex. The outer and inner hair cells are separated by the outer and inner pillar cells, the phalangeal processes of which form the tunnel of Corti, the outer pillar cell buttressing against the inner pillar cell (Fig 3B)[48]. The inner hair cell itself is closely surrounded by supporting cells. To the outside of the OHC are Hensen's cells which, especially in the more apical coils of the organ of Corti, contain large lipid droplets. These are thought to provide a mechanical loading to the cells that influences the mechanical properties of the organ of Corti and its motion in response to sound stimulation.

The Deiters' and pillar cells are thought to provide mechanical support that has a significant role in mechanical activity that leads to stimulation of the hair cells in response to sound. They contain large numbers of microtubules in parallel arrays running from the base to apex of the cell[6]. These arrays are some of the largest microtubule bundles in the entire body[48], and would act like scaffolding poles to provide rigidity. The tubulin composing the microtubules of these supporting cells is in a form that is resistant to de-polymerisation suggesting that the microtubules are long-lived structures[49]. The rigidity of the supporting cells provides a means to couple basilar membrane motion to movement of the entire organ of Corti to produce the relative motion between the apical surface of the sensory epithelium and the overlying tectorial membrane that results in deflection of the hair bundles. Loss of supporting cell rigidity would, therefore, result in decoupling of basilar membrane motion from the tectorial membrane motion and loss of hearing acuity. It has been suggested that this may occur with ageing[50].

The basilar membrane

The basilar membrane (BM), upon which the organ of Corti sits, is a sheet of predominantly extracellular matrix structure composed of filaments within a ground substance, with a discontinuous layer of thin, elongated tympanic border cells on the underside facing the perilymph of the scala tympani[6]. The fibrils of the basilar membrane run predominantly radially, and are composed of collagen, mostly collagen type IV α1–α5 chains (COL4A1–COL4A5)[51]. In addition, fibronectin[52] and laminin type 11[53], adhesive-type molecules common to extracellular matrices, are localised to the basilar membrane and presumably compose the ground substance in which the collagen fibrils reside. The composition of the BM does not appear to be unique in comparison with basement membranes elsewhere in the body, but a novel extracellular matrix protein (named 'usherin') has been identified through the genetic mutation that is associated with Usher's syndrome type IIa[54], in which there is high frequency hearing loss. Mutations in the genes for the proteins composing the basilar membrane might be expected to affect the mechanical responses of the organ of Corti in response to sound and thereby cause hearing impairment. X-linked Alport's syndrome has been attributed to mutations in the gene for the COL4A5 gene. It has been suggested that the loss of this protein from the basilar membrane affects the ability to create tension through interactions with the tension fibrocytes in the cochlear lateral wall resulting in the high frequency hearing loss associated with this condition[55].

Tectorial membrane

The tectorial membrane (TM) is a structured sheet of extracellular matrix material that overlies the organ of Corti. It is attached to the interdental cells of the spiral limbus at its inner edge, but appears not to be attached to the surface of the organ of Corti at its outer edge. The longest stereocilia of each OHC are embedded in the underside of the TM. Through this coupling, relative movement between the TM and the apical surface of the organ of Corti in response to sound-induced motion of the basilar membrane produces deflections of the OHC stereocilia. IHC stereocilia may contact and be deflected by Hensen's stripe, a ridge running along the middle of the underside of the TM just outside the position of the IHC stereocilia. The body of the TM is formed of fibre bundles running approximately radially, embedded within a matrix composed of striated sheets formed of fine cross-linked fibrils[56]. The fibre bundles are formed of collagen types II, V and IX[57,58], which are different types from those in the BM. Associated with the collagen bundles is a glycoprotein unique to the inner ear, otogelin[59], defects in which result in the 'Twister' mouse phenotype[60]. The matrix of the TM also is composed of glycoproteins that are unique to the inner ear, α- and β-tectorin[61,62]. Tectorins and otogelin are also present in the otolithic membranes that cover the saccular and utricular maculae and otogelin is present in the cupulae of the cristae, but none of these glycoproteins are found elsewhere in the body. Consequently, mutations in the genes for these proteins are associated with non-syndromic hearing loss in humans[59,63]. Expression of the mRNAs for otogelin[64] and the tectorins[65] is detected only during development of the cochlea; they are not expressed in the organ of Corti of adults. Thus, the tectorial membrane is a life-long structure produced only during cochlear development and there is no turn-over of the proteins. This would imply that if the tectorial membrane were damaged it would not be repaired.

Ion transporting epithelia

The stria vascularis (SV) lines the lateral wall of the scala media (Fig. 3A). It is responsible for the production and maintenance of both the high endolymphatic K^+ concentration and the EP[1]. The SV encloses a complex capillary network and is composed of three cell types: (i) the marginal cells which line the endolymphatic compartment; (ii) intermediate cells in a discontinuous layer enclosed entirely within the body of the epithelium; and (iii) the basal cells that separate the SV from the underlying spiral ligament (Fig. 3D). Endolymph composition in the vestibular system is maintained by the dark cells. The dark cells form a single layer resting on top of pigmented cells at the base of the skirts of each crista in the semi-circular canals and around the utricular macula. There is no dark cell region in the saccule. The dark cells are essentially identical morphologically and functionally to the marginal cells of the stria.

Marginal cells of stria vascularis and dark cells of the vestibular system

The marginal cells of the SV and vestibular dark cells are primarily involved with the transport of K^+. Their basolateral membranes are extensively infolded, enclosing numerous large mitochondria and they contain high levels of Na^+/K^+-ATPase, both α- and β-isoforms[66], which transports K^+ into the cell in exchange for Na^+. The infoldings provide a large surface area over which ion exchange can occur and the numerous large mitochondria enclosed within them provides the energy source (ATP) for the active ion transport. The basolateral membranes contain in addition a $Na^+/K^+/Cl^-$-co-transporter (NKCC1)[67] that transports the three ions into the cell. The uptake of Na^+ enhances ATPase activity by stimulating the outward transport of Na^+ and, thus, the inward transport of K^+[1]. NKCC1 is the therapeutic target of action for loop diuretics in the kidney and loop diuretics have rapid, acute ototoxic side-effects through an action on the co-transporter in the strial marginal cells (and vestibular dark cells) inhibiting ion transport resulting in accumulation of ions in the extracellular spaces of the stria and a consequent oedema.

The apical membranes of the marginal cells and the dark cells contain a K^+ channel which is formed of two subunits, the KCNE1 regulatory protein and the KCNQ1 channel proteins[68] (these subunits were formally named IsK and KvQLT1, respectively). This channel provides the pathway through which K^+ is secreted into endolymph[69]. Mutations in the KCNE1 gene disrupt endolymph production leading, in the cochlea, to collapse of Reissner's membrane and deafness, and in the vestibular system to collapse of the epithelia of the roof of the utricle, saccule and ampullae and shaker/waltzer-type behaviours in mice indicating dysfunction of the vestibular sensory organs[68].

During development, high levels of K^+ are found in cochlear endolymph, and strial marginal cells show high Na/K-ATPase activity, before an EP can be recorded[70]. In the vestibular system, there is no high positive potential equivalent to EP recordable in the vestibular endolymphatic compartment yet dark cells and marginal cells appear to have almost identical morphology and physiology. These, and other physiological data[1], indicate that strial marginal cells, and dark cells, are primarily concerned with active K^+ transport to maintain the concentration of that ion in endolymph, but the generation of EP is a separate phenomenon. The absence of any other cell type from the ion transporting tissue of the vestibular system suggests that the intermediate and/or basal cells in the stria play a role in EP generation.

Intermediate cells of SV

The intermediate cells are melanocytes – melanin pigment-containing cells – that arise during development from cells that migrate from the neural crest. They are entirely enclosed within the corpus of the stria, interdigitating with the other two cell types. They contain a variety of enzymes that enable energy production from alternative substrates such as lipids as well as enzymes that detoxify oxidative wastes[71]. Coupled with the presence of melanin, that can act as a free radical scavenger, this suggests that one role for intermediate cells is to protect the stria under conditions of stress and perhaps also to provide alternative energy sources to maintain activity during periods of reduced blood supply. Intermediate cells also appear to have a role in the generation and maintenance of EP. In the *viable dominant spotting* mouse mutant, there is a neural crest defect, intermediate cells are highly reduced in number or completely absent, and there is no EP generated[72]; other than the absence of intermediate cells, the stria appears normal and the marginal cells possess ATPase activity[73].

Basal cells

The basal cells are flattened and elongated, forming 1–3 layers delimiting the basal aspect of the stria. They arise during development from the mesenchymal cells that also form the spiral ligament. Basal cells closely appose each other and tight junctions are present between the adjacent cells across the entire region of contact. During development, the initial formation of the tight junctions and the increase in their complexity coincides with the initial onset of EP, suggesting that these junctions are necessary to provide the electrical insulation required for the potential to be generated and maintained.

In addition, large numbers of gap junctions are associated with basal cells[74]. They are present between adjacent basal cells, basal and intermediate cells and basal cells and fibrocytes in the spiral ligament[33,34,75]. Thus, basal cells appear to be the central element in a coupled unit consisting of basal cells, intermediate cells, and spiral ligament fibrocytes. Marginal cells are excluded from this syncitium; they do not form gap junctions either with each other or with either basal or intermediate cells[33,34] and are thus separated, functionally, from each other and from the basal cell/intermediate cell/ligament fibrocyte coupled unit.

As gap junctions provide for direct cell-to-cell communication, the coupling between basal cells and ligament fibrocytes potentially provides a pathway for access of ions into stria cells from the ligament that bypasses the tight junctional sealing. Fibrocytes of the spiral ligament possess Na^+/K^+-ATPase activity[66] and thus probably function to take up K^+ from the perilymph. The gap junctions between fibrocytes would, therefore, provide an intracellular route for K^+ to those fibrocytes beneath the SV, which are coupled to strial basal cells and, in turn, for K^+ entry into strial cells. This gap junction system, therefore, provides a route for re-cycling of K^+: from endolymph, through hair cells to perilymph in the spaces in the organ of Corti, into supporting cells and then to the spiral ligament; into fibrocytes, then to stria and back to endolymph. The intercellular communication provided by gap junctions may, therefore, be important for the maintenance of EP. During development, the initial onset and subsequent rise in EP corresponds with the initial formation and subsequent increase in size and number of gap junctions associated with basal cells[70]. The gap junctions in the cochlear lateral wall – stria vascularis and spiral ligament – in rodents are all composed of both cx26 and cx30[76]. Thus, mutations in the Cx26 gene might be expected to affect K^+ recycling and EP generation.

Concluding remarks

Analysis of the structure and function of the inner ear has lagged behind that of many other body tissues. This was due, in part, to the relative inaccessibility of the inner ear tissues and the small number of specialised cells they contain (~15,000 hair cells in total in a single cochlea[35]). However, our understanding of the complexities of the architectural organisation necessary for cochlear and vestibular function has advanced so rapidly that the inner ear is becoming a major model for post-genomic studies, the attempt to discover for what all the genes identified in the human genome actually code. More specifically, the continuing identification of the molecular basis of inner ear function is laying the basis for developing rational new approaches to diagnosis, management and treatment of auditory and vestibular disorders.

References

1   Wangemann P, Schacht J. Homeostatic mechanisms in the cochlea. In: Dallos P, Popper AN, Fay RR. (eds) *The Cochlea*. New York: Springer, 1996; 130–85

2   Hudspeth AJ. How the ear's works work. *Nature* 1989; **341**: 397–404

3   Tilney LG, Tilney MS, DeRosier DJ. Actin filaments, stereocilia, and hair cells: how cells count and measure. *Annu Rev Cell Biol* 1992; **8**: 257–74

4   Flock A, Bretscher A, Weber K. Immunohistochemical localization of several cytoskeletal proteins in inner ear sensory and supporting cells. *Hear Res* 1982; **7**: 75–89

5   Zheng J, Shen W, He DZ, Long KB, Madison LD, Dallos P. Prestin is the motor protein of cochlear outer hair cells. *Nature* 2000; **405**: 149–55

6   Slepecky NB. Structure of the mammalian cochlea. In: Dallos P, Popper AN, Fay RR. (eds) *The Cochlea*. New York: Springer, 1996; 44–129

7   Ylikoski J, Pirvola U, Lehtonen E. Distribution of F-actin and fodrin in the hair cells of the guinea pig cochlea as revealed by confocal fluorescence microscopy. *Hear Res* 1992; **60**: 80–8

8   Hirokawa N, Tilney LG. Interactions between actin filaments and between actin filaments and membranes in quick-frozen and deeply etched hair cells of the chick ear. *J Cell Biol* 1982; **95**: 249–61

9   Steel KP, Kros CJ. A genetic approach to understanding auditory function. *Nat Genet* 2001; **27**: 143–9

10 Self T, Sobe T, Copeland NG, Jenkins NA, Avraham KB, Steel KP. Role of myosin VI in the differentiation of cochlear hair cells. *Dev Biol* 1999; **214**: 331–41

11 Wright A. Giant cilia in the human organ of Corti. *Clin Otolaryngol* 1982; **7**: 193–9

12 Probst FJ, Fridell RA, Raphael Y *et al.* Correction of deafness in shaker-2 mice by an unconventional myosin in a BAC transgene. *Science* 1998; **280**: 1444–7

13 Weil D, Blanchard S, Kaplan J *et al.* Defective myosin VIIA gene responsible for Usher syndrome type 1B. *Nature* 1995; **374**: 60–1

14 Self T, Mahony M, Fleming J, Walsh J, Brown SD, Steel KP. Shaker-1 mutations reveal roles for myosin VIIA in both development and function of cochlear hair cells. *Development* 1998; **125**: 557–66

15 Pickles JO. Early events in auditory processing. *Curr Opin Neurobiol* 1993; **3**: 558–62

16 Pickles JO, Comis SD, Osborne MP. Cross-links between stereocilia in the guinea pig organ of Corti, and their possible relation to sensory transduction. *Hear Res* 1984; **15**: 103–12

17 Markin VS, Hudspeth AJ. Gating-spring models of mechanoelectrical transduction by hair cells of the internal ear. *Annu Rev Biophys Biomol Struct* 1995; **24**: 59–83

18 Kachar B, Parakkal M, Kurc M, Zhao Y, Gillespie PG. High-resolution structure of hair-cell tip links. *Proc Natl Acad Sci USA* 2000; **97**: 13336–41

19 Tsuprun V, Santi P. Helical structure of hair cell stereocilia tip links in the chinchilla cochlea. *J Assoc Res Otolaryngol* 2000; **1**: 224–31

20 Gillespie PG. Molecular machinery of auditory and vestibular transduction. *Curr Opin Neurobiol* 1995; **5**: 449–55

21 Steyger PS, Gillespie PG, Baird RA. Myosin Ibeta is located at tip link anchors in vestibular hair bundles. *J Neurosci* 1998; **18**: 4603–15

22 Holt JR, Gillespie SK, Provance DW *et al.* A chemical-genetic strategy implicates myosin-1c in adaptation by hair cells. *Cell* 2002; **108**: 371–81

23 Kros CJ, Marcotti W, van Netten SM *et al.* Reduced climbing and increased slipping adaptation in cochlear hair cells of mice with Myo7a mutations. *Nat Neurosci* 2002; **5**: 41–7

24 Goodyear RJ, Gates R, Lukashkin AN, Richardson GP. Hair-cell numbers continue to increase in the utricular macula of the early posthatch chick. *J Neurocytol* 1999; **28**: 851–61

25 Richardson GP, Bartolami S, Russell IJ. Identification of a 275-kD protein associated with the apical surfaces of sensory hair cells in the avian inner ear. *J Cell Biol* 1990; **110**: 1055–66

26 Alagramam KN, Murcia CL, Kwon HY, Pawlowski KS, Wright CG, Woychik RP. The mouse Ames waltzer hearing-loss mutant is caused by mutation of Pcdh15, a novel protocadherin gene. *Nat Genet* 2001; **27**: 99–102

27 Alagramam KN, Yuan H, Kuehn MH *et al.* Mutations in the novel protocadherin PCDH15 cause Usher syndrome type 1F. *Hum Mol Genet* 2001; **10**: 1709–18

28 Di Palma F, Holme RH, Bryda EC *et al*. Mutations in Cdh23, encoding a new type of cadherin, cause stereocilia disorganization in waltzer, the mouse model for Usher syndrome type 1D. *Nat Genet* 2001; **27**: 103–7

29 Kussel-Andermann P, El-Amraoui A, Safieddine S *et al*. Vezatin, a novel transmembrane protein, bridges myosin VIIA to the cadherin-catenins complex. *EMBO J* 2000; **19**: 6020–9

30 Eatock RA, Rusch A. Developmental changes in the physiology of hair cells. *Semin Cell Dev Biol* 1997; **8**: 265–75

31 Kuijpers W, Tonnaer EL, Peters TA, Ramaekers FC. Expression of intermediate filament proteins in the mature inner ear of the rat and guinea pig. *Hear Res* 1991; **52**: 133–46

32 Schulte BA, Adams JC. Immunohistochemical localization of vimentin in the gerbil inner ear. *J Histochem Cytochem* 1989; **37**: 1787–97

33 Forge A, Becker D, Casalotti S *et al*. Gap junctions and connexin expression in the inner ear. *Novartis Found Symp* 1999; **219**: 134–50, discussion 151–6

34 Kikuchi T, Kimura RS, Paul DL, Adams JC. Gap junctions in the rat cochlea: immunohistochemical and ultrastructural analysis. *Anat Embryol (Berl)* 1995; **191**: 101–18

35 Wright A, Davis A, Bredberg G, Ulehlova L, Spencer H. Hair cell distributions in the normal human cochlea. *Acta Otolaryngol Suppl* 1987; **444**: 1–48

36 Spoendlin H. Anatomy of cochlear innervation. *Am J Otolaryngol* 1985; **6**: 453–67

37 Pujol R, Lavigne-Rebillard M, Lenoir M. Development of the sensory and neural structures in the mammalian cochlea. In: Rubel EW, Popper AN, Fay RR. (eds) *Development of the Auditory System*. New York: Springer, 1998; 146–93

38 Wright A. Dimensions of the cochlear stereocilia in man and the guinea pig. *Hear Res* 1984; **13**: 89–98

39 Ashmore JF. The electrophysiology of hair cells. *Annu Rev Physiol* 1991; **53**: 465–76

40 Ashmore JF, Kolston PJ. Hair cell based amplification in the cochlea. *Curr Opin Neurobiol* 1994; **4**: 503–8

41 Forge A. Structural features of the lateral walls in mammalian cochlear outer hair cells. *Cell Tissue Res* 1991; **265**: 473–83

42 Souter M, Nevill G, Forge A. Postnatal development of membrane specialisations of gerbil outer hair cells. *Hear Res* 1995; **91**: 43–62

43 Oliver D, He DZ, Klocker N *et al*. Intracellular anions as the voltage sensor of prestin, the outer hair cell motor protein. *Science* 2001; **292**: 2340–3

44 Holley MC, Ashmore JF. Spectrin, actin and the structure of the cortical lattice in mammalian cochlear outer hair cells. *J Cell Sci* 1990; **96**: 283–91

45 Kalinec F, Holley MC, Iwasa KH, Lim DJ, Kachar B. A membrane-based force generation mechanism in auditory sensory cells. *Proc Natl Acad Sci USA* 1992; **89**: 8671–5

46 Forge A, Zajic G, Li L, Nevill G, Schacht J. Structural variability of the sub-surface cisternae in intact, isolated outer hair cells shown by fluorescent labelling of intracellular membranes and freeze-fracture. *Hear Res* 1993; **64**: 175–83

47 Schulte BA. Immunohistochemical localization of intracellular Ca-ATPase in outer hair cells, neurons and fibrocytes in the adult and developing inner ear. *Hear Res* 1993; **65**: 262–73

48 Tucker JB, Mogensen MM, Henderson CG, Doxsey SJ, Wright M, Stearns T. Nucleation and capture of large cell surface-associated microtubule arrays that are not located near centrosomes in certain cochlear epithelial cells. *J Anat* 1998; **192**: 119–30

49 Slepecky NB, Henderson CG, Saha S. Post-translational modifications of tubulin suggest that dynamic microtubules are present in sensory cells and stable microtubules are present in supporting cells of the mammalian cochlea. *Hear Res* 1995; **91**: 136–47

50 Saha S, Slepecky NB. Age-related changes in microtubules in the guinea pig organ of Corti. Tubulin isoform shifts with increasing age suggest changes in micromechanical properties of the sensory epithelium. *Cell Tissue Res* 2000; **300**: 29–46

51 Cosgrove D, Kornak JM, Samuelson G. Expression of basement membrane type IV collagen chains during postnatal development in the murine cochlea. *Hear Res* 1996; **100**: 21–32

52 Cosgrove D, Samuelson G, Pinnt J. Immunohistochemical localization of basement membrane collagens and associated proteins in the murine cochlea. *Hear Res* 1996; **97**: 54–65

53 Rodgers KD, Barritt L, Miner JH, Cosgrove D. The laminins in the murine inner ear: developmental transitions and expression in cochlear basement membranes. *Hear Res* 2001; **158**: 39–50

54 Bhattacharya G, Miller C, Kimberling WJ, Jablonski MM, Cosgrove D. Localization and expression of usherin: a novel basement membrane protein defective in people with Usher's syndrome type IIa. *Hear Res* 2002; **163**: 1–11

55 Harvey SJ, Mount R, Sado Y *et al*. The inner ear of dogs with X-linked nephritis provides clues to the pathogenesis of hearing loss in X-linked Alport syndrome. *Am J Pathol* 2001; **159**: 1097–104

56 Hasko JA, Richardson GP. The ultrastructural organization and properties of the mouse tectorial membrane matrix. *Hear Res* 1988; **35**: 21–38

57 Richardson GP, Russell IJ, Duance VC, Bailey AJ. Polypeptide composition of the mammalian tectorial membrane. *Hear Res* 1987; **25**: 45–60

58 Slepecky NB, Savage JE, Cefaratti LK, Yoo TJ. Electron-microscopic localization of type II, IX, and V collagen in the organ of Corti of the gerbil. *Cell Tissue Res* 1992; **267**: 413–8

59 Cohen-Salmon M, El-Amraoui A, Leibovici M, Petit C. Otogelin: a glycoprotein specific to the acellular membranes of the inner ear. *Proc Natl Acad Sci USA* 1997; **94**: 14450–5

60 Simmler MC, Zwaenepoel I, Verpy E *et al*. Twister mutant mice are defective for otogelin, a component specific to inner ear acellular membranes. *Mamm Genome* 2000; **11**: 960–6

61 Legan PK, Lukashkina VA, Goodyear RJ, Kossi M, Russell IJ, Richardson GP. A targeted deletion in alpha-tectorin reveals that the tectorial membrane is required for the gain and timing of cochlear feedback. *Neuron* 2000; **28**: 273–85

62 Legan PK, Rau A, Keen JN, Richardson GP. The mouse tectorins. Modular matrix proteins of the inner ear homologous to components of the sperm-egg adhesion system. *J Biol Chem* 1997; **272**: 8791–801

63 Verhoeven K, Van Laer L, Kirschhofer K *et al*. Mutations in the human alpha-tectorin gene cause autosomal dominant non-syndromic hearing impairment. *Nat Genet* 1998; **19**: 60–2

64 El-Amraoui A, Cohen-Salmon M, Petit C, Simmler MC. Spatiotemporal expression of otogelin in the developing and adult mouse inner ear. *Hear Res* 2001; **158**: 151–9

65 Rau A, Legan PK, Richardson GP. Tectorin mRNA expression is spatially and temporally restricted during mouse inner ear development. *J Comp Neurol* 1999; **405**: 271–80

66 McGuirt JP, Schulte BA. Distribution of immunoreactive alpha- and beta-subunit isoforms of Na,K-ATPase in the gerbil inner ear. *J Histochem Cytochem* 1994; **42**: 843–53

67 Crouch JJ, Sakaguchi N, Lytle C, Schulte BA. Immunohistochemical localization of the Na-K-Cl co-transporter (NKCC1) in the gerbil inner ear. *J Histochem Cytochem* 1997; **45**: 773–8

68 Vetter DE, Mann JR, Wangemann P *et al*. Inner ear defects induced by null mutation of the *isk* gene. *Neuron* 1996; **17**: 1251–64

69 Sunose H, Liu J, Shen Z, Marcus DC. cAMP increases apical IsK channel current and K$^+$ secretion in vestibular dark cells. *J Membr Biol* 1997; **156**: 25–35

70 Souter M, Forge A. Intercellular junctional maturation in the stria vascularis: possible association with onset and rise of endocochlear potential. *Hear Res* 1998; **119**: 81–95

71 Spector GJ, Carr C. The ultrastructural cytochemistry of peroxisomes in the guinea pig cochlea: a metabolic hypothesis for the stria vascularis. *Laryngoscope* 1979; **89**: 1–38

72 Steel KP, Barkway C. Another role for melanocytes: their importance for normal stria vascularis development in the mammalian inner ear. *Development* 1989; **107**: 453–63

73 Schulte BA, Steel KP. Expression of alpha and beta subunit isoforms of Na,K-ATPase in the mouse inner ear and changes with mutations at the *Wv* or *Sld* loci. *Hear Res* 1994; **78**: 65–76

74 Forge A. Gap junctions in the stria vascularis and effects of ethacrynic acid. *Hear Res* 1984; **13**: 189–200

75 Carlisle L, Steel K, Forge A. Endocochlear potential generation is associated with intercellular communication in the stria vascularis: structural analysis in the viable dominant spotting mouse mutant. *Cell Tissue Res* 1990; **262**: 329–37

76 Forge A, Becker D, Casalotti S, Edwards J, Marziano N, Nickel R. Gap junctions and connexins in the inner ear. *Audiol Neurootol* 2002; 7: 141–5

Cochlear pathology, sensory cell death and regeneration

Yehoash Raphael

KHRI, The University of Michigan Medical School, Ann Arbor, Michigan, USA

Loss of cochlear hair cells leads to permanent hearing loss. Hair cells may degenerate due to hereditary or environmental causes, or a combination of the two. Cochlear supporting cells actively participate in the process of hair cell elimination and scar formation by rapidly expanding and sealing the reticular lamina, the barrier between endolymph and perilymph. This scarring process helps preserve the remaining hair cells and hearing. Anti-apoptotic agents, anti-oxidants and several growth factors have been shown to protect hair cells and hearing against environmental insults. Characterization of the genes that regulate the development of the inner ear and its response to trauma has been helpful in designing strategies for enhancing protection of the inner ear and for inducing hair cell regeneration. This chapter discusses the potential for some of these approaches.

The hair cells in the human inner ear are born in the first trimester of embryonic development. These cells are expected to survive, without renewal, for life. Intuitively, it seems that the expectation for a cell to survive over nearly a century is rather demanding and imposing. However, several other cell types in the human body are capable of such long service, including, most notably, muscle cells and neurons. What makes the inner ear different is the fact that, unlike neurons, the total number of hair cells is very small and there is very little (if any) redundancy in this population. Thus, considering that every region in the cochlea is optimized for best function at a given frequency, loss of a single hair cell is associated with compromised hearing in a specific frequency.

Hair cell loss is the leading cause of hearing loss. Hair cell death can be caused by lack of essential growth factors, exogenous toxins (such as ototoxic drugs), overstimulation by noise or sound, viral or bacterial infections, autoimmune conditions or hereditary disease. The reader is familiar with the devastating outcome of hearing loss and with the prevalence of this sensory impairment. Sensorineural hearing loss is irreversible. This chapter describes our knowledge of the events that lead to hair cell loss and replacement, and presents possible strategies that may yield potential therapies in the future. While the proposed strategies

Correspondence to:
Dr Yehoash Raphael,
KHRI, The University of Michigan Medical School,
MSRB III Room-9303,
Ann Arbor,
MI 48109-0648, USA

are based on current biological and technological data and concepts, some of the proposed interventions are visionary and should serve as a working plan for future research and development rather than a promise to the current population of patients.

Hair cell degeneration

Cell elimination and scar formation

As in any classical drama, the death of a hair cell is staged in a complex array of considerations involving time and space. The immediate surrounding environment is of great importance. Consider that the apical surface of a hair cell is bathed in endolymph, a fluid so rich in K^+ ions that it is toxic to neuronal endings that innervate the basal-lateral portion of the hair cell membrane. Thus, if a hair cell were to disappear and leave behind an open space, even for a short time, the hearing of the entire ear could be compromised. Nevertheless, most adult humans have lost some hair cells without having lost their entire hearing reserve. This can only be explained by a highly regulated and complex mechanism of cell death and scar formation in the organ of Corti.

The term 'scar' is used to describe replacement of the original cell type (hair cell) by a 'filling' cell, a supporting cell. The use of the term scar in the organ of Corti is justified because the scar is permanent. The immediate role of the scarring process is to prevent fluid mixing. It is especially important to prevent endolymph leakage into the fluid bathing the basal domain of inner hair cells where terminals of the auditory nerve reside. Potassium-rich endolymph would depolarize the neurons, and abolish hearing and lead to further tissue damage.

The mechanism of scar formation depends to a great extent on another important element in the immediate surroundings of the hair cell, namely, the neighbouring supporting cells. Supporting cells co-ordinate neat and organized scar formation following damage by ototoxic drugs and noise trauma[1]. Early responses of supporting cells were detected in response to hair cell trauma, as two of the four supporting cells which surround a hair cell execute a dying hair cell and seal the reticular lamina against a leak of fluids, thus preventing the mixing of perilymph and endolymph[2,3]. The involvement of supporting cells in hair cell loss, therefore, results in rapid expansion of the apical domain of two supporting cells, constricting the hair cell beneath its apical membrane, and sealing the reticular lamina prior to formation of a fluid leak (Fig. 1). Conspicuous actin cables are seen in the scarring region, suggesting that an actin–myosin system is involved in the removal of the dying hair cell (see Fig. 1).

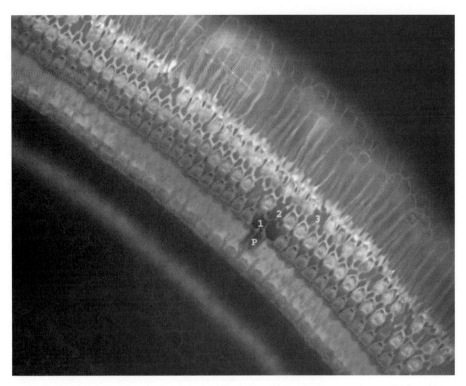

Fig. 1 A whole-mount (surface preparation) of the guinea pig organ of Corti (3rd cochlear turn) labelled with rhodamine phalloidin (a specific F-actin stain) and photographed using epifluorescence. One pillar cell is missing in the row of pillars (p). Scars made by supporting cells are seen in several sites where hair cells are missing (1, scar in the first row of outer hair cells; 2, scar in the second row of hair cells; 3, scar in the third row of hair cells) but the overall structure of the organ of Corti is preserved.

Studies on epithelial cell death in other systems have demonstrated similar mechanism to that described above[4]. At the molecular level, inhibition of Rho, one of the members of a family of small GTPases, blocks the scarring[4]. The formation of the actin–myosin rings and the process of cellular replacement (scarring) was shown to occur very early in the apoptotic cascade, prior to procaspase activation and cell changes in morphology of the dying cells. Interestingly, similar to the observation in the organ of Corti, the epithelial surface remained intact during the scarring, as determined by constant electrical resistance measured in the face of extensive cell death[4].

This scarring mechanism implies that the hair cell or, at least, most of the hair cell body remains within the epithelium. The hair cell body can be eliminated by phagocytosis, either by macrophages or by supporting cells. Evidence for macrophages is provided by their occasional presence in the auditory epithelium after lesions. However, the small number and infrequent identification of macrophages implicates supporting cells as phagocytes for dead hair cells. Evidence from other epithelial tissues such as the retinal pigment epithelium point to similar mechanisms whereby supporting elements eliminate sensory cells that die within the epithelium[5].

An insult can lead to sub-lethal pathology in hair cells, resulting in morphological and functional changes that can be defined as hair cell injury. While some hair cells gradually degenerate, others are likely to recover and regain normal function. This implies that supporting cells do not create a scar to replace injured hair cells. It is unclear at present how supporting cells chose their action: thumbs-up to allow the survival of an injured hair cell versus thumbs-down to order and perform its execution. Regardless of the mechanism, the possibility that injured hair cells survive under the reticular lamina has important implications for hair cell regeneration. Reports of hair cells that are injured by an insult and remain under the reticular laminar surface among the supporting cells came from studies of lesions in the developing organ of Corti in culture[6].

So far, diseases associated with impaired scarring mechanism in supporting cells have not been described. However, such impairment would certainly be detrimental to the organ of Corti during hair cell degeneration. I propose, hypothetically, that some forms of sudden deafness may be related to faulty scarring, during which the integrity of the reticular lamina is compromised. Accordingly, treatment of such hearing loss should be based on manipulating supporting cells and their ability to form scars rapidly and effectively.

Apoptosis and necrosis

The study of cell death is not a new one; yet, it has received much attention and effort in the last decade[7]. Of significant importance is the impressive enhancement in our understanding of active cell death, or apoptosis, including genes that encode necessary participants in the active cell death cascade, and other proteins that may inhibit active cell death. Understanding the molecular mechanism of cell death should help us design the means to manipulate active cell death.

Active cell death is a physiological process important for normal development and tissue homeostasis as well as in cell removal in response to a variety of pathological conditions. The initial signal for active cell death can be stress (of several types), absence of a trophic factor or a diffusible molecule that binds to a specific cell-surface receptor. The receptors are called death receptors. One of the better studied receptors mediating cell death is Fas. This is a transmembrane receptor found in a variety of cell types[8]. Once activated, the Fas receptor leads to direct activation of caspase-3, or to activation of caspase-8 which, in turn, leads to the release of cytochrome c from mitochondria. Cytochrome c then activates caspase-3. Mitochondria have an alternative pathway for participating in the active cell death cascade, in which they release Smac/Diablo, which in turn activates caspase-3[9]. Molecules from the Bcl-2 family can inhibit apoptosis at this stage by preventing mitochondrial changes[10].

The main pathway of active cell death terminates by activation of specific proteases from the caspase family which serve as the cell 'executioners'[11]. The apoptotic initiators act upstream and include caspase-2, caspase-8 and caspase-9 while the downstream executioners are caspase-3, caspase-6 and caspase-7[12]. Caspase-3 is the most common molecule for inducing active cell death. Once activated, it acts on several targets, each of which leads to break-up of a different cellular compartment. To degrade chromatin, caspase-3 acts on a set of DNAses and nucleases[13]. To degrade the cell membrane and the cytoskeleton, caspase-3 acts on gelsolin and fodrin[14].

Natural inhibitors of caspases have been shown to exist in mammalian cells. These inhibitors can serve as agents for cell protection against death. For instance, a protein named X-linked inhibitor of apoptosis (XIAP) has been show to have robust anti-apoptotic activity[15]. Active cell death inhibition is accomplished by binding of the XIAP to the caspase, and inhibiting its function.

In many types of cells, identification of active cell death in terms of the criteria above is conclusive. However, in other tissues and conditions leading to cell death, the distinction between active cell death and necrosis is not perfectly clear[16]. Overlap in molecular and morphological manifestations between active cell death and necrosis, along with artefacts inherent in the technology for detection of active cell death complicate our ability to distinguish between these two types of cell death.

The degeneration of hair cells in the organ of Corti has not been easy to study. The paucity of cells precludes most biochemical analyses. TUNEL staining and other types of DNA labelling have been performed by several laboratories, identifying organ of Corti hair cells that are presumably undergoing active cell death[17,18]. Other studies clearly demonstrate false-positive apoptosis staining in hair cells and warn of the inability of present technology to distinguish reliably between active cell death and necrosis[19].

To complicate the picture further, there is a growing body of evidence that TUNEL-positive cells in several tissues are undergoing necrosis. In practical terms, the identification of proteins that are involved in the demise of the hair cells is important because this knowledge can lead to the development of preventive measures. Thus, while the distinction between active cell death and necrosis is not always clear, the similarities between them enable use of a common set of intervention means to prevent cell death (see below).

Prevention of cell death

Three major agents have been investigated for preventing hair cell loss due to ototoxic and acoustic insults. These agents are molecules that belong to the families of neurotrophic factors, anti-oxidants or anti-apoptotic agents. All three types of molecules have the potential to become clinically applicable for similar types of trauma. However, such therapy is usually effective for preventive medicine and not helpful for treating a lesion that has already occurred.

Neurotrophic factors

Neurotrophic factors are relatively small peptides that are secreted to act in a paracrine or autocrine fashion. Upon binding with specific receptors on the membrane of the target cell, they activate an intracellular signalling cascade leading to one or more of their functions. These include signals that are necessary for development, maintenance of the differentiated state, survival in the face of insults and re-growth or axonal regeneration. The term neurotrophic factor implies an influence on neurons, but in reality most neurotrophic factors have been shown to also influence a large variety of non-neuronal tissues, including the auditory epithelium. The two neurotrophic factors found to be important for normal development of auditory neurons are brain derived neurotrophic factor (BDNF) and neurotrophin 3 (NT-3)[20]. NT-3 is also important for the developing auditory sensory epithelium[21]. Both BDNF and NT-3 were found to be protective against trauma in mature auditory hair cells, as were other neurotrophic factors such as glial cell-line derived neurotrophic factor (GDNF)[22-24].

While neurotrophin protection of hair cells and hearing against drug and noise trauma appears to be statistically significant, the extent of protection is less than ideal. However, because they act on early stages up the cascade of cell degeneration, neurotrophic factors have the potential to be excellent protective agents. It is, therefore, necessary to optimize their use by developing protective interventions via combined use of several neurotrophic factors or in combination with other protective agents. The visionary future therapy for prevention of hair cell loss may be based on application of a combination of neurotrophic factors with anti-oxidants, NMDA type of glutamate receptor antagonists, nitric oxide (NO) blockers and/or anti-apoptotic agents[25]. The use of a large array of protective agents will cover several stages in the cascade of molecular events leading to cell degeneration.

Anti-oxidants

Reactive oxygen species (ROS) have been shown to play a role in several tissues in the response to a variety of insults, resulting in cell death and replacement. Increase in ROS has been found in the inner ear following both noise and drug trauma. It was, therefore, intuitive that free radical scavengers or other anti-oxidants could be used to protect hair cells and hearing against lesions caused by environmental inner ear insults. Indeed, iron chelators such as deferoxamine or dihydroxybenzoate were shown to reduce significantly the lesion and the functional deficit caused by several aminoglycosides in the inner ear[26]. Cisplatin ototoxicity was also significantly reduced by protective agents that enhanced the antioxidant defence of the cochlea[27]. Similarly, anti-oxidant therapy has been shown to be effective for protection against acoustic trauma[28,29]. Safe and effective antioxidant therapy needs to be developed for clinical use. One of the most promising candidates which is inexpensive, safe and widely available is aspirin[30].

Anti-apoptotic agents

The active cell death cascade involves a relatively limited number of pathways and the molecules that participate in signalling in each part of the cascade are rapidly being identified. The identification of signalling molecules in this cascade can help design ways to prevent cell death. For instance, hair cell death due to gentamicin-induced ototoxicity has been shown to involve JNK activation and hair cell apoptosis. The degeneration of hair cells can be attenuated by administration of CEP-134731, a potent inhibitor of JNK signalling.

The identification of several caspase inhibitors has paved the way to rescue experiments in many types of tissues, including the organ of Corti. One general caspase inhibitor that has been used in several rescue experiments in the inner ear is N-benzyloxycarbonyl-Val-Ala-Asp(OMe)-fluoromethylketone (Z-VAD-FMK). Z-VAD-FMK has provided protection against hair cell degeneration following cisplatin[32]. In recent experiments, chinchillas were exposed to intense noise then stained with carboxyfluorescein labelled Z-VAD-FMK. This helped identify caspase-3 as the mediator of apoptosis in the organ of Corti. Interestingly, caspase-3 dependent apoptosis is necessary for normal development of the organ of Corti[33].

In the inner ear, caspase inhibitors seem effective in rescuing hair cells that are exposed to a variety of insults[32,34]. It remains to be determined if anti-apoptotic agents can also rescue hair cells from death due to genetic disease. Based on the success in hair cell rescue by pan-caspase inhibitors, it is important to develop more specific inhibitors for use in the clinic, based on knowledge of the specific caspases that are activated following insult in the human organ of Corti. Such agents should also be cell-permeable and non-toxic.

Role of the immune system

In most tissues, there are several important roles for cells and signalling of the immune system, such as phagocytosis of pathogens and of degenerating cells or cellular debris. In addition, cytokines and other molecules provide signalling that mediates the initial response to the insult and the reparative processes. Phagocytes and immune-mediated signals, especially cytokines, play important roles in the response of the inner ear to trauma. Most significantly, cytokines have been shown to participate in the signalling for hair cell turnover and regeneration in the avian basilar papilla[35], and to influence survival of inner ear neurons[36–38]. Excessive inflammatory response can be detrimental to the structure and function of the cochlea. Thus, the beneficial as well as negative roles played by the immune system in the homeostasis of the inner ear need to be understood better so as to facilitate the design of relevant therapies for protection and repair in the cochlea[39].

Repair of injured cells

It is likely that some hair cells injured by acoustic trauma or aminoglycoside ototoxicity remain in the organ of Corti for a certain time and may be induced to heal or recover structurally and functionally. Some repair of injured cells may take place spontaneously, but the extent of such repair is difficult to measure[40]. Although it is difficult to observe tissue changing *in vivo*, functional assays may be indicative of the extent of recovery, especially within the outer hair cell population. There is an urgent need for studies that will determine what kind of therapy may enhance repair of injured hair cells in the organ of Corti.

Hearing loss and ageing

Not all hair cells survive for the full life-span of the animal and their loss gradually contributes to the general deterioration in hearing shown in ageing individuals. Presbycusis, in its more severe form, may be linked to a hereditary basis, as shown in mice with mutations in the *Ahl* gene[41]. However, humans have compromised hearing at an advanced age regardless of mutations in the *Ahl* gene. A combination of environmental factors with the extracellular environment may influence the demise of those hair cells that degenerate throughout our life[42]. Protective mechanisms discussed above versus acoustic trauma and aminoglycoside toxicity may also have relevance, at least in part, for enhancing the preservation of hearing through ageing. Considering that a large portion of the patients who seek help with hearing suffer from presbycusis, it is extremely important to determine what type of diet, chronic low-level medications or other preventive means may prevent of reduce ageing-related hearing loss[25]. It is likely that at least some of the therapies mentioned above for protection against drug and noise inner ear trauma may also be active against presbycusis. One example is ROS antagonists which have been shown to reduce age-related hearing loss[43] either directly on hair cells or indirectly by improving circulation.

Hair cell regeneration

Once cochlear hair cells are lost, they are not replaced. The term 'regeneration' is commonly used for describing generation of new hair cells. In the scientific and medical disciplines dealing with neural repair and re-growth, nerve regeneration is used to describe repair of a pre-existing cell, not necessarily implying generation of a new cell. A clear distinction between these two mechanisms, re-growth and generation of new cells, would prevent confusion.

Conceptually, there are several possible ways to attempt generation (or introduction of) new hair cells to restore function of the organ of Corti. These include generation of new cells by mitosis of supporting cells (with some of the progeny differentiating into new hair cells), conversion of the phenotype of supporting cells to hair cells (without mitosis), or implantation of stem cells or other types of cell that will be enticed to differentiate to new hair cells. At present, none of these approaches are possible in the adult mammalian organ of Corti *in vivo*. However, several lines of research are rapidly enhancing our arsenal for possible interventions to accomplish these goals (see Holley, this volume). Most importantly, genes that regulate the proliferation of hair cell progenitors and the differentiation of hair cells and supporting cells are being discovered rapidly. The genes belong to several families, which participate in cell-cycle regulation, surface receptors and several transcription factors.

The potential for cell-cycle genes to facilitate regeneration

Cells in complex organisms constantly receive multiple signals from their environment, either from soluble extracellular factors such as growth factors and hormones, which bind to their respective receptors and activate various intracellular signalling pathways, or by physical signals provided by interaction with other cells or the extracellular matrix. Among the most important signals are those that influence a cell in its decision to commit to another round of cell division, or to remain in a quiescent state. To enter the cell cycle, cells require the appropriately regulated activities of various cyclins and cyclin-dependent kinases (CDKs)[44]. Upon activation, the cyclin–CDK complex phosphorylates and inactivates the pRb tumour suppressor protein, thus promoting entry into the cell cycle. *In vivo*, CDK molecules exist in complex with various inhibitor molecules, which inhibit CDK activity, and thereby prevent cells from entering the cell cycle. The Cip/Kip family (for CDK interacting protein/ kinase inhibitory protein) includes p21[Cip1], p27[Kip1] and p57[Kip2]. p27[Kip1] has been shown to inhibit several CDK molecules and regulate the decision to divide[44].

Recently, expression of p27[Kip1] protein was demonstrated in the supporting cells of the organ of Corti[45], consistent with the notion that p27[Kip1] may play a critical role in cell cycle arrest and in maintaining the differentiated phenotype. In developing p27[Kip1–/–] mice, the cells of the organ of Corti continue to proliferate for more than 2 weeks after proliferation would normally have ceased[46]. Moreover, supporting cells in the p27[Kip1–/–] mice can generate new hair cells after trauma-induced hair cell loss. These findings demonstrate that overcoming or releasing the inhibition of the cell cycle in these knockout mice allows the generation of excessive number of hair cells. It is necessary to design somatic cell interventions *in vivo* to remove p27[Kip1] inhibition of cell cycle in a way that will be specific and restricted to supporting cells in the organ of Corti. It is also necessary to identify other families of molecules that may influence proliferation of supporting cells. The vestibular epithelium is a good source of information for such searches[47]. Once the important molecules that signal mitosis in the epithelium are identified, the next major step toward accomplishing hair cell regeneration will be introducing and regulating expression of these genes in supporting cells of the cochlea.

Phenotypic conversion

One potential way to generate new hair cells is by conversion of the phenotype of supporting cells without cell division (see Richardson, this volume). Such conversion likely occurs as a secondary mechanism of hair cell regeneration in the avian basilar papilla[48,49]. The genes that mediate conversion in the inner ear are unknown. Identification of this set of genes and the ability to over-express them in supporting cells of the organ of Corti may lead to means for restoring the hair cell population, without the risk of malignancy that may accompany any change in cell cycle regulation.

Genes that specify the hair cell phenotype

During embryonic development, the fate of otocyst cells is determined in a sequence of events governed by intercellular signalling and expression sequence of specific genes. Among these genes are *Math1*[50], *Hes1*[51], *Brn-3.1*[52] *GATA3*[53] and genes from the *Notch* family[54] (see Richardson, this volume). Manipulation of the level of expression of genes that encode hair cell differentiation may influence the fate of remaining supporting cells in the organ of Corti and possibly lead to hair cell regeneration following inner ear trauma.

Cell lines and stem cell therapy

The use of cultured cells for replacing lost hair cells is a relatively new concept with exciting potential (see Holley, this volume). Candidate culture cells are hair cell lines and stem cells. Hair cell lines are cell lines that may be generated by specific selection of sub-populations from dissociated otocysts. Currently, available hair cell lines are derived from otocyst of immortomouse[55–57]. The other source of cells is multipotent self-renewing stem cells. These clonal cells keep proliferating until they receive signals that induce their differentiation. In the absence of basal cells or stem cells in the organ of Corti, it is necessary to develop the technology to introduce stem cells into the area of the organ of Corti and provide the necessary signals for their differentiation and innervation[58]. One major challenge in any introduction of foreign cells into the cochlea will be the incorporation of transplanted cells into the correct site.

Hereditary hearing losses

Approximately half of congenital deafness is thought to be due to hereditary causes. Genetics also influences the disposition of individuals to progressive hearing loss later in life. Identification of the genes involved in deafness in humans has important implications for diagnostics and prognosis. One of the major challenges we face is the development of a cure for genetic inner ear disease. Such a cure will depend on our knowledge of the mutated genes and the technology for gene transfer. The intervention (gene transfer) should be based on substituting the mutated gene (or the missing or faulty gene product) with the normal gene. A proof of the principle that such replacement may reverse the phenotype and rescue hearing and hair cells was recently provided. Specifically, germ-line insertion of a wild-type *Myo15* transgene (in a bacterial artificial chromosome) into a zygote destined to develop into an affected shaker 2 mutant mouse (deaf and circling), resulted in a phenotypic rescue. The mouse that developed was hearing and did not circle[59]. At present, as physicians refer patients for genetic counselling and diagnostic testing, the number of known families with hereditary inner ear disease is increasing, leading to an intensive effort by the research community to identify the mutated genes. Along with development of the technology for gene transfer, the likelihood that therapy for hereditary disease will become a real option is increasing.

Conclusions and key points for clinical practice

- Better understanding of cell death mechanism may help prevent hair cell loss in the inner ear.

- Several types of molecules have been shown to have protective effects against cochlear trauma.

- Once lost, hair cells cannot be replaced. However, the expanding knowledge of the molecular basis cell cycle and differentiation, along with advances in gene transfer technology, may help develop methods for gene therapy aimed at hair cell regeneration.

- Use of stem cells or cell lines as cell replacement therapy may also contribute to restoration of inner ear function.

- Identification of the genes that are mutated in hereditary inner ear disease, along with the development of vectors that will allow gene introduction into the specific cells of the auditory system, will help develop cure for genetic disease.

Acknowledgements

I thank Matthew Holley for constructive suggestions, and Graham Atkin, Lisa Beyer and Christopher Zurenka for helpful comments on the manuscript. Supported by NIH NIDCD Grant DC01634.

References

1   Hawkins Jr JE, Johnsson LG, Stebbins WC, Moody DB, Coombs SL. Hearing loss and cochlear pathology in monkeys after noise exposure. *Acta Otolaryngol* 1976; **81**: 337–43
2   Raphael Y, Altschuler RA. Reorganization of cytoskeletal and junctional proteins during cochlear hair cell degeneration. *Cell Motil Cytoskel* 1991; **18**: 215–27
3   Lenoir M, Daudet N, Humbert G *et al*. Morphological and molecular changes in the inner hair cell region of the rat cochlea after amikacin treatment. *J Neurocytol* 1999; **28**: 925–37
4   Rosenblatt J, Raff MC, Cramer LP. An epithelial cell destined for apoptosis signals its neighbors to extrude it by an actin- and myosin-dependent mechanism. *Curr Biol* 2001; **11**: 1847–57
5   Bok D. The retinal pigment epithelium: a versatile partner in vision. *J Cell Sci Suppl* 1993; **17**: 189–95
6   Sobkowicz HM, August BK, Slapnick SM. Post-traumatic survival and recovery of the auditory sensory cells in culture. *Acta Otolaryngol* 1996; **116**: 257–62

7   Jacobson MD, Weil M, Raff MC. Programmed cell death in animal development. *Cell* 1997; **88**: 347–54

8   Cheng J, Zhou T, Liu C *et al*. Protection from Fas-mediated apoptosis by a soluble form of the Fas molecule. *Science* 1994; **263**: 1759–62

9   Carson JP, Behnam M, Sutton JN *et al*. Smac is required for cytochrome c-induced apoptosis in prostate cancer LNCaP cells. *Cancer Res* 2002; **62**: 18–23

10 Nunez G, Merino R, Simonian PL, Grillot DA. Regulation of lymphoid apoptosis by Bcl-2 and Bcl-XL. *Adv Exp Med Biol* 1996; **406**: 75–82

11 Nunez G, Benedict MA, Hu Y, Inohara N. Caspases: the proteases of the apoptotic pathway. *Oncogene* 1998; **17**: 3237–45

12 Ashkenazi A, Dixit VM. Death receptors: signaling and modulation. *Science* 1998; **281**: 1305–8

13 Liu X, Zou H, Slaughter C, Wang X. DFF, a heterodimeric protein that functions downstream of caspase-3 to trigger DNA fragmentation during apoptosis. *Cell* 1997; **89**: 175–84

14 Kothakota S, Azuma T, Reinhard C *et al*. Caspase-3-generated fragment of gelsolin: effector of morphological change in apoptosis. *Science* 1997; **278**: 294–8

15 Roy N, Deveraux QL, Takahashi R, Salvesen GS, Reed JC. The c-IAP-1 and c-IAP-2 proteins are direct inhibitors of specific caspases. *EMBO J* 1997; **16**: 6914–25

16 McCarthy NJ, Evan GI. Methods for detecting and quantifying apoptosis. *Curr Top Dev Biol* 1998; **36**: 259–78

17 Hu BH, Guo W, Wang PY, Henderson D, Jiang SC. Intense noise-induced apoptosis in hair cells of guinea pig cochleae. *Acta Otolaryngol* 2000; **120**: 19–24

18 Zheng Y, Ikeda K, Nakamura M, Takasaka T. Endonuclease cleavage of DNA in the aged cochlea of Mongolian gerbil. *Hear Res* 1998; **126**: 11–8

19 Nishizaki K, Yoshino T, Orita Y, Nomiya S, Masuda Y. TUNEL staining of inner ear structures may reflect autolysis, not apoptosis. *Hear Res* 1999; **130**: 131–6

20 Fritzsch B, Farinas I, Reichardt LF. Lack of neurotrophin 3 causes losses of both classes of spiral ganglion neurons in the cochlea in a region-specific fashion. *J Neurosci* 1997; **17**: 6213–25

21 Fritzsch B, Barbacid M, Silos-Santiago I. Nerve dependency of developing and mature sensory receptor cells. *Ann NY Acad Sci* 1998; **855**: 14–27

22 Gao WQ. Therapeutic potential of neurotrophins for treatment of hearing loss. *Mol Neurobiol* 1998; **17**: 17–31

23 Marzella PL, Gillespie LN, Clark GM, Bartlett PF, Kilpatrick TJ. The neurotrophins act synergistically with LIF and members of the TGF-beta superfamily to promote the survival of spiral ganglia neurons *in vitro*. *Hear Res* 1999; **138**: 73–80

24 Keithley EM, Ma CL, Ryan AF, Louis JC, Magal E. GDNF protects the cochlea against noise damage. *Neuroreport* 1998; **9**: 2183–7

25 Seidman MD. Effects of dietary restriction and antioxidants on presbycusis. *Laryngoscope* 2000; **110**: 727–38

26 Song BB, Anderson DJ, Schacht J. Protection from gentamicin ototoxicity by iron chelators in guinea pig *in vivo*. *J Pharmacol Exp Ther* 1997; **282**: 369–77

27 Rybak LP, Somani S. Ototoxicity. Amelioration by protective agents. *Ann NY Acad Sci* 1999; **884**: 143–51

28 Kopke RD, Weisskopf PA, Boone JL *et al*. Reduction of noise-induced hearing loss using L-NAC and salicylate in the chinchilla. *Hear Res* 2000; **149**: 138–46

29 Henderson D, McFadden SL, Liu CC, Hight N, Zheng XY. The role of antioxidants in protection from impulse noise. *Ann NY Acad Sci* 1999; **884**: 368–80

30 Sha SH, Schacht J. Antioxidants attenuate gentamicin-induced free radical formation *in vitro* and ototoxicity *in vivo*: D-methionine is a potential protectant. *Hear Res* 2000; **142**: 34–40

31 Ylikoski J, Xing-Qun L, Virkkala J, Pirvola U. Blockade of c-Jun N-terminal kinase pathway attenuates gentamicin-induced cochlear and vestibular hair cell death. *Hear Res* 2002; **163**: 71–81

32 Liu W, Staecker H, Stupak H, Malgrange B, Lefebvre P, Van De Water TR. Caspase inhibitors prevent cisplatin-induced apoptosis of auditory sensory cells. *Neuroreport* 1998; **9**: 2609–14

33 Takahashi K, Kamiya K, Urase K *et al*. Caspase-3-deficiency induces hyperplasia of supporting cells and degeneration of sensory cells resulting in the hearing loss. *Brain Res* 2001; **894**: 359–67

34 Rybak LP, Husain K, Morris C, Whitworth C, Somani S. Effect of protective agents against cisplatin ototoxicity. *Am J Otol* 2000; **21**: 513–20

35 Warchol ME. Immune cytokines and dexamethasone influence sensory regeneration in the avian vestibular periphery. *J Neurocytol* 1999; **28**: 889–900

36 Warchol ME, Kaplan BA. Macrophage secretory products influence the survival of statoacoustic neurons. *Neuroreport* 1999; **10**:665-8

37 Komeda M, Roessler BJ, Raphael Y. The influence of interleukin-1 receptor antagonist transgene on spiral ganglion neurons. *Hear Res* 1999; **131**: 1–10

38 Marzella PL, Clark GM, Shepherd RK, Bartlett PF, Kilpatrick TJ. LIF potentiates the NT-3-mediated survival of spiral ganglia neurones *in vitro*. *Neuroreport* 1997; **8**: 1641–4

39 Ryan AF, Pak K, Low W *et al*. Immunological damage to the inner ear: current and future therapeutic strategies. *Adv Otorhinolaryngol* 2002; **59**: 66–74

40 Engstrom B, Flock A, Borg E. Ultrastructural studies of stereocilia in noise-exposed rabbits. *Hear Res* 1983; **12**: 251–64

41 Willott JF, Erway LC. Genetics of age-related hearing loss in mice. IV. Cochlear pathology and hearing loss in 25 BXD recombinant inbred mouse strains. *Hear Res* 1998; **119**: 27–36

42 Jennings CR, Jones NS. Presbycusis. *J Laryngol Otol* 2001; **115**: 171–8

43 Seidman MD, Quirk WS, Shirwany NA. Mechanisms of alterations in the microcirculation of the cochlea. *Ann NY Acad Sci* 1999; **884**: 226–32

44 Vidal A, Koff A. Cell-cycle inhibitors: three families united by a common cause. *Gene* 2000; **247**: 1–15

45 Chen P. Segil N. p27(Kip1) links cell proliferation to morphogenesis in the developing organ of Corti. *Development* 1999; **126**: 1581–90

46 Lowenheim H, Furness DN, Kil J *et al*. Gene disruption of p27(Kip1) allows cell proliferation in the postnatal and adult organ of Corti. *Proc Natl Acad Sci USA* 1999; **96**: 4084–8

47 Montcouquiol M, Corwin JT. Intracellular signals that control cell proliferation in mammalian balance epithelia: key roles for phosphatidylinositol-3 kinase, mammalian target of rapamycin, and S6 kinases in preference to calcium, protein kinase C, and mitogen-activated protein kinase. *J Neurosci* 2001; **21**: 570–80

48 Adler HJ, Raphael Y. New hair cells arise from supporting cell conversion in the acoustically damaged chick inner ear. *Neurosci Lett* 1996; **205**: 17–20

49 Roberson DW, Kreig CS, Rubel EW. Light microscopic evidence that direct transdifferentiation gives rise to new hair cells in regenerating avian auditory epithelium. *Aud Neurosci* 1996; **2**: 195–205

50 Bermingham NA, Hassan BA, Price SD *et al*. Math1: an essential gene for the generation of inner ear hair cells. *Science* 1999; **284**: 1837–41

51 Zheng JL, Shou J, Guillemot F, Kageyama R, Gao WQ. Hes1 is a negative regulator of inner ear hair cell differentiation. *Development* 2000; **127**: 4551–60

52 Keithley EM, Erkman L, Bennett T, Lou L, Ryan AF. Effects of a hair cell transcription factor, Brn-3.1, gene deletion on homozygous and heterozygous mouse cochleas in adulthood and aging. *Hear Res* 1999; **134**: 71–6

53 Rivolta MN, Holley MC. GATA3 is downregulated during hair cell differentiation in the mouse cochlea. *J Neurocytol* 1998; **27**: 637–47

54 Lanford PJ, Lan Y, Jiang R *et al*. Notch signalling pathway mediates hair cell development in mammalian cochlea [see comments]. *Nat Genet* 1999; **21**: 289–92

55 Barald KF, Lindberg KH, Hardiman K *et al*. Immortalized cell lines from embryonic avian and murine otocysts: tools for molecular studies of the developing inner ear. *Int J Dev Neurosci* 1997; **15**: 523–40

56 Lawlor P, Marcotti W, Rivolta MN, Kros CJ, Holley MC. Differentiation of mammalian vestibular hair cells from conditionally immortal, postnatal supporting cells. *J Neurosci* 1999; **19**: 9445–58

57 Rivolta MN, Grix N, Lawlor P, Ashmore JF, Jagger DJ, Holley MC. Auditory hair cell precursors immortalized from the mammalian inner ear. *Proc R Soc Lond B Biol Sci* 1998; **265**: 1595–603

58 Ito J, Kojima K, Kawaguchi S. Survival of neural stem cells in the cochlea. *Acta Otolaryngol* 2001; **121**: 140–2

59 Probst FJ, Fridell RA, Raphael Y *et al*. Correction of deafness in shaker-2 mice by an unconventional myosin in a BAC transgene *Science* 1998; **280**: 1444–7

Sensory organ development in the inner ear: molecular and cellular mechanisms

Jane Bryant, Richard J Goodyear and **Guy P Richardson**

School of Biological Sciences, University of Sussex, Brighton, UK

The molecular mechanisms underlying the specification of sensory organs in the inner ear and the development of hair and supporting cells within these organs are described. The different organs are all derived from a common pro-sensory region, and may be specified by their proximity to the boundaries between compartments – broad domains within the otocyst defined by the asymmetric expression patterns of transcription factors. Activation of Notch may specify the pro-sensory region, and lateral inhibition mediated by Notch signalling influences whether cells of common lineage in a sensory patch differentiate as either hair cells or supporting cells. The transcription factors Math1 and Brn3.1 are required for hair cell differentiation, and supporting cells express negative regulators of neurogenesis, Hes1 and Hes5. Retinoic acid and thyroid hormone influence early aspects and timing of hair cell differentiation, respectively. Development of the hair cell's mechanosensory hair bundle involves interactions between the cytoskeleton, cell-surface adhesion molecules, receptors and associated extracellular matrix.

There are six distinct sensory organs in the mammalian inner ear: the three cristae of the semicircular canals, the two maculae of the saccule and utricle, and the organ of Corti of the cochlea (Fig. 1). The cristae and the maculae are vestibular organs that respond to angular and linear acceleration, respectively. The organ of Corti is the organ of hearing. These three types of organ differ in their function, and in the fine details of their cellular architecture, but they all conform to the same basic plan. They are relatively simple epithelia composed of two basic cell types, the sensory hair cells and their surrounding, non-sensory supporting cells. These epithelia lie upon a sheet of extracellular matrix, a basal lamina, and also have a prominent extracellular structure, a cupula, an otoconial membrane or a tectorial membrane, associated with their apical surface. The supporting cells sit on the basal lamina, and their lateral membranes surround the hair cells, projecting up to the surface of the epithelium. The hair cells do not contact the basal lamina, and they are isolated from one another by the supporting cells. At the apical surface of the epithelium, the supporting cell processes form tight and adherens junctions with each

Correspondence to:
Dr Guy P Richardson,
School of Biological
Sciences, University of
Sussex, Falmer,
Brighton BN1 9QG, UK

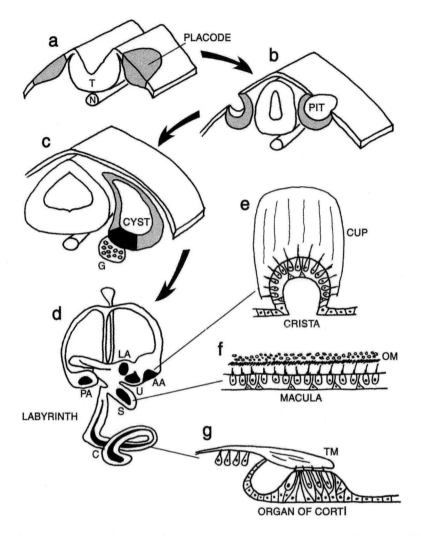

Fig. 1 Diagram illustrating the main steps in the development of the inner ear (a–d), and the structure of the three types of sensory organ (e–g). The inner ear develops from the otic placode (a) an ectodermal thickening that invaginates to form the otic pit (b) which in turns pinches off from the ectoderm to form the otic vesicle (c). The different sensory organs are derived from a common pro-sensory patch (black) in the ventromedial wall of the otocyst (c). A complex series of morphogenetic events transforms the otic vesicle (c) into the labyrinth (d) containing three cristae (e), two maculae (f), and an organ of Corti (g). Abbreviations: G, VIIIth ganglion; AA, anterior ampulla; LA, lateral ampulla; PA, posterior ampulla;, U, utricle; S, saccule; C, cochlea; CUP, cupula; OM, otoconial membrane; TM, tectorial membrane.

other and with the hair cells. The hair cells have a highly specialized bundle of modified microvilli on their apical surface, a hair bundle, and it is this feature that enables them to detect mechanical stimuli and transduce them into electrical signals.

These sensory organs of the inner ear are all derived during development from the wall of the otocyst, a hollow, pear-shaped structure that forms, just after neural tube closure, from a thickening of the head ectoderm that lies adjacent to the rhombencephalon and is known as the otic placode. The neurones that innervate the hair cells in each organ of the ear are also derived from the otocyst, by a process of delamination, prior to the formation the sensory organs. Although these neurones become critically dependent on trophic support from the hair cells[1,2], there is little evidence that they influence the development of hair and supporting cells. In this brief review, we will focus specifically on the sequence of molecular and cellular events that leads to the differentiation of hair and supporting cells within these epithelial organs, rather than the process of synaptogenesis. We will describe the origin of the different sensory organs, the lineage relationships of hair and supporting cells, and how the two cell types come to adopt different fates. The roles of retinoic acid and thyroid hormone will be discussed, and recent evidence indicating that a complex interplay between the cytoskeleton, components of the hair cell surface and the associated extracellular matrix controls the process of hair bundle development will be reviewed.

Much of our understanding about the development of the inner ear comes from a number of different systems, and not just from the experiments done with mammalian species. Studies on the developing chick inner ear, and more recently that of the zebrafish, provide considerable information on basic mechanisms and principles that are likely to be applicable to the process of hair and supporting cell development in both mice and humans. For certain aspects, detailed data are only available for the chick and, when necessary, these will be used to illustrate how the sensory patches in the inner ear are formed.

Generation and specification of sensory organs

Histological studies[3] originally suggested that the different sensory organs of the chick inner ear are all derived from a single patch of cells in the ventromedial wall of the otocyst. Molecular studies have recently revived support for this suggestion, and have revealed that there is a pro-sensory area in the ventromedial region of the otocyst that can be defined by the expression patterns of *Serrate1*[4], *Lunatic fringe*[4] and BEN[5]. Serrate1 (known as Jagged1 in mammals) is a transmembrane ligand for Notch, a membrane receptor that is involved in many aspects of development[6]. Lunatic fringe is a protein that modulates interaction between Notch and its ligands[7]. BEN is a cell–cell adhesion molecule of the Ig superfamily[8]. Notch is widely expressed throughout the otocyst[9], and Serrate1 may serve to maintain a high level of Notch activation within the pro-sensory patch, endowing this region with the capacity to form sensory organs, and preventing the premature differentiation of hair cells[10]. The role of Lunatic fringe in the pro-sensory patch is uncertain. *Lfng*[-/-] mice do not have any inner ear abnormalities[11], and it may only act as a weak inhibitor of Notch signalling[10]. As a cell–cell adhesion molecule, BEN may serve to stop the cells of the pro-sensory patch from mixing with cells in other regions of the otocyst, *i.e.* those that are destined to become non-sensory parts of the ear[5]. Although these studies provide evidence for the existence of a common pro-sensory patch and reveal molecular constituents with potential roles, it is not yet known what signals determine the formation of this region, or from where these signals emanate.

A boundary model has been proposed to account for how the different sensory organs of the inner ear are specified[12]. This model postulates that the different sensory organs of the inner ear form at, or in proximity to, the boundaries between a small number of different compartments. These compartments are defined by the asymmetric expression patterns of a few genes and may, for example, correspond to the ventral and dorsal halves, or the anterior and posterior segments of the otocyst. Genes for transcription factors such as Pax2, Dlx5, Otx1 and Hmx3 are expressed in such broad domains in the otocyst, and data from knockout mice are consistent with the boundary model (see Brigande *et al*[13] and Cantos *et al*[14] for reviews). For example, anterior and posterior cristae along with their associated canals are missing in *Dlx5*[-/-] mice[15]. Also *Pax2*[-/-] mice fail to form a cochlear duct[16]. Compartment boundary intersection points may, therefore, define where a sensory organ forms within the ventromedial pro-sensory patch, and whether it becomes a crista, a macula, or a hearing organ.

The expression of *BMP4* in spatially discrete regions within the ventromedial pro-sensory patch marks the first appearance of individual sensory organs[17,18]. BMP4 is a member of the TGF-β family of secreted growth factors and, in the chick otocyst, *BMP4* is expressed in all of the sensory organs as they first emerge[17]. However, BMP4 is not a good marker for every sensory organ in the mouse otocyst[18], and it is only expressed in some of the organs in the zebrafish ear[19]. Although BMP4 could autonomously regulate the development of hair and supporting cells within the organs within which it is expressed, it may actually play a major role in controlling the development of the accessory structures that form adjacent to the sensory patches. For example, the BMP4 antagonist Noggin severely disrupts semicircular canal formation but has comparatively little effect on the development and differentiation of hair cells[20,21]. FGF10 is also expressed by the presumptive sensory epithelia of the mouse otocyst, and it too may operate in a paracrine fashion, signalling through the IIIb isoform of FGFR-2 to control the development of adjacent non-sensory tissues[22]. A number of other genes are also expressed in sensory patches at the very early stages of their development. These include *BMP5* and *BMP7*[23], *p75NGFR*[24,25], *Msx1*[17], *NT3*[18,24], *bmp2b*[19], and *MsxC*[19,26]. Some of these, like *MsxC*, are only expressed in certain sensory patches, and may specify the type of organ that develops.

Lineage and birth of hair and supporting cells

Hair and supporting cells in the mammalian inner ear are born over a brief period of development after the sensory patches have been specified[27,28]. The cells then differentiate and remain mitotically inactive. In the cochlea of the mouse, the cyclin-dependent kinase inhibitor, $p27^{Kip1}$, is expressed by cells of the organ of Corti as soon as they withdraw from the cell cycle[29,30]. The pattern of $p27^{Kip1}$ expression precisely delineates the region of the cochlear duct within which the hair and supporting cells of the organ of Corti will differentiate. The expression of $p27^{Kip1}$ is down-regulated in hair cells as they begin overt cytodifferentiation, but in supporting cells it persists into adulthood[29]. In $p27^{Kip1-/-}$ mice, cell proliferation within the organ of Corti continues, and an excess of hair and supporting cells is found[29,31]. These data indicate $p27^{Kip1}$ negatively regulates cell proliferation in the organ of Corti. However, other molecules must also control this process as many hair and supporting cells do leave the cell cycle and differentiate in the cochleae of $p27^{Kip1}$ knockout mice.

In the hearing organs of both mammals[27] and birds[32], hair and supporting cells at any one place within the structure are born simultaneously, suggesting they may share a common lineage. Retroviral tracing studies in the chick auditory organ have provided firm experimental evidence for this suggestion[33,34]. Furthermore, it has been shown that the potential to become either a hair or a supporting cell is retained by a progenitor cell until it has passed through its final mitotic division, as two-cell clones were found that contained either two supporting cells, two hair cells or both cell types[33].

The differentiation of hair and supporting cells

The decision to become either a hair cell or a supporting cell most probably involves lateral inhibition[35,36], a process by which cells of common origin adopt different fates. Lateral inhibition is usually mediated by Notch signalling, and a number of studies have now shown that the products of the neurogenic genes of the Notch signalling pathway play a key role in mediating the differentiation of hair and

Table 1 Expression patterns of transcription factors and components of the Notch signalling pathway observed during sensory organ development in the inner ear, and the effects of experimentally manipulating their expression

Name of gene or protein	Nature of protein	Expression pattern	Mutant/experimental phenotype	References
Math1	bHLH transcription factor	Mouse vestibule at E12, cochlea at E13.5; expressed transiently by hair cells and down-regulated by P3	Complete absence of hair cells in the inner ear of *Math1*$^{-/-}$ mice by P1	30, 42, 50, 54
Brn3.1	POU domain transcription factor	Mouse vestibule E12.5, cochlea at E14.5; expressed specifically by hair cells	Loss of hair cells by P14 in *Brn3.1*$^{-/-}$ mice	46–48
GATA3	C4 zinc finger transcription factor	Mouse auditory epithelium at E14; down-regulates in hair cells, then in supporting cells		49
Hes1	bHLH transcription factor	Greater and lesser epithelial ridges of rat (E17.5) and mouse (E18.5) cochlea; supporting cells of rat utricle by E17.5	Increase in inner hair cells and utricular hair cells in *Hes1*$^{-/-}$ mice	52, 53
Hes5	bHLH transcription factor	Mouse cochlea at E15, restricted to Deiter's cells by E17	Increased in outer hair cells and macular hair cells in *Hes5*$^{-/-}$ mice	53, 54
Notch1	Transmembrane receptor	Wide-spread in epithelium of otocyst from early stages, becomes restricted to supporting cells as they differentiate	Increase in OIICs in *Notch1*$^{+/-}$ mice. Increased rows of IHCs and OHCs in rat cochlear cultures treated with Notch1 antisense oligonucleotides	9, 37–40, 42, 43
Delta1	Transmembrane ligand for Notch	Mouse vestibular hair cells at E12.5, mouse cochlear hair cells at 14.5. In sensory patches of chick otocyst from E3.5 onwards, and zebrafish otocyst at 14 hpf	Large increase in hair cells numbers in zebrafish dominant negative DeltaA^{dx2} mutants. Retroviral expression of dominant negative Dl1^{dn} in chick down-regulates *Ser1* expression	9, 10, 38, 39
Serrate1 (Jagged1)	Transmembrane ligand for Notch	In all sensory organs of the mouse inner ear by E12.5, and becomes restricted to supporting cells as hair cells differentiate In pro-sensory patch of chick otocyst from E2.5 (stage 19)	Extra IHCs but loss of third row OHCs along with loss of cristae in mice with dominant missense Jag1 mutations. Extra rows of IHCs and OHCs in rat cochlear cultures treated with Jag1 antisense oligonucleotides	4, 9, 38, 39, 43–45
Serrate2 (Jagged2)	Transmembrane ligand for Notch	In hair cells of mouse vestibule at E13.5, and cochlea at E14.5. In rat IHCs at E18, and OHCs at E20. In zebrafish from 18 hpf	Extra rows of IHCs and OHCs in Jag2 null mutant mice	37, 40, 43
Lunatic fringe	Glycosyl transferase that modifies Notch extracellular domain	In sensory organs of mouse inner ear by E11.5, restricted to supporting cells in organ of Corti by E16. In pro-sensory patch of chick otocyst by E2.5	No obvious phenotype in inner ear of Lfng deficient mice, but the extra rows of IHCs seen in Jag2 null mutant are suppressed on a Lfng null mutant background	4, 11, 18
Numb	Intracellular protein that blocks Notch activation	In all cells of chick sensory patch at E3, restricted to hair cells at E12		10

Abbreviations: IHC, inner hair cell; OHC, outer hair cell; E, embryonic day; P, postnatal day; hpf, hours post-fertilisation.

supporting cells in the inner ear[9,10,37–45]. The expression patterns of these genes in the ear, and the phenotypes of the different mutants that have been examined, are summarised in Table 1. In addition, a number of transcription factors have been shown to be involved in the process of hair and supporting-cell differentiation[46–54], some of which may directly interact with the Notch signalling pathway. These are also listed in Table 1. The expression patterns of both the neurogenic genes and the transcription factors, the consequences of experimentally manipulating their expression, are now described and discussed in detail.

Math1

Math1, a mouse homologue of the *Drosophila* proneural gene *atonal*, encodes a basic, helix-loop-helix (bHLH) transcription factor. It is expressed in the primordium of the organ of Corti after the cells in this region have withdrawn from the cell cycle and have begun to express $p27^{Kip1}$, but before hair cells have started to express myosin VIIa, a marker of overt differentiation[30]. Math1 is initially expressed by thin bands of cells that span the entire thickness of the epithelium, and expression becomes restricted to hair cells located at the lumenal surface of the epithelium as they differentiate[30,54]. These thin bands of Math1-expressing cells that initially span the thickness of the epithelium may be bi-potential progenitor cells[54]. Alternatively, they may be vertical stacks of hair cells that subsequently undergo movement within the thickness of the epithelium and spread out along the longitudinal axis of the cochlea as it elongates[30].

Hair cells are absent from the inner ears of *Math1*[−/−] mice by birth[50], and the ectopic expression of Math1 in the non-sensory cells of the greater epithelial ridge that lie adjacent to the organ of Corti results in the formation of supernumerary hair cells[51]. These results indicate that Math1 is both 'necessary and sufficient' for hair cell differentiation[30]. Early markers of overt hair cell differentiation, myosin VI and calretinin, are never expressed during inner ear development in *Math1*[−/−] mice[50]. The sensory epithelia are thinner and non-stratified, but have an overlying extracellular matrix suggesting the supporting cells may have differentiated. An apparent overcrowding of supporting-cell nuclei and a failure to observe apoptosis in the sensory epithelia of *Math1*[−/−] mice was originally interpreted as indicating that a fate switch had occurred, leading to an overproduction of supporting cells[50]. However, apoptotic cells have recently been reported in the organ of Corti of *Math1*[−/−] mice, so the hair cells may be produced, fail to express any known markers of differentiation, and then die[30]. Sensory epithelia, albeit eventually devoid of hair cells, do form in *Math1*[−/−] mice, so it is unlikely that *Math1* is acting as a true proneural gene like its invertebrate homologue *atonal*[50]. A proneural gene required for sensory organ specification in the inner ear has, therefore, yet to be discovered.

Delta1, Jagged2 and Notch1

Delta1 and *Jagged2* (known as *Serrate2* in chick) are expressed by hair cells in the mouse cochlea approximately 1 day after the onset of Math1 expression[38,40]. In *Jagged2* null mutant mice, there is an increase in the linear density of inner and outer hair cells in the cochlea, with a nearly complete duplication of the normal, single row of inner hair cells, and many stretches where there are four instead of three rows of outer hair cells[40]. Delta mutants have not been studied in the mouse, but a dominant negative allele of the zebrafish *deltaA* gene, *deltaA*[dx2], results in a 5–6-fold increase in hair cell numbers in the inner ear, and a loss of most of the supporting cells[41]. Notch expression is initially widely distributed throughout the inner ear epithelium and the sensory patches, and becomes restricted to the supporting-cell layer as the hair cells differentiate[9,39,40,42,43]. *Notch1*[-/-] mice are early embryonic lethals, but in heterozygotes with presumably reduced levels of Notch1, a significant increase is observed in the numbers of regions along the cochlea where there are four instead of three rows of outer hair cells[11]. Treating rat cochlear cultures with antisense Notch oligonucleotides causes the production of extra rows of both inner and outer hair cells[43]. The expression of *Delta1* and *Jagged2* in hair cells, and the overproduction of hair cells seen in corresponding mutants and with antisense oligonucleotides to *Notch1*, all indicate that hair cells use Notch signalling to inhibit laterally their neighbouring cells and thereby prevent them from adopting the same fate.

Serrate1/Jagged1

Serrate1/Jagged1 is expressed throughout the pro-sensory patch initially[4,9,38], but becomes progressively restricted to the supporting cells as they differentiate[38,39]. The expression of Serrate1/Jagged1 by supporting cells may not appear to be consistent with the idea that hair cells inhibit their neighbours. However, there is evidence from the chick that hair cells express Numb, a protein that blocks Notch signalling[10]. These hair cells would, therefore, be deaf to signals delivered by Serrate1 from adjacent supporting cells. Furthermore, there is also evidence from the chick inner ear that the expression of *Serrate 1* in supporting cells is positively regulated by Notch signalling via lateral induction[10]. This would serve to increase the level of Notch activation amongst the supporting cells, and ensure that they do not differentiate as hair cells. The overproduction of hair cells in late embryonic rat cochlear cultures caused by Jagged1 antisense oligonucleotides[43] is consistent with this, as reduced Notch activation should lead to an excess of hair cells. However, in mouse mutants[44,45], Jagged1 mutations that are assumed to be dominant negative lead to the complete loss of some sensory organs (cristae) and only perturb hair cell patterning in others (cochlea). This could be because Serrate1/Jagged1 has an early role in specifying sensory

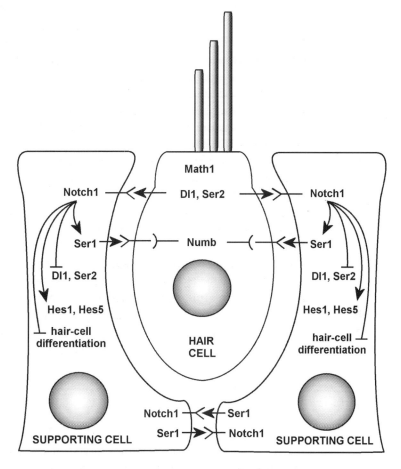

Fig. 2 Diagram illustrating the regulatory interactions occurring between components of the Notch signalling pathway that lead to the differentiation of hair and supporting cells in the sensory organs of the inner ear. A single hair cell is shown that is surrounded by two supporting cells. Activation of Notch1 stimulates Serrate1/Jagged1 (Ser1) production, represses expression of Delta1 (Dl1) and Serrate2/Jagged2 (Ser2), positively regulates expression of Hes1/5 and inhibits hair cell differentiation. Hair cells express Delta1 (Dl1), Serrate2/Jagged2 (Ser2) and Numb. Numb prevents Serrate1/Jagged1 (Ser1) expressed by supporting cells from activating Notch. A high level of Notch activation leads to cells adopting the secondary fate, *i.e.* they become supporting cells. Cells with low levels of Notch activation adopt the primary, default state and become hair cells. Modified from Eddison *et al*[10] with permission from the author.

patches and/or preventing their premature differentiation, and a later role in regulating the development of hair and supporting cells within the patch[44]. Whilst this may partially explain why the mutations, which are effective throughout development, and antisense treatment, which has only been applied at relatively late developmental stages, have different effects, it does not explain why the different organs in the ears of *Jagged1* mutant mice respond differently to the same mutation. However, the loss of cristae may occur secondarily to the truncation of the canals, which in turn may be due to diminished BMP4 signalling from the sensory patch resulting from reduced Notch activation.

The expression patterns of the neurogenic genes described above and the phenotypes of the different mutants that have been examined are generally in accordance with the theory that hair cells laterally inhibit their neighbours and force them to become supporting cells. However, the situation is clearly more complex than originally envisioned[35,36]. Although a stochastic fluctuation in Notch signalling in a field of cells initially expressing uniform levels of Notch and Delta can theoretically lead, as a result of negative feedback, to the production of regular mosaics of hair and supporting cells[55,56], Delta1 is not uniformly expressed[38], there are two other Notch ligands operating in the ear, and the signalling pathway can be modulated at many levels, making the simple scenario, although attractive, less likely. Furthermore, an active re-arrangement of hair and supporting cells relative to one another may contribute to the formation of a precise cellular mosaic, and refine the imperfect patterns that are initially observed during the early stages of development[57], indicating that lateral inhibition with feedback is not the only mechanism contributing to pattern formation in the sensory epithelia. The expression patterns for the neurogenic genes and the experimental findings described above are largely consistent with a system of regulatory interactions (see Fig. 2) recently proposed by Lewis and colleagues[10].

Hes1 and Hes5

Hes1 and *Hes5*, mammalian homologues of the *Drosophila hairy* and *enhancer of Split* genes, are expressed in patterns that are both complementary and overlapping in the developing cochlea and utricle of the mammal[52,53]. The products of these genes act as negative regulators of neurogenesis in vertebrates[58]. Expression of *Hes5* is first observed in the supporting cells of the organ of Corti after the expression of *Math1* has begun in differentiating hair cells, and probably slightly after the onset of expression of Delta1 and Jagged2[54]. The expression of Hes5 may be positively regulated by Notch activation as it is much reduced in the supporting cells (Deiter's cells) of *Jag2*[-/-] mice[54]. Additional inner hair cells are observed in *Hes1*[-/-] mutant mice, and additional outer hair cells are observed in *Hes5*[-/-] mutants[52,53], generally consistent with the expression patterns of these genes and their proposed role as negative regulators of hair cell differentiation. Hes1 may directly antagonize the activity of Math1, as co-transfecting cells in cochlear cultures with Hes1 and Math1, blocks the effects of ectopic Math1 expression[52], reducing the production of supernumerary hair cells.

Brn3.1 and GATA3

Brn3.1 (also called Brn3c) is a POU domain transcription factor that is specifically expressed by hair cells within the adult mouse inner ear[46,47]. Brn3.1 is expressed by postmitotic hair cells at approximately the same time as Jagged2 and Delta1, 1 day before the hair cell markers myosin VI and myosin VIIa[48]. In *Brn3.1*[-/-] mice, hair cells are generated and express myosin VI, myosin VIIa and calretinin, but they never develop sensory hair bundles and are lost from the inner ear by P14[46,47]. The ectopic overexpression of Brn3.1 does not lead to the production of hair cells[51], indicating Brn3.1 is only required for the later aspects of hair cell differentiation. GATA3 is another transcription factor that may be involved in cell differentiation within the sensory patches. All epithelial cells in the dorsal wall of the cochlear duct express GATA3, and its expression selectively decreases in both hair and supporting cells as they differentiate, indicating it may act as a negative regulator of hair and supporting-cell differentiation[49].

Roles of thyroid hormone and retinoic acid in hair cell differentiation

Nuclear receptors for thyroid hormone and retinoic acid are expressed in the developing sensory epithelia of the inner ear and their respective ligands are known to play roles in hair cell development (see Raz and Kelley[59] for recent review). Retinoic acid is produced by the embryonic, but not adult, organ of Corti, and treating cochlear cultures from early, but not late, embryonic stages of development with retinoic acid leads to the production of extra rows of inner and outer hair cells[60]. The RARα/RXRα heterodimer is the most likely hair cell receptor for retinoic acid, and application of the RARα antagonist Ro-41-5253 to cochlear cultures leads to a reduction in the number of hair cells that eventually develop[61]. However Ro-41-5253 does not block the initial differentiation of hair cells, as judged by the expression of Brn3.1 and myosin VI[61], so it has been suggested that retinoic acid induces certain early aspects of hair cell differentiation rather than determining the size of the pro-sensory cell population[61].

The three functional thyroid hormone receptors, TRα1, TRβ1 and TRβ2, and the non-ligand binding TRα2 are expressed in the sensory epithelia of the inner ear from early stages, with the expression of TRβ1 and TRβ2 being restricted to the cochlear epithelium[62]. Chemically induced hypothyroidism results in a delay in the maturation of most elements in the organ of Corti, and the same effect is observed in transgenic mice that lack all known thyroid hormone receptors[63]. TRβ is essential for the development of hearing[64] and in $Thrb^{-/-}$ mice there is a delay in the onset of the fast potassium conductance ($I_{K,f}$) in inner hair cells, but the onset of outer hair cell motility is unaffected[65]. Although $I_{K,f}$ is eventually expressed by inner hair cells in $Thrb^{-/-}$ mice, hearing does not recover, possibly due to a permanent impairment of the tectorial membrane[63]. In $Thra^{-/-}/Thrb^{-/-}$ compound null mutant mice both the onset of $I_{K,f}$ and outer hair cell motility is delayed[63], and a recent study has shown that the gene encoding prestin, the outer hair cell motor[66], is regulated by thyroid hormone[67].

Development of the sensory hair bundle

The sensory hair bundle, a precisely determined array of actin-filled stereocilia located on the hair cell's apical surface, is a distinguishing characteristic of the hair cell and is essential for the process of mechanotransduction. The development of the hair bundle is a complex process and, for the auditory organ of the avian inner ear, the morphological details have been described thoroughly (see Tilney and Tilney[68] for review). For the mammal, this process has been best characterized in the mouse vestibular system[69,70], and the cochlea of the hamster[71] and the rat[72]. For the mouse cochlea, information is somewhat limited.

Although there are some inter-species and inter-organ differences, the general features of the process of hair bundle development can be described as follows. First, small stereocilia sprout up over the entire apical surface of the hair cell, clustering around a centrally located kinocilium to form a short bundle of uniform height. Second, the kinocilium migrates to one side of the cell and the stereocilia nearest the kinocilium begin to elongate and generate the staircase pattern in which adjacent rows of stereocilia become arranged in increasing height with the tallest row lying next to the now eccentrically placed kinocilium. The position of the kinocilium, therefore, defines the planar polarity of the hair cell and its bundle. Third, rootlets project down from the stereocilia, anchoring them into the cuticular plate, and the excess supernumerary stereocilia that have not been incorporated into the ranked rows of the bundle are re-absorbed. Finally, the stereocilia within the bundle grow to their final width and height, and the bundle achieves its mature shape and form. In the chick auditory organ, increases in the width and height of stereocilia occur over different time periods[68], whereas in mammals both processes, thickening and lengthening, occur concurrently[71]. Also, differences in bundle height in the avian hearing organ may be governed by regulating the period over which the growth of stereocilia occurs at a constant rate[68], whereas in the mammalian cochlea they may be generated by differences in growth rate[71].

Surprisingly little is known about the molecular basis of hair bundle development in any species. Clearly, it will involve molecules and pathways that direct the assembly of the actin cytoskeleton, like the Rho-GTPases along with their upstream effectors and their downstream targets, and two recent reviews have suggested how this may be accomplished[73,74]. However, thus far, studies on mouse mutants and human deafness genes have provided the greatest insight into the molecular processes that may be involved in hair bundle development.

Mice with mutations in the genes that underlie deaf-blindness in three of the genetic forms of the human Usher type I syndrome, USHIB, USHID and USHIF, exhibit defects in hair-bundle development. These genes encode the unconventional myosin, myosin VIIa (*shaker-1* mouse[75]), and two cell adhesion molecules, cadherin 23 (*waltzer* mouse[76]) and protocadherin 15 (*Ames waltzer* mouse[77]). Bundles with ranked rows of stereocilia form in all three mouse mutants, but by the early stages of postnatal development, they show varying degrees of disruption and are often fragmented into several smaller units[75–77], suggesting there may be defects in the mechanisms of inter-stereociliary adhesion. The *USHIC* gene encodes a PDZ domain protein that is present in stereocilia and could act as an interface between the cytoskeleton and the plasma membrane[78], although it is not yet known how mutations in this gene affect hair bundle development. Interactions between the actin cytoskeleton, unconventional myosins, PDZ domain proteins and cell-surface adhesion molecules may, therefore, play a pivotal role in the development of hair bundle integrity. Mutations in two other unconventional myosins, cause non-syndromic human hereditary deafness and cause defects in hair bundle development in the corresponding mouse mutants. Defects in myosin VI (*Snell's waltzer* mouse[79]) lead to the fusion of stereocilia and the formation of giant bundles in the early postnatal period[80]. Myosin VI is unusual as it is a minus-end directed actin motor[81], unlike most other myosins that move towards the plus, or barbed, ends of actin filaments. It is not found in stereocilia and it has been proposed[80] that it tethers the apical membrane around the base of each stereocilium to the rootlet or the cuticular plate, thereby stabilising the stereocilium. Defects in myosin XV (*shaker-2* mouse[82]) lead to the production of hair bundles that are abnormally short, although of normal shape and with height-ranked rows of stereocilia. Abnormally long actin filament bundles, cytocauds, are found in these hair cells that project many microns from the base of the cell[83], suggesting a mis-regulated deployment of a limited supply of actin monomers may account for the reduction in bundle height observed.

Integrins are cell surface receptors for extracellular matrix molecules and a recent study[84] has shown that the $\alpha 8$ integrin subunit specifically localizes to the apical pole of developing utricular hair cells along with focal adhesion kinase (FAK), and that the extracellular matrix molecules fibronectin and collagen type IV are associated with the apical surface of the developing epithelium. Transgenic inactivation of the $\alpha 8$ integrin subunit leads to the malformation of a subset of utricular hair bundles, a loss of FAK from the apical pole of the hair cell and a disappearance of fibronectin from the apical epithelial surface. The growth of sensory hair bundles may, therefore, involve reciprocal interactions between hair bundle receptors and matrix molecules associated with the apical surface of the sensory epithelia.

Conclusions and key points for clinicians

The evidence reviewed suggests the following sequence of molecular events occurs during the differentiation of sensory organs in the inner ear (Fig. 3). The different sensory organs all originate from a single common patch in the otocyst that can be defined by the expression of *Serrate1*, *Lunatic fringe*, and BEN. Notch is present throughout the otocyst, and is maintained in an activated state within the pro-sensory patch by Serrate1. Notch activation can also laterally induce Serrate1/Jagged1, re-inforcing the expression of Serrate1/Jagged1 in cells with activated Notch. Notch activation may make the patch sensory-competent, and prevent the premature differentiation of hair cells. Discrete regions within this pro-sensory patch then become specified to form different types of organs, cristae, maculae or a cochlea, possibly by virtue of their position relative to compartment boundaries within the inner ear. Hair and supporting cells share a common lineage, and express p27[Kip1], a cyclin-dependent kinase inhibitor, as soon as they withdraw from the cell cycle. Once postmitotic, the hair cells express Math1, followed by Delta1, Jagged2/Serrate2 and Brn3.1 At some stage during this process, possibly during the final round of cell division, the presumptive hair cells acquire Numb, thereby rendering them deaf to Jagged1/Serrate1 signalling from the supporting cells. This decreases Notch activation in the presumptive hair cells, further promoting their

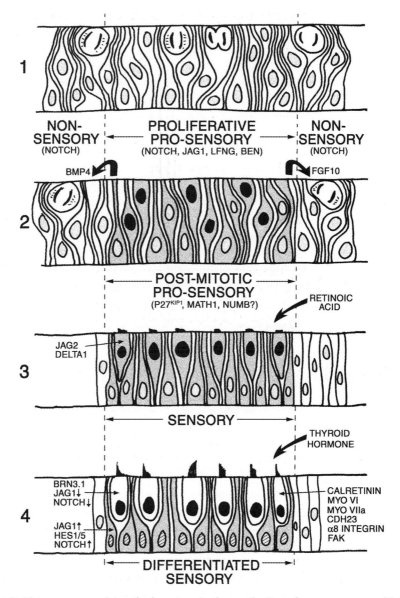

Fig. 3 Diagram summarizing the key steps in the production of a sensory organ. (**1**) A proliferative pro-sensory region is defined by the expression Jagged1/Serrate1 (JAG1), Lunatic fringe (LFNG) and BEN. Notch1 (NOTCH) is expressed throughout the epithelial wall of the otocyst. (**2**) Cells within a future sensory organ withdraw from the cell cycle and express p27^{Kip1} (grey cytoplasm). Hair cell progenitors may inherit Numb at this stage, via asymmetric division. Shortly after, a subset of cells begins to express Math1 (black nuclei). (**3**) Math1 expressing cells express Jagged2/Serrate2 (JAG2) and Delta1 as they differentiate as hair cells, forcing their neighbours to become supporting cells. (**4**) Hair cells down-regulate Notch1 and Jagged1/Serrate1, and express Brn3.1 followed by a number of hair cell markers including myosin VI, myosin VIIa and calretinin. Notch 1, Jagged1/Serrate1 and Lunatic fringe become restricted to the supporting cells, and these cells begin to express Hes1/5 (hatched nuclei).

differentiation along the hair cell pathway. Delta1 and Jagged2/Serrate2 signalling from hair cells increases the levels of Notch activation in supporting cells, preventing them from expressing Delta1 and Jagged2/Serrate2, and inhibiting hair cell differentiation, probably by positively regulating the expression of Hes1/5. Levels of Notch activation, therefore, determine whether a cell becomes a hair cell (low levels) or a supporting cell (high levels); intermediate levels may maintain cells as pro-sensory progenitors. Retinoic acid may control an early event in the differentiation of hair cells, but probably does not determine the size of the pro-sensory cell population. Brn3.1 is required for the later stages of hair cell differentiation, including the appearance of a sensory hair bundle, the full and complete development of which may involve interactions between the cytoskeleton, cell adhesion molecules, cell-surface receptors and surface associated extracellular matrix. Finally, thyroid hormone controls the timing of certain aspects of hair cell differentiation, including the expression of ion channels and, in cochlear outer hair cells, the motor protein, prestin.

Acknowledgements

Jane Bryant is an MRC postgraduate student. Richard Goodyear and Guy Richardson are supported with funds from The Wellcome Trust. The authors would like to thank Stuart Johnson for his help with figure preparation.

References

1   Rubel EW, Fritzsch B. Auditory system development: primary auditory neurons and their targets. *Annu Rev Neurosci* 2002; **25**: 51–101
2   Fritzsch B, Pirvola U, Ylikowski J. Making and breaking the innervation of the inner ear: neurotrophic support during ear development and its clinical implications. *Cell Tissue Res* 1999; **295**: 369–82
3   Knowlton VY. Correlation of the development of membranous and bony labyrinths, acoustic ganglia, nerves, and brain centers of chick embryos. *J Morphol* 1967; **121**: 179–208
4   Cole LK, Le Roux I, Nunes B, Laufer E, Lewis J, Wu DK. Sensory organ generation in the chick inner ear: contributions of bone morphogenetic protein 4, Serrate1, and Lunatic Fringe. *J Comp Neurol* 2000; **424**: 509–20
5   Goodyear RJ, Kwan T, Oh S-H, Raphael Y, Richardson GP. The cell adhesion molecule BEN defines a prosensory patch in the developing avian otocyst. *J Comp Neurol* 2001; **434**: 275–88
6   Bray S. Notch signalling in *Drosophila*: three ways to use a pathway. *Semin Cell Dev Biol* 1998; **9**: 591–7
7   Moloney DJ, Panin VM, Johnston SH *et al*. Fringe is a glycosyl transferase that modifies Notch. *Nature* 2000; **406**: 369–75
8   Pourquié O, Corbel C, Le Caer J-P, Rossier J, Le Douarin NM. BEN, a surface glycoprotein of the immunoglobulin superfamily, is expressed in a variety of developing systems. *Proc Natl Acad Sci USA* 1992; **89**: 5261–5
9   Adam J, Myat A, Le Roux I *et al*. Cell fate choices and the expression of Notch, Delta and Serrate homologues in the chick inner ear: parallels with *Drosophila* sense-organ development. *Development* 1998; **125**: 4645–54

10   Eddison M, Le Roux I, Lewis J. Notch signalling in the development of the inner ear: lessons from *Drosophila*. *Proc Natl Acad Sci USA* 2000; **97**: 1692–9

11   Zhang N, Martin GV, Kelley MW, Gridley T. A mutation in the Lunatic fringe gene suppresses the effects of a Jagged2 mutation on inner hair cell development in the cochlea. *Curr Biol* 2000; **10**: 659–62

12   Fekete DM. Cell fate specification in the inner ear. *Curr Opin Neurobiol* 1996; **6**: 533–41

13   Brigande JV, Kiernan AE, Gao X, Iten LE, Fekete DM. Molecular genetics of pattern formation in the inner ear: Do compartment boundaries play a role. *Proc Natl Acad Sci USA* 2000; **97**: 11700–6

14   Cantos R, Cole LK, Acampora D, Simeone A, Wu DK. Patterning of the mammalian cochlea. *Proc Natl Acad Sci USA* 2000; **97**: 1170713

15   Acampora D, Merlo GR, Paleari L *et al*. Craniofacial, vestibular and bone defects in mice lacking the Distal-less-related gene Dlx5. *Development* 1999; **126**: 3795–809

16   Torres M, Gomez-Pardo E, Gruss P. Pax2 contributes to inner ear patterning and optic nerve trajectory. *Development* 1996; **122**: 3381–91

17   Wu DK, Oh S-H. Sensory organ generation in the chick inner ear. *J Neurosci* 1996; **16**: 6454–62

18   Morsli H, Choo D, Ryan A, Johnson R, Wu DK. Development of the mouse inner ear and origin of its sensory organs. *J Neurosci* 1998; **18**: 3327–35

19   Mowbray C, Hammerschmidt M, Whitfield TT. Expression of BMP signalling pathway members in the developing zebrafish inner ear and lateral line. *Mech Dev* 2001; **108**: 179–84

20   Chang W, Numes FD, De Jesus-Escobar JM, Harland R, Wu DK. Ectopic noggin blocks sensory and nonsensory organ morphogenesis in the chicken inner ear. *Dev Biol* 1999; **216**: 369–81

21   Gerlach LM, Hutson MR, Germiller JA, Nguyen-Luu D, Victor JC, Barald KF. Addition of the BMP4 antagonist, noggin, disrupts avian inner ear development. *Development* 2000; **127**: 45–54

22   Pirvola U, Spencer-Dene B, Xing-Qun L *et al*. FGF/FGFR-2(IIIb) signalling is essential for inner ear morphogenesis. *J Neurosci* 2000; **20**: 6125–34

23   Oh S-H, Johnson R, Wu DK. Differential expression of bone morphogenetic proteins in the developing vestibular and auditory sensory organs. *J Neurosci* 1996; **16**: 6463–75

24   Von Bartheld CS, Patterson SL, Heuer JG, Wheeler EF, Bothwell M, Rubel EW. Expression of nerve growth factor (NGF) receptors in the developing inner ear of chick and rat. *Development* 1991; **113**: 455–70

25   Pirvola U, Arumäe U, Moshnyakov M, Palgi J, Saarma M, Ylikoski J. Coordinated expression and function of neurotrophins and their receptors in the rat inner ear during target innervation. *Hear Res* 1994; **75**: 131–44

26   Ekker M, Akimenko MA, Bremiller R, Westerfield M. Regional expression of three homeobox transcripts in the inner ear of zebrafish embryos. *Neuron* 1992; **9**: 27–35

27   Ruben RJ. Development of the inner ear of the mouse: a radioautographic study of terminal mitoses. *Acta Otolaryngol Suppl* 1967; **220**: 1–44

28   Sans A, Chat M. Analysis of temporal and spatial patterns of rat vestibular hair cell differentiation by tritiated thymidine radioautography. *J Comp Neurol* 1982; **206**: 1–8

29   Chen P, Segil N. p27[Kip1] links cell proliferation to morphogenesis in the developing organ of Corti. *Development* 1999; **126**: 1581–90

30   Chen P, Johnson JE, Zoghbi HY, Segil N. The role of Math1 in inner ear development: uncoupling the establishment of the sensory primordium from hair cell fate determination. *Development* 2002; **129**: 2495–505

31   Lowenheim H, Furness DN, Kil J *et al*. Gene disruption of p27[Kip1] allows cell proliferation in the postnatal and adult organ of Corti. *Proc Natl Acad Sci USA* 1999; **96**: 4084–8

32   Katayama A, Corwin JT. Cell production in the chicken cochlea. *J Comp Neurol* 1989; **81**: 129–35

33   Fekete DM, Muthukumar S, Karagogeos D. Hair and supporting cells share a common progenitor in the avian inner ear. *J Neurosci* 1998; **18**: 7811–21

34   Lang H, Fekete DM. Lineage analysis in the chicken inner ear shows differences in clonal dispersion for epithelial, neuronal, and mesenchymal cells. *Dev Biol* 2001; **234**: 120–37

35   Lewis J. Rules for the production of sensory hair cells. *Ciba Found Symp* 1991; **160**: 25–39

36   Corwin JT, Jones JE, Katayama A, Kelley MW, Warchol ME. Hair cell regeneration: the identities of progenitor cells, potential triggers and instructive cues. *Ciba Found Symp* 1991; **160**: 103–20

37   Haddon C, Jiang Y-J, Smithers L, Lewis J. Delta-Notch signalling and the patterning of sensory cell differentiation in the zebrafish ear: evidence from the mind bomb mutant. *Development* 1998; **125**: 4637–44

38 Morrison A, Hodgetts C, Gossler A, Hrabé de Angelis M, Lewis J. Expression of *Delta1* and *Serrate1 (Jagged1)* in the mouse inner ear. *Mech Dev* 1999 **84**: 169–72

39 Stone JS, Rubel EW. Delta1 expression during avian hair cell regeneration. *Development* 1999; **126**: 961–73

40 Lanford PJ, Lan Y, Jiang R *et al*. Notch signalling pathway mediates hair cell development in mammalian cochlea. *Nat Genet* 1999; **21**: 289–92

41 Riley B, Chiang M-Y, Farmer L, Heck R. The *deltaA* gene of zebrafish mediates lateral inhibition of hair cells in the inner ear and is regulated by *pax2.1 Development* 1999; **126**: 5669–78

42 Shailam R, Lanford PJ, Dolinsky CM, Norton C, Gridley T, Kelley MW. Expression of proneural and neurogenic genes in the embryonic mammalian vestibular system. *J Neurocytol* 1999; **28**: 809–19

43 Zine A, Van de Water TR, de Ribaupierre F. Notch signalling regulates the pattern of auditory hair cell differentiation in mammals. *Development* 2000; **127**: 3373–83

44 Kiernan AE, Ahituv N, Fuchs H *et al*. The Notch ligand *Jagged1* is required for inner ear sensory development. *Proc Natl Acad Sci USA* 2001; **98**: 3873–8

45 Tsai H, Hardisty RE, Rhodes C *et al*. The mouse *slalom* mutant demonstrates a role for Jagged1 in neuroepithelial patterning in the organ of Corti. *Hum Mol Genet* 2001; **10**: 507–12

46 Erkman L, McEvilly RJ, Luo L *et al*. Role of transcription factors Brn-3.1 and Brn-3.2 in auditory and visual system development. *Nature* 1996; **381**: 603–6

47 Xiang M, Gan L, Li D *et al*. Essential role of POU-domain transcription factor Brn-3c in auditory and vestibular hair cell development. *Proc Natl Acad Sci USA* 1997; **94**: 9445–50

48 Xiang M, Gao W-Q, Hasson T, Shin JJ. Requirement for Brn-3c in maturation and survival, but not in fate determination of inner ear hair cells. *Development* 1998; **125**: 3935–46

49 Rivolta MN, Holley MC. GATA3 is downregulated during hair cell differentiation in the mouse cochlea. *J Neurocytol* 1998; **27**: 637–47

50 Bermingham NA, Hassan BA, Price SD *et al*. Math1: an essential gene for the generation of inner ear hair cells. *Science* 1999; **284**: 1837–41

51 Zheng JL, Gao W-Q. Overexpression of *Math1* induces robust production of extra hair cells in postnatal rat inner ears. *Nat Neurosci* 2000; **3**: 580–6

52 Xheng JL, Shou J, Guillemot F, Kageyama F, Gao W-Q. Hes1 is a negative regulator of inner ear hair cell differentiation. *Development* 2000; **127**: 4551–60

53 Zine A, Aubert A, Qiu J *et al*. Hes1 and Hes5 activities are required for the normal development of the hair cells in the mammalian inner ear. *J Neurosci* 2001; **21**: 4712–20

54 Lanford PJ, Shailam R, Norton CR, Gridley T, Kelley MW. Expression of *Math1* and *Hes5* in the cochlea of wild type and Jag2 mutant mice. *J Assoc Res Otolaryngol* 2000; **1**: 161–71

55 Collier JR, Monk NA, Maini PK, Lewis JA. Pattern formation by lateral inhibition: a mathematical model of Delta-Notch intercellular signalling. *J Theor Biol* 1996; **183**: 429–46

56 Pickles JO, van Heumen WRA. Lateral interactions account for the pattern of the hair cell array in the chick basilar papilla. *Hear Res* 2000; **145**: 65–74

57 Goodyear R, Richardson G. Pattern formation in the basilar papilla: evidence for cell rearrangement. *J Neurosci* 1997; **17**: 6289–301

58 Ohtsuka T, Ishibashi M, Gradwohl G, Nakanishi S, Guillemot F, Kageyama R. Hes1 and Hes5 as notch effectors in mammalian neuronal differentiation. *EMBO J* 1999; **18**: 2196–207

59 Raz Y, Kelley MW. Effects of retinoid and thyroid receptors during development of the inner ear. *Semin Cell Dev Biol* 1997; **8**: 257–64

60 Kelley MW, Xu XM, Wagner MA, Warchol ME, Corwin JT. The developing organ of Corti contains retinoic acid and forms supernumerary hair cells in response to exogenous retinoic acid in culture. *Development* 1993; **119**: 1041–53

61 Raz Y, Kelley MW. Retinoic acid signalling is necessary for the development of the organ of Corti. *Dev Biol* 1999; **213**: 180–93

62 Bradley DJ, Towle HC, Young III WS. α and β thyroid hormone receptor (TR) gene expression during auditory neurogenesis: evidence for TR isoform-specific transcriptional regulation *in vivo*. *Proc Natl Acad Sci USA* 1994; **91**: 439–43

63 Rüsch A, Ng L, Goodyear R *et al*. Retardation of cochlear maturation and impaired hair cell function caused by deletion of all known thyroid hormone receptors. *J Neurosci* 2001; **21**: 9792–800

64 Forrest D, Erway LC, Ng L, Altschuler R, Curran T. Thyroid hormone receptor β is essential for development of auditory function. *Nat Genet* 1996; **13**: 354–7

65 Rüsch A, Erway LC, Oliver D, Vennstrom B, Forrest D. Thyroid hormone receptor β-dependent expression of a potassium conductance in inner hair cells at the onset of hearing. *Proc Natl Acad Sci USA* 1998; **95**: 15758–62

66 Zheng J, Shen W, He DZZ, Long KB, Madison LD, Dallos P. Prestin is the motor protein of cochlear hair outer hair cells. *Nature* 2000; **405**: 149–55

67 Weber T, Zimmerman U, Winter H *et al*. Thyroid hormone is a critical determinant for the regulation of the cochlear motor protein prestin. *Proc Natl Acad Sci USA* 2002; **99**: 2901–6

68 Tilney LG, Tilney MS. Actin filaments, stereocilia, and hair cells: how cells count and measure. *Annu Rev Cell Biol* 1992; **8**: 257–74

69 Mbiene J-P, Sans A. Differentiation and maturation of the sensory hair bundles in the fetal and postnatal vestibular receptors of the mouse: a scanning electron microscope study. *J Comp Neurol* 1996; **254**: 271–8

70 Denman-Johnson K, Forge A. Establishment of hair bundle polarity and orientation in the developing vestibular system of the mouse. *J Neurocytol* 1999; **28**: 821–35

71 Kaltenbach JA, Falzarano PR, Simpson TH. Postnatal development of the hamster cochlea. II. Growth and differentiation of stereocilia bundles. *J Comp Neurol* 1994; **350**: 187–98

72 Zine A, Romand R. Development of the auditory receptors of the rat: a SEM study. *Brain Res* 1996; **721**: 49–58

73 Kollmar R. Who does the hair cell's do? Rho GTPase and hair-bundle morphogenesis. *Curr Opin Neurobiol* 1999; **9**: 394–8

74 Muller U, Littlewood-Evans A. Mechanisms that regulate mechanosensory hair cell differentiation. *Trends Cell Biol* 2001; **11**: 334–42

75 Self T, Mahoney M, Fleming J, Walsh J, Brown SDM, Steel KP. Shaker-1 mutations reveal roles for myosin VIIA in both development and function of cochlear hair cells. *Development* 1996; **125**: 557–66

76 Di Palma F, Holme RH, Bryda EC *et al*. Mutations in Cdh23, encoding a new type of cadherin, cause stereocilia disorganization in waltzer, the mouse model for Usher syndrome type 1D. *Nat Genet* 2001; **27**: 103–7

77 Alagramam KN, Murcia CL, Kwon HY, Pawlowski KS, Wright CG, Woychik B. The mouse Ames waltzer hearing-loss mutant is caused by a mutation of *Pdch15*, a novel protocadherin gene. *Nat Genet* 2001; **27**: 99–102

78 Verpy E, Leibovici M, Zwaenpoel I *et al*. A defect in harmonin, a PDZ domain-containing protein expressed in the inner ear sensory hair cells, underlies Usher syndrome type 1c. *Nat Genet* 2000; **26**: 51–5

79 Avraham KB, Hasson T, Steel KP *et al*. The mouse Snells waltzer deafness gene encodes an unconventional myosin required for structural integrity of the inner ear hair cells. *Nat Genet* 1995; **11**: 369–75

80 Self T, Sobe T, Copeland NG, Jenkins NA, Avraham KB, Steel KP. Role of myosin VI in the differentiation of cochlear hair cells. *Dev Biol* 1999; **214**: 331–41

81 Wells AL, Lin AW, Chen LQ *et al*. Myosin VI is an actin-based motor that moves backwards. *Nature* 1999; **401**: 505–8

82 Probst FJ, Fridell RA, Raphael Y *et al*. Correction of deafness in shaker-2 mice by an unconventional myosin in a BAC transgene. *Science* 1998; **280**: 1444–7

83 Beyer LA, Odeh H, Probst FJ *et al*. Hair cells in the inner ear of the pirouette and shaker 2 mutant mice. *J Neurocytol* 2000; **29**: 227–40

84 Littlewood-Evans A, Muller U. Stereocilia defects in the sensory hair cells of the inner ear in mice deficient in integrin α8β1. *Nat Genet* 2000; **24**: 424–8

Biophysics of the cochlea – biomechanics and ion channelopathies

Jonathan Ashmore

Department of Physiology, University College London, London, UK

Understanding how the cochlea works as a system has become increasingly important. We need to know this before integrating new information from genetic, physiological and clinical sources. This chapter will show how the cochlea should be seen as a device for carrying out a frequency analysis built from cells that have been adapted for specialist purposes. Sensory hair cells convert mechanical displacements into the neural code. The transducer channel remains to be identified. The biomechanics of the cochlear duct depends on an energy-dependent feedback from the sensory outer hair cells. The molecular basis for outer hair cell feedback depends on a protein that has recently been identified. The auditory signal encoded by the cochlea is further modified by membrane properties of the hair cells and cochlear supporting cells. The interplay between techniques of genetics, molecular biology and cell physiology has started to reveal which ion channels and transporters in the cochlea are mutated in certain forms of deafness. The interpretation of these mutations requires the cell physiology of the cochlear partition to be better characterised in the future.

There have been significant steps in the way in which we understand the cochlea. Over the past decade, the question of which molecules participate in hearing has been brought from speculation to the laboratory bench. Although some of the techniques for studying cellular physiology were starting to producing new insights when the last *British Medical Bulletin* survey of the field was made in 1987, the introduction of molecular biology techniques into hearing research has driven many developments. The barrier of limited tissue sample quantities in hearing no longer seems to be so insurmountable as 10 years ago. Modern molecular techniques aided by genomic searches now have the ability to identify the small numbers of molecules present in the inner ear.

Correspondence to:
Prof. Jonathan Ashmore,
Department of
Physiology, University
College London,
Gower Street,
London WC1E 6BT, UK

Cochlear mechanics

It has long been appreciated that the mammalian cochlea is designed to analyse the frequency components present in complex sounds. It does this using the mechanical properties of the cochlear partition. The principles have been understood for well over 60 years when the physics was first encapsulated by simple mathematical models. In the majority of these models, the cochlea is simplified to a fluid-filled tube with a membrane, the basilar membrane, dividing it lengthwise. As explored by von Békésy in the 1940s, the stiffness gradient along the partition sets up a frequency map so that differing frequencies are associated with different resonant excitation sites. The wave motion along the basilar membrane induced by sound entering the inner ear can now be modelled with reasonable accuracy on a small computer[1]. The cochlea thus behaves as a mechanical spectrum analyser over the full auditory range.

The resulting design works reliably and with stability at frequencies that may extend above 10 kHz. For some mammals, the upper auditory range may extend 2–3 octaves above this frequency. Over the past 15 years, methods for measuring basilar membrane mechanics have improved considerably, mainly due to the appearance of a new generation of interferometers for measuring the nanometre scales of basilar membrane displacements[2-4]. Some of these instruments have been designed to measure motions of relatively low reflecting surfaces[4,5]. Experiments in *in vivo* animal models show that at the threshold of hearing (0 dB SPL) the amplitude of the basilar membrane vibration is about 0.3 nm.

Active versus passive cochlear biomechanics

If the cochlea were simply a fluid-filled tube (the coiling does not affect the physics), the amplitude evoked by a sound on the basilar membrane would be highly damped down. Such 'passive' cochleas are indeed the type studied by von Békésy and would now be classified as exhibiting severe sensorineural hearing loss. Both psycho-acoustics and auditory nerve recording *in vivo* lead one to expect much higher degrees of frequency selectivity. Vibration in the cochlear partition is intrinsically damped down by viscous forces, originating in part from the fluid within the duct and in part from viscous forces from within the organ of Corti. Extensive studies from a variety of animal models show that *in vivo* the basilar membrane amplitude is enhanced by over 100 times (*i.e.* by 40 dB) at low sound levels (for a review, see Robles and Ruggero[4]). The removal of the viscous damping forces requires a power input to the biomechanics and this is often described by saying that the cochlea is 'active'. The problem was identified by Gold in 1948[6], but resisted elaboration until the instrumentation improved. The underlying cellular mechanisms have only become clearer over the past decade. The source of active amplification is, with little doubt, the cochlear outer hair cells. For each input sound frequency, a cluster of about 300 outer hair cells amplify the basilar membrane vibration, a process named 'cochlear amplification'[7].

Although traceable to Helmholtz in the 1860s, the idea that every section of the cochlea might behave like a lightly damped mechanical resonator went out of fashion in the early modelling attempts, as the propagating nature of the basilar membrane travelling wave was emphasised. The high damping in the cochlear duct was also seen as an insurmountable impediment to an explanation of cochlear tuning that depended on the mechanical properties of the cochlear cells even thought the literature contained suggestions to the contrary[8]. The advent of better measurements and clear improvement of cochlear preparation techniques re-opened this question and focused interest on mechanisms by which viscous damping could be reduced[9]. The dominant view now is that the outer hair cells both detect and feed forces back into the cochlear partition so that the frequency selectivity is essentially a property of the mechanics of the cochlea.

With the inclusion of outer hair cell forces, computer models can be made which match quite well measurements made with laser-based motion detection systems. More recently, there has been a revived interest in the cochlea as a two dimensional structure[3,5]. This work shows that a complete model of the cochlea may also have to pay attention to the variation of mechanical properties across the partition as well as along it. As is known from auditory nerve recordings[10], the relative sharpness of tuning (on a logarithmic frequency scale) varies along the length of the cochlea, with the basal tuning curves being sharper than those at the apex.

Converting sound into electricity: mechano-electric transduction

At each site along the cochlea, the basilar membrane motion is signalled to the auditory nerve by the primary sensory cells of the cochlea, the inner hair cells. The primary cellular event is the deflection of the hair cell bundle. Such deflections occur at the same rate as the sound frequency and hence a primary requirement is that the mechano-electrical transduction step is rapid. In channel language, the transduction channel gating is too fast to involve intermediate biochemical steps.

Despite considerable effort, the molecular identity of the transducer in mammalian cochlear hair cells is unknown. This must represent one of the key unsolved problems of the cellular mechanisms of hearing. It is certainly associated with apical stereocilia (as reviewed recently by Gillespie and Walker[11]). It seems increasingly clear that the transducer mechanism is a complex of proteins, containing linkage and anchoring subunits. The functional assay for any potential candidates, normally so simple for ligand gated receptors, is complicated by this complexity. Most of the information about hair cell transduction is derived from much simpler model systems, particularly in lower vertebrates such as the frog and the turtle. By far the largest body of biophysical information about the mammalian transducer is derived from early stage (mainly postnatal days 0–8) mouse cochlear explants where the stimulus can be applied directly to the hair cell bundle[12,13]). There are few biophysical recordings from hair cells in the adult mammalian cochlea and this is a serious gap in the data. The technical reasons are not clear, although it is possible that the mature hair cell transducer requires factors that are hard to duplicate under *in vitro* recording conditions. Although there has been recent progress in recording from adult vestibular cells in the mouse[14], there may be differences between auditory and vestibular transduction mechanisms. Although vestibular cells adapt, sensory hair cells within the cochlea contain channels modified for ultrafast response times and show little adaptation. Whether this means that different hair cell types differ in their transducer channel remains an open question.

A number of possible candidates for the transducer have been identified in other systems. In the nematode worm, a cluster of degenerin genes has been implicated in mechanosensitivity, but as yet no mammalian homologues have been convincingly shown to act as mechanically gated channels[15]. In the fruitfly, loss of bristle mechanosensitivity has been associated with mutations in the gene *nompC* (standing for no mechano-receptor potential)[16]. This gene has generated a great deal of interest as it is a member of the TRP (standing for 'transient receptor potential') superfamily of membrane receptors that were originally identified in insect photoreceptors. This superfamily also contains a number of vertebrate stretch-sensitive proteins. The protein in the fruitfly is a transmembrane protein with a long C-terminal repeat of ankyrin binding sites. It is clear that mutations leading to deafness and hair cell loss are well worth exploring. There are recent examples where channel-like proteins, identified by genome searches, have shown considerable promise for the study of hearing[17], but as yet the mammalian homologue of the mechano-electrical transduction channel has not been identified.

Converting electricity into sound: electromechanical transduction

The argument for an amplifying cell system in the cochlea depends on physics alone. The selectivity of the cochlea is greater than would be predicted from a knowledge of the materials and of the structure of the cochlea. The cochlea travelling wave would normally propagate along the basilar membrane under conditions where it would be highly damped by the viscosity of the cochlear fluid and of the organ of Corti. To overcome such dissipative forces, two alternative suggestions have been made.

The first originates with an idea that was first reported in 1985 when it was shown that turtle hair bundles undergo 'active' deflections[18]. There has been a recent revival of interest in the idea that the hair bundle is the source of cochlear amplification. In lower vertebrates, the bundle undergoes mechanical motions in excess of those induced by thermal fluctuations alone. Although this phenomenon was found originally in turtle hair cells, the more recent evidence comes from a re-investigation both in turtle[19] and in frog hair cells[20] of bundle forces that are generated when the stereocilia are pushed. Two mechanisms producing bundle motion have been described. The first is a force arising from the myosin-dependent motor responsible for tensioning of the tip link at the end of the stereocilia; this mechanism is unlikely to operate at frequencies above 100 Hz. The second is a consequence of calcium entering through the transducer channel, leading to channel reclosing and generating a force[21]. Both of these mechanisms are found in turtle hair cells, a system where the frequency range is limited to below about 700 Hz. The current discussion centres around whether either of these mechanisms can provide the right forces with correct bandwidth to contribute to mammalian hearing. The experimental evidence for either of these mechanisms operating in mammalian hair cells is not strong.

In the mammalian cochlea, the more probable cellular mechanism depends on the basolateral membrane of the hair cells. Reported in 1985 by Brownell and co-workers[22], outer hair cells generate forces along their length when their membrane potential is altered. Although the original measurement was limited to relatively low frequencies to be captured at video rates, the use of patch clamp stimulating methods[23] and the most recent techniques have shown that these length changes can be driven at frequencies in excess of 80 kHz[24].

The hypothesis that outer hair cells can cancel viscous damping is supported by many pieces of experimental evidence. Outer hair cells are force generating elements that are stimulated by opening of the mechano-electric transducer channels in their apical pole. The cells are also positioned to feed back energy into the basilar membrane vibration. When outer hair cells are stimulated electrically in the intact organ of Corti, these forces are large enough to distort structures in the cochlear partition[25].

The molecular basis of cochlear amplification

Given that the outer hair cell acts as a force generator, there has been considerable interest in the molecular nature of the force generating step. The cell's basolateral membrane exhibits properties that might be termed 'piezo-electric'. The molecular basis for this force is a dense array of motor molecules in the basolateral membrane of the outer hair cells which are able to extract energy from the electric field across the membrane. This still remains a contentious issue, since the process has to operate at acoustic frequencies in excess of 10 kHz.

High resolution freeze-fracture studies show that the lateral membrane of outer hair cells contains a high density of particles about 8–11 nm in diameter with an estimated density in excess of 4000 per sq micron[26,27]. These lateral membrane particles can also be detected by electro-physiological signs, for when the membrane potential is changed there is a rapid transient current in the outer hair cell membrane that corresponds to a movement of charge[28]. This phenomenon is similar to the gating charges that can be detected when ion channels undergo a conformational change. However, the charge movement is larger by over an order of magnitude than can readily be seen in other cell types. In fact, the density is such that it can be measured in individual patches either as a charge movement or, equivalently, as a voltage-dependent capacitance of the membrane (since by definition of electrical capacitance, $C = dQ/dV$). Thus individual patches of membrane, explored with a patch pipette 1–2 µm in diameter, show both non-linear capacitance and movement[29,30]. For each of the 10^7 particles in the outer hair cell lateral membrane, between 1 and 2 electronic charges are required to transit through the membrane to account for the charge transient. The approximate match between the electrophysiology, the time course of the movement of the cell, and the observed freeze-fracture pattern in the outer hair cell membrane lead to the most economical explanation: that the particles form the 'motor' of the outer hair cell.

The simplest biophysical explanation for how the motor works is that it is an area motor[26]. When the membrane potential changes, each molecule undergoes a conformational change in the plane of the membrane. The high packing density ensures that a small change in protein area becomes a cell length change that can be observed under a microscope, since all the motors are in series. The area change need only be a few percent: this would theoretically be equivalent to a slight re-orientation of the molecule. It is also worth noting that an area change of the motor is likely to be intrinsically faster than a major structural re-organisation of the protein, as happens, for example, when an ion channel gates between open and closed states.

A recent significant advance has been the identification of a protein expressed in outer, but not inner, hair cells and which behaves like the predicted area motor[31]. A subtractive cDNA library was constructed by separating inner hair cells and outer hair cells and subtractively identifying genes expressed preferentially in outer hair cells. One of the 10 unique library clones identified was a 744 amino acid protein. When expressed in a kidney cell line, the protein exhibited the biophysical properties of a hair cell motor, conferring a (restricted) electromotility on the cells. It also conferred a voltage-dependent capacitance on the transfected cell, the second characteristic of the outer hair cell motor. The protein has been named 'prestin' in recognition of the speed of movement that outer hair cells possess. Subsequent protein analysis suggests that prestin contains 12 α-helices that form a hydrophobic core embedded in the membrane. Genomic analysis shows that prestin is the fifth member (SLC26A5) of an anion transporter superfamily SLC26 that includes a number of bicarbonate transporters expressed in the membranes of other epithelial systems[32]. On the basis of this family membership, prestin is likely to be a modified anion bicarbonate transporter. Therefore, the model is that, as part of its transport cycle, the protein is able to change its area.

A further step forward has been to combine electrophysiology and mutation analysis to suggest an economical explanation for prestin's ability to detect changes in the electrical field[30]. When prestin is mutated, by replacing charged with neutral amino acids, at sites around the hydrophobic core, major changes occur in the voltage dependence, but not to the charge movement. The voltage-dependent capacitance is, however, dependent on the presence of intracellular chloride in outer hair cells and in expression systems. An economical explanation is that the charge movement arises from the induced movement of intracellular anions into a deep pore of the protein structure on the cytoplasmic surface of the molecule. The motor thus appears to be a transporter that exhibits an incomplete transport cycle, but whose operation is exploited by the outer hair cell to generate a cellular force.

An earlier study using both immunohistochemistry and functional studies had suggested that the motor in outer hair cells had some affinities to a sugar transporter[33,34]. This result depends, in part, on the specificity of the antibody used. Surprisingly, there is more recent physiological evidence that members of the SLC26 family do transport other solutes. Thus prestin may share some properties of a sugar transporter. From the viewpoint of a cell biologist, the high density of this transporter in hair cells makes this an attractive system in which to study the interplay between molecular structure, cell function and system properties. As well as its growing interest to sensory physiologists, the cochlea thus has the potential to be a laboratory for testing proposals about how transport molecules work. When a mouse is made with the prestin gene 'knocked out', as it will undoubtedly be soon, then we will have much clearer view of prestin's contribution to auditory function.

Experimentally, outer hair cells removed from the cochlea can be stimulated to change length at frequencies in excess of 70 kHz. There has been a long-running debate about whether the membrane potential changes in the cells would be large enough at acoustic frequencies to activate the motor, since intracellular potentials will be attenuated by the cell's own low-pass electrical characteristics. For this reason it has been suggested that cochlear amplification could arise through the reaction of the hair cell stereocilia during deflection[20]. There must also be doubts about this scheme, as any stereocilial feedback force needs precise timing to work at any cochlear position. The resolution of this issue requires further experimental data on how adult mammalian hair cell mechano-transduction works.

Channelopathies

The cellular structure of the mammalian cochlea is well conserved between species, so that homologous populations of hair cells and supporting cells can be reliably identified. This has provided a basis for extrapolating between many animal systems (and in particular mouse models) and human hearing. There are differences of detail, however, which reflect the slightly different hearing ranges found between species. The region of the cochlea that seems to be most susceptible to insult is the basal end. At this end, cells have proved the most difficult to study. Data from several laboratories have indicated that there are also gradients of cell morphology and of channel species along the length of the cochlea that may correlate with selective hearing losses of both genetic and environmental origin.

Stereocilia and their associated transducer channels face into scala media, a high potassium and low calcium containing compartment. The K^+ levels are maintained by active pumps in the stria vascularis that result in the efflux of K^+ into scala media through a potassium channel that is also associated with the long QT syndrome in the heart (see Bitner-Glindzicz, this volume). Although the transducer channels themselves are intrinsically cation selective, they appear to be functional potassium channels as K^+ is the majority cation that carries charge into the cell. K^+ exits through the basolateral membrane of the hair cells and determines all changes of voltage in the cell. Potassium channels thus play a key role in the responses to sound.

Hair cell potassium channels

Inner hair cells have at least two distinct K^+ channels in their basolateral membrane[35] which together determine how the cell membrane potential responds to stereocilial deflection. In addition, inner hair cells express calcium channels (now characterised as an L-type calcium current) that are part of the triggering mechanism for synaptic release. Figure 1 summarizes a number of the known channel types found in mammalian hair cells.

Outer hair cells have at least three types of K^+ channel[36]. The main and novel outer hair cell current is carried through a channel that was originally termed I_{Kn}. It is active at negative potentials and serves to keep the outer hair cell hyperpolarised. This channel contains subunits of the KCNQ family of potassium channels. Other members of this family

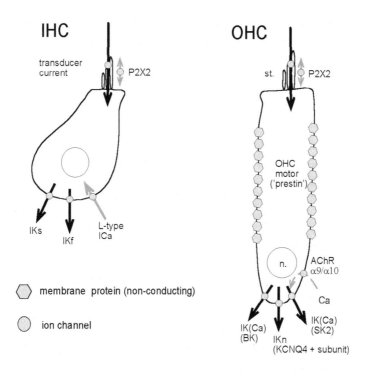

Fig. 1 Main channel types in mammalian cochlear hair cells. Currents enter the cells through the mechano-electrical transducer channel in the stereocilia (st.) and are carried mainly by K⁺ ions. Channels gated by external ATP (a purinergic receptor P2X2) are distributed along the stereocilia. The currents exit at the hair cell base, through cell specific channels, near the nucleus, n. Inner hair cells (IHC) have two K⁺ channel types, a fast (IKf) and a slow (IKs) channel type[35]. Outer hair cells (OHC) have different, cochlear position-dependent sets of potassium channels as labelled (see text).

include KCNQ1, a channel expressed in the stria vascularis, and KCNQ2 and KCNQ3 which together form a channel that generates the M-current, an important modulatory potassium current of the CNS controlled by acetylcholine[37]. The hair cell member channel in this family is KCNQ4. This is a voltage gated potassium channel discovered only recently[38,39]. The channel is expressed prominently in outer hair cells and mutations result in a non-syndromic, autosomal dominant, progressive hearing loss (identified as one of the components of DFNA2 in humans). There is molecular and electrophysiological evidence to show that KCNQ4 expresses itself in a gradient along the cochlea[40]. The negative activation of I_{Kn} suggests that KCNQ4 may be acting in concert with some other, as yet undiscovered, subunit. One of the more intriguing questions is how this gradient (or indeed any cochlear gradient) might be set up. There is little indication of the answer, although there is evidence that channel properties in hair cells change during cochleogenesis[41] and so a complex orchestration of changes of channel type occurs during development. Such gradients of channels are found throughout hearing organs. For example, there is a higher density of potassium channels expressed in outer hair cells from the basal coils of the cochlea[42]. The mammalian cochlea is not unique in this property, as other lower vertebrates show differential channel expression along the hearing organ. The turtle hearing organ depends on individual cells being electrically tuned, and differential expression of K^+ channels provides the mechanism for the range of electrical tuning along the turtle's auditory organ[43]. However, there is no evidence for electrical tuning in the mammalian cochlea. The observed gradient must, therefore, reflect other features of cochlear function.

One of the curious receptor types found ubiquitously in the cochlea is a receptor for extracellular ATP. Such purinergic receptors have been found in a wide variety of tissues. They are cation channels and, in the cochlea, are localised on the apical (stereocilial) end of the cell[44]. Notably, non-sensory cells and basal cochlear hair cells express higher levels of the ATP receptor P2X2 than do apical cochlear hair cells. The gradient may be correlated with the larger transducer currents found in cells encoding higher frequencies, as the receptor is found on the stereocilia. The function of such purinergic receptors in the cochlea is unclear. ATP levels in the bathing endolymph appear to be very low. The higher expression level, experimentally, goes some way towards explaining why basal cells are experimentally more difficult to study since purinergic receptors, once activated by external ATP, are cation permeable. This may lead to calcium loading of the cells and consequent cell death.

Hair cell ligand-gated channels

Hair cells are under descending control from the central nervous system. A long-standing problem in cochlear physiology has been the precise role of the cholinergic efferent system: its behavioural effects appear to be subtle and hard to detect[45]. The medial component of the olivocochlear efferent pathway originates from cells near the lateral superior olive and terminates on the OHCs. A distinct branch terminates on the inner hair cell afferent terminals. There has been a long-running debate as to whether the efferents protect against noise damage[46], or even enhance signals in a noisy background. Postnatal de-efferentation does not significantly alter cochlear development[47]. Molecular biological techniques have not clarified the efferent function role although they have identified the hair cell receptors. The receptor on outer hair cells for acetylcholine (ACh), liberated from the efferent terminals, is a novel one. It is now known to be composed of two subunits termed $\alpha 9$ and $\alpha 10$.

It can be can be expressed as a functional channel in oocyte membranes[48]. It is highly permeable to calcium[49,50]. This permeability leads to the ACh-induced calcium rises that can be detected in outer hair cells[51]. Nevertheless, knockout of the α9 ACh receptor, the presumed OHC receptor, does not yield a phenotype showing major hearing abnormalities[52]. The possibility that the native ACh receptor is really not a homomer but a heteromer of two specialised cochlear receptor units, α9 + α10, leaves the case unsettled until the double knockout is performed. At the moment it is not known whether nature has already carried out this experiment for us and provided a mutation with the pathway functionally removed.

When the efferent pathway is activated, it releases ACh onto the outer hair cells. The action of acetylcholine thus can lead to opening of potassium channels and hyperpolarization of the cell membrane. The channel is presumed be the member SK2 of the small K channel family because of its sensitivity to apamin[53]. The channel is functional early in development[54]. Activation of the efferents produces a hyperpolarization and could serve to clamp OHCs at a hyperpolarized potential so removing outer hair cells from the feedback loop where they affect the mechanics. More subtle and slower effects of efferent activity can be detected as consequences of cytoskeletal alterations induced within the OHC[55]. There is likely to be much more activity in this field, as the ACh signalling pathway includes Rho and other small GTPases studied extensively by cell biologists[56]. Since these signalling molecules have already made an appearance in bundle morphogenesis, we can anticipate that the control pathways within the cell to maintain cochlear gain are going to become a good deal more complex that we appreciate at present.

Conclusions

Looking to the future is always hazardous. Looking back over the work on single cell physiology, considerable strides in understanding the cell biophysics have been made, but there are many nagging questions remaining about the precise distribution of membrane ion channels and transporters on hair cells and supporting cells. The outstanding question in the field in the identity of the hair cell transducer. There is no guarantee that its identification in a lower vertebrate system will answer the question of its identity in the mammalian cochlea. The issue in understanding mammalian hearing has been that the frequency range strains the measurement technology. However, one area that is emerging, driven in part by a desire to understand genomic complexity, is the development of large-scale computational frameworks in biology. These may allow a synthesis of molecular and cellular data into a systems model of the cochlea where the contribution of each part can be understood in the working of the whole.

Key points for clinical practice

- The physiology of the cochlea needs characterisation before we understand the way in which specific mutations in cochlear proteins lead to hearing losses.

- There is now little doubt that cochlear structure allows the inner ear to perform like a multichannel mechanical spectrum analyser.

- The essential cellular components of this machine are now known and these are the targets for specific interventions in the future albeit, on a scale much smaller than found in current practice.

References

1   Nobili R, Mammano F, Ashmore J. How well do we understand the cochlea? *Trends Neurosci* 1998; **21**: 159–67
2   Cooper NP. An improved heterodyne laser interferometer for use in studies of cochlear mechanics. *J Neurosci Methods* 1999; **88**: 93–102
3   Nilsen KE, Russell IJ. Timing of cochlear feedback: spatial and temporal representation of a tone across the basilar membrane. *Nat Neurosci* 1999; **2**: 642–8
4   Robles L, Ruggero MA. Mechanics of the mammalian cochlea. *Physiol Rev* 2001; **81**: 1305–52
5   Nilsen KE, Russell IJ. The spatial and temporal representation of a tone on the guinea pig basilar membrane. *Proc Natl Acad Sci USA* 2000; **97**: 11751–8
6   Gold T. Hearing II: the physical basis of the action of the cochlea. *Proc R Soc Lond B Biol Sci* 1948; **135**: 492–8
7   Davis H. An active process in cochlear mechanics. *Hear Res* 1983; **9**: 79–90
8   Huxley AF. Is resonance possible in the cochlea after all? *Nature* 1969; **221**: 935–40
9   Neely ST, Kim DO. A model for active elements in cochlear biomechanics. *J Acoust Soc Am* 1986; **79**: 1472–80
10 Evans EF, Pratt SR, Spenner H, Cooper NP. Comparisons of physiological and behavioural properties: auditory and frequency selectivity. In: Cazals Y, Horner K, Demany L. (eds) *Auditory Physiology and Perception*. Oxford: Pergamon, 1992; 159–69
11 Gillespie PG, Walker RG. Molecular basis of mechanosensory transduction. *Nature* 2001; **413**: 194–202
12 Rusch A, Kros CJ, Richardson GP. Block by amiloride and its derivatives of mechano-electrical transduction in outer hair cells of mouse cochlear cultures. *J Physiol (Lond)* 1994; **474**: 75–86
13 Gale JE, Marcotti W, Kennedy HJ, Kros CJ, Richardson GP. FM1-43 dye behaves as a permeant blocker of the hair-cell mechanotransducer channel. *J Neurosci* 2001; **21**: 7013–25
14 Holt JR, Gillespie SK, Provance DW *et al*. A chemical-genetic strategy implicates myosin-1c in adaptation by hair cells. *Cell* 2002; **108**: 371–81
15 Garcia-Anoveros J, Garcia JA, Liu JD, Corey DP. The nematode degenerin UNC-105 forms ion channels that are activated by degeneration- or hypercontraction-causing mutations. *Neuron* 1998; **20**: 1231–41
16 Walker RG, Willingham AT, Zuker CS. A *Drosophila* mechanosensory transduction channel. *Science* 2000; **287**: 2229–34

17   Vreugde S, Erven A, Kros CJ et al. Beethoven, a mouse model for dominant, progressive hearing loss DFNA36. Nat Genet 2002; 30: 257–8

18   Crawford AC, Fettiplace R. The mechanical properties of ciliary bundles of turtle cochlear hair cells. J Physiol (Lond) 1985; 364: 359–79

19   Ricci AJ, Crawford AC, Fettiplace R. Active hair bundle motion linked to fast transducer adaptation in auditory hair cells. J Neurosci 2000; 20: 7131–42

20   Martin P, Hudspeth AJ. Active hair-bundle movements can amplify a hair cell's response to oscillatory mechanical stimuli. Proc Natl Acad Sci USA 1999; 96: 14306–11

21   Fettiplace R, Fuchs PA. Mechanisms of hair cell tuning. Annu Rev Physiol 1999; 61: 809–34

22   Brownell WE, Bader CR, Bertrand D, de Ribaupierre Y. Evoked mechanical responses of isolated cochlear outer hair cells. Science 1985; 227: 194–6

23   Ashmore JF. A fast motile response in guinea-pig outer hair cells: the cellular basis of the cochlear amplifier. J Physiol (Lond) 1987; 388: 323–47

24   Frank G, Hemmert W, Gummer AW. Limiting dynamics of high-frequency electromechanical transduction of outer hair cells. Proc Natl Acad Sci USA 1999; 96: 4420–5

25   Mammano F, Ashmore JF. Reverse transduction measured in the isolated cochlea by laser Michelson interferometry. Nature 1993; 365: 838–41

26   Kalinec F, Holley MC, Iwasa KH, Lim DJ, Kachar B. A membrane-based force generation mechanism in auditory sensory cells. Proc Natl Acad Sci USA 1992; 89: 8671–5

27   Forge A. Structural features of the lateral walls in mammalian cochlear outer hair cells. Cell Tissue Res 1991; 265: 473–83

28   Ashmore JF. Mammalian hearing and the cellular mechanisms of the cochlear amplifier. In: Corey D, Roper S. (eds) Sensory Transduction. New York: Rockefeller University Press, 1992; 396–412

29   Gale JE, Ashmore JF. The outer hair cell motor in membrane patches. Eur J Physiol (Pflügers Arch) 1997; 434: 267–71

30   Oliver D, He DZ, Klocker N et al. Intracellular anions as the voltage sensor of prestin, the outer hair cell motor protein. Science 2001; 292: 2340–3

31   Zheng J, Shen W, He DZ, Long KB, Madison LD, Dallos P. Prestin is the motor protein of cochlear outer hair cells [see comments]. Nature 2000; 405: 149–55

32   Lohi H, Kujala M, Kerkela E, Saarialho-Kere U, Kestila M, Kere J. Mapping of five new putative anion transporter genes in human and characterization of SLC26A6, a candidate gene for pancreatic anion exchanger. Genomics 2000; 70: 102–12

33   Ashmore JF, Geleoc GS, Harbott L. Molecular mechanisms of sound amplification in the mammalian cochlea. Proc Natl Acad Sci USA 2000; 97: 11759–64

34   Geleoc GS, Casalotti SO, Forge A, Ashmore JF. A sugar transporter as a candidate for the outer hair cell motor. Nat Neurosci 1999; 2: 713–9

35   Kros CJ, Crawford AC. Potassium currents in inner hair cells isolated from the guinea-pig cochlea. J Physiol (Lond) 1990; 421: 263–91

36   Housley GD, Ashmore JF. Ionic currents of outer hair cells isolated from the guinea-pig cochlea. J Physiol (Lond) 1992; 448: 73–98

37   Selyanko AA, Hadley JK, Brown DA. Properties of single M-type KCNQ2/KCNQ3 potassium channels expressed in mammalian cells. J Physiol (Lond) 2001; 534: 15–24

38   Kharkovets T, Hardelin JP, Safieddine S et al. KCNQ4, a K⁺ channel mutated in a form of dominant deafness, is expressed in the inner ear and the central auditory pathway. Proc Natl Acad Sci USA 2000; 97: 4333–8

39   Kubisch C, Schroeder BC, Friedrich T et al. KCNQ4, a novel potassium channel expressed in sensory outer hair cells, is mutated in dominant deafness. Cell 1999; 96: 437–46

40   Beisel KW, Nelson NC, Delimont DC, Fritzsch B. Longitudinal gradients of KCNQ4 expression in spiral ganglion and cochlear hair cells correlate with progressive hearing loss in DFNA2. Brain Res Mol Brain Res 2000; 82: 137–49

41   Marcotti W, Kros CJ. Developmental expression of the potassium current $I_{K,n}$ contributes to maturation of mouse outer hair cells. J Physiol (Lond) 1999; 520: 653–60

42   Mammano F, Ashmore JF. Differential expression of outer hair cell potassium currents in the isolated cochlea of the guinea-pig. J Physiol (Lond) 1996; 496: 639–46

43   Jones EM, Gray-Keller M, Fettiplace R. The role of Ca^{2+}-activated K⁺ channel spliced variants in the tonotopic organization of the turtle cochlea. J Physiol (Lond) 1999; 518: 653–65

44 Housley GD. Physiological effects of extracellular nucleotides in the inner ear. *Clin Exp Pharmacol Physiol* 2000; **27**: 575–80

45 Prosen CA, Bath KG, Vetter DE, May BJ. Behavioral assessments of auditory sensitivity in transgenic mice. *J Neurosci Methods* 2000; **97**: 59–67

46 Rajan R. Centrifugal pathways protect hearing sensitivity at the cochlea in noisy environments that exacerbate the damage induced by loud sound. *J Neurosci* 2000; **20**: 6684–93

47 Liberman MC, O'Grady DF, Dodds LW, McGee J, Walsh EJ. Afferent innervation of outer and inner hair cells is normal in neonatally de-efferented cats. *J Comp Neurol* 2000; **423**: 132–9

48 Katz E, Verbitsky M, Rothlin CV, Vetter DE, Heinemann SF, Belen EA. High calcium permeability and calcium block of the alpha9 nicotinic acetylcholine receptor. *Hear Res* 2000; **141**: 117–28

49 Blanchet C, Erostegui C, Sugasawa M, Dulon D. Gentamicin blocks ACh-evoked K^+ current in guinea-pig outer hair cells by impairing Ca^{2+} entry at the cholinergic receptor. *J Physiol (Lond)* 2000; **525**: 641–54

50 Jagger DJ, Griesinger CB, Rivolta MN, Holley MC, Ashmore JF. Calcium signalling mediated by the 9 acetylcholine receptor in a cochlear cell line from the immortomouse. *J Physiol (Lond)* 2000; **527**: 49–54

51 Evans MG, Lagostena L, Darbon P, Mammano F. Cholinergic control of membrane conductance and intracellular free Ca^{2+} in outer hair cells of the guinea pig cochlea. *Cell Calcium* 2000; **28**: 195–203

52 Vetter DE, Liberman MC, Mann J *et al*. Role of alpha9 nicotinic ACh receptor subunits in the development and function of cochlear efferent innervation. *Neuron* 1999; **23**: 93–103

53 Oliver D, Klocker N, Schuck J, Baukrowitz T, Ruppersberg JP, Fakler B. Gating of Ca^{2+}-activated K^+ channels controls fast inhibitory synaptic transmission at auditory outer hair cells. *Neuron* 2000; **26**: 595–601

54 Glowatzki E, Fuchs PA. Cholinergic synaptic inhibition of inner hair cells in the neonatal mammalian cochlea. *Science* 2000; **288**: 2366–8

55 Szonyi M, Csermely P, Sziklai I. Acetylcholine-induced phosphorylation in isolated outer hair cells. *Acta Otolaryngol* 1999; **119**: 185–8

56 Kalinec F, Zhang M, Urrutia R, Kalinec G. Rho GTPases mediate the regulation of cochlear outer hair cell motility by acetylcholine. *J Biol Chem* 2000; **275**: 28000–5

Hereditary deafness and phenotyping in humans

Maria Bitner-Glindzicz

Unit of Clinical and Molecular Genetics, Institute of Child Health, London, UK

Hereditary deafness has proved to be extremely heterogeneous genetically with more than 40 genes mapped or cloned for non-syndromic dominant deafness and 30 for autosomal recessive non-syndromic deafness. In spite of significant advances in the understanding of the molecular basis of hearing loss, identifying the precise genetic cause in an individual remains difficult. Consequently, it is important to exclude syndromic causes of deafness by clinical and special investigation and to use all available phenotypic clues for diagnosis. A clinical approach to the aetiological investigation of individuals with hearing loss is suggested, which includes ophthalmology review, renal ultrasound scan and neuro-imaging of petrous temporal bone. Molecular screening of the *GJB2* (*Connexin 26)* gene should be undertaken in all cases of non-syndromic deafness where the cause cannot be identified, since it is a common cause of recessive hearing impairment, the screening is straightforward, and the phenotype unremarkable. By the same token, mitochondrial inheritance of hearing loss should be considered in all multigeneration families, particularly if there is a history of exposure to amino-glycoside antibiotics, since genetic testing of specific mitochondrial genes is technically feasible.

Most forms of non-syndromic autosomal recessive hearing impairment cause a prelingual hearing loss, which is generally severe to profound and not associated with abnormal radiology. Exceptions to this include DFNB2 (*MYO7A*), DFNB8/10 (*TMPRSS3*) and DFNB16 (*STRC*) where age of onset may sometimes be later on in childhood, DFNB4 (*SLC26A4*) where there may be dilated vestibular aqueducts and endolymphatic sacs, and DFNB9 (*OTOF*) where there may also be an associated auditory neuropathy. Unusual phenotypes in autosomal dominant forms of deafness, include low frequency hearing loss in DFNA1 (*HDIA1*) and DFNA6/14/38 (*WFS1*), mid-frequency hearing loss in DFNA8/12 (*TECTA*), DFNA13 (*COL11A2*) and vestibular symptoms and signs in DFNA9 (*COCH*) and sometimes in DFNA11 (*MYO7A*). Continued clinical evaluation of types and course of hearing loss and correlation with genotype is important for the intelligent application of molecular testing in the next few years.

Correspondence to:
Dr Maria Bitner-Glindzicz,
Unit of Clinical and
Molecular Genetics,
Institute of Child Health,
30 Guilford Street,
London WC1N 1EH, UK

Hearing impairment is the most common sensory disorder world-wide. When present in an infant, it may have dramatic effects on language

---

Table 1 Causes of hearing impairment

Genetic (syndromic and non-syndromic)
Autosomal recessive
Autosomal dominant
X-linked
Mitochondrial
Chromosomal, *e.g.* Down syndrome and trisomies 13 and 18, Turner syndrome, 22q11 deletions, mosaic trisomy 8
Environmental
Ototoxic medication, *e.g.* aminoglycosides, platinum derivatives
Prematurity
Neonatal hypoxia
Low birth weight
Severe neonatal jaundice
Head trauma
Infection: prenatal, *e.g.* CMV, toxoplasmosis, rubella; postnatal, *e.g.* meningitis
Noise exposure

acquisition and educational progress. Hearing loss which becomes apparent in later childhood or in adult life may have profound effects upon the social and working lives of those affected.

Causes of hearing impairment are numerous (Table 1) and, in a particular population, the relative contribution of genetic and environmental causes may be determined by social factors such as population structure and consanguinity, infection control and immunisation, and provision of neonatal and postnatal medical care[1]. Thus, in non-industrialised countries, environmental causes of hearing loss may outnumber those that are genetically determined whereas in industrialised countries the importance of the genetic contribution to hearing loss has become more apparent.

Epidemiological surveys of the deaf have consistently shown that about 50% of childhood deafness can be attributed to genetic causes, but all of the surveys have pointed out that the cause cannot be determined in a considerable proportion of individuals[1]. Recent molecular work has demonstrated that in this group of 'cause unknown' deafness, genetic causes are common and extremely heterogeneous. Many deaf individuals and their families want to know the cause of their deafness and particularly whether it is genetic. Proven genetic diagnosis may allow for accurate genetic counselling and family planning, carrier testing for relatives, and may provide essential information about environmental risk factors (*e.g.* aminoglycoside antibiotics in those with the A1555G mtDNA mutation, or risk of progression of hearing loss in those with dilated vestibular aqueducts). In addition, precise molecular diagnosis may be important for planning and assessing success of therapies such as cochlear implant[2] or future gene therapy.

The increasing knowledge of the molecular basis of hearing impairment will raise expectations among deaf people and their families that the exact cause of their hearing impairment may be determined and understood by genetic analysis. While this may be possible for some families with common causes of genetic hearing impairment or extensive family histories, the complexity of hearing, demonstrated by the underlying molecular heterogeneity, poses considerable problems in aetiological diagnosis in the majority. The aim of this chapter is not to provide an exhaustive description of genes implicated in hereditary deafness, but to describe a clinical approach to diagnosis and genetic testing, with the interested non-specialist in mind.

Epidemiology of hearing impairment

About 1 per 1000 children in the UK is born with a permanent hearing impairment and a similar number develop this during early childhood[3]. As age increases so too does the prevalence of hearing impairment; by the age of 40–50 years, 2.3% of the population experience a hearing loss of greater than 40 dB, and nearly 30% of those over 70 years are similarly affected[4]. Genetic factors are likely to be important in all of these age groups.

About 30% of those with a genetic form of hearing loss present with other clinical features in addition to hearing impairment, as part of a

Table 2 Aetiological investigation of hearing impairment

History

Prenatal, perinatal and postnatal factors, infection, prematurity, *etc*
Family history (at least 3 generations with specific enquiry about consanguinity)

Examination

Dysmorphic features
Special attention to external ears and neck, skin, hair, eyes and digits

Investigations *(including those which might reveal a syndromic cause)*

- Serology and culture for congenital infection if child presents early
- Ophthalmology examination with visual acuity and dilated fundoscopy to look for pigmentary retinopathy, signs of congenital infection or developmental malformation. ERG if pigmentary retinopathy, or history or vestibular examination suggests vestibular failure
- Urinalysis for blood and protein suggestive or nephritis or nephrotic syndrome
- Renal ultrasound scan to reveal renal dysplasia (BOR and HDR syndromes[46,95–97])
- Neuro-imaging CT and/or MRI, to exclude dilated vestibular aqueducts and Mondini malformations or other appearances suggestive of syndrome diagnoses[45–47,98,99]
- ECG if hearing loss is congenital and severe/profound, to look for prolonged QT interval (especially if there are delayed motor milestones)
- Audiometry on first degree relatives, to determine whether more than one generation is affected
- Consider vestibular investigations (hypofunction seen in Usher syndrome type 1, Jervell and Lange-Nielsen syndrome, Pendred syndrome, DFNA9 (*COCH*), DFNA11 (*MYO7A*), DFNB2 (*MYO7A*), DFNB4 (*SLC26A4*), DFNB12 (*CDH23*))

Table 3 Some of the genes underlying syndromic forms of hearing impairment

Syndrome	Inheritance	Gene	Type of molecule encoded	Clinical features.
Waardenburg type 1	Autosomal dominant	PAX3	Transcription factor	Abnormal pigmentation of hair, skin and eyes. Dystopia canthorum, hypoplastic alae nasi, short philtrum, synophrys. Deafness in 20%, unilateral or bilateral.
Waardenburg type 2	Autosomal dominant	MITF and others	Transcription factor	Abnormal pigmentation of hair, skin and eyes. Deafness in 40%, unilateral or bilateral. No dysmorphic features.
Waardenburg type 3	Autosomal dominant	PAX3	Transcription factor	Features of type 1 with limb anomalies.
Waardenburg type 4	Autosomal dominant	EDN3, EDNRB SOX10	Endothelin ligand and receptor Transcription factor	Abnormal pigmentation of hair, skin and eyes in addition to Hirschprung's disease.
Treacher Collins	Autosomal dominant	TCOF	Nuclear cytoplasmic transport protein	Down-slanting palpebral fissures, malformation of external (microtia, stenosis and tags) and middle ears, sparse lower eyelashes and colobomata of lower eyelids, malar hypoplasia, cleft palate in some. Deafness may be conductive, sensorineural or mixed.
Branchio-oto-renal	Autosomal dominant	EYA1	Transcriptional activator	Branchial cysts and fistulae, external ear malformations (cup, lop ear or microtia, ear pits) renal dysplasia or hypoplasia. Deafness may be conductive, sensorineural or mixed.
Jervell and Lange-Nielsen	Autosomal recessive	KCNQ1, KCNE1	Ion channel	Profound congenital deafness and prolonged QT interval on ECG leading to syncope and possible sudden death.
Pendred syndrome	Autosomal recessive	SLC26A4	Anion transporter	Congenital deafness and goitre. Thyroid dysfunction, dilated vestibular aqueduct and endolymphatic sacs, Mondini malformation of cochlea may co-exist.
Alport	X-linked dominant Autosomal recessive	COL4A5/6 COL4A3/COL4A4	Structural collagens	Progressive high frequency deafness and nephritis. Anterior lenticonus and macular flecks.
Muckle Wells	Autosomal dominant	CIAS1	Pyrin-like protein involved in apoptosis and inflammation	Arthritis, abdominal pain and urticaria. Progressive deafness. Amyloidosis of AA type causing renal failure.
Non-muscle myosin heavy chain IIA diseases	Autosomal dominant	MYHIIA	Non-muscle myosin heavy chain	Giant platelets and thrombocytopaenia, nephritis, cataracts and hearing loss. Hearing loss is childhood onset, bilateral and progressive.
Norrie	X-linked recessive	NDP	Extracellular matrix protein	Pseudotumour, retinal detachment leading to infantile or congenital blindness. Progressive mental retardation in some and progressive childhood onset hearing loss.

(continued on next page)

Table 3 *(cont'd from previous page)* Some of the genes underlying syndromic forms of hearing impairment

Syndrome	Inheritance	Gene	Type of molecule encoded	Clinical features
Stickler	Autosomal dominant	COL2A1, COL11A1 COL11A2	Structural collagen	Short stature, myopia, arthropathy, mid-face hypoplasia. High frequency progressive sensorineural hearing loss.
Usher type 1B	Autosomal recessive	MYO7A	Motor molecule	Profound congenital deafness, retinitis pigmentosa, vestibular arreflexia.
Usher type 1C	Autosomal recessive	USH1C	PDZ domain protein	Profound congenital deafness, retinitis pigmentosa, vestibular arreflexia.
Usher type 1D	Autosomal recessive	CDH23	Cadherin	Profound congenital deafness, variable retinitis pigmentosa, and variable vestibular function.
Usher type 1E	Autosomal recessive	PCD15	Protocadherin	Profound congenital deafness, retinitis pigmentosa, vestibular arreflexia.
Usher type 2A	Autosomal recessive	USH2A	Extracellular matrix protein	Congenital moderate-to-severe sensorineural hearing loss (normal vestibular function) and retinitis pigmentosa.
Usher type 3	Autosomal recessive	USH3A	Transmembrane protein	Progressive sensorineural hearing loss, normal or absent vestibular function and retinitis pigmentosa.
Bartter syndrome and deafness	Autosomal recessive	BSND	Chloride channel	Polyhydramnios, weight loss, failure to thrive, hypokalaemic hypochloraemic metabolic alkalosis and congenital deafness.
Hypoparathyroidism, deafness and renal dysplasia	Autosomal dominant	GATA3	Transcription factor (zinc finger)	Hypoparathyroidism (hypocalcaemia may be asymptomatic). Renal dysplasia or hypoplasia, but kidneys may rarely be normal. Hearing loss is usually bilateral symmetrical and non-progressive.
Piebaldism and deafness	Autosomal dominant	c-KIT	Tyrosine kinase receptor	Variable frequency of deafness and characteristic depigmentation of skin.
Renal tubular acidosis and deafness	Autosomal recessive	ATP6B1	Ion pump	Distal renal tubular acidosis, presenting with acute dehydration, vomiting and failure to thrive. Hearing loss is present in a subset of families and is progressive, tending to be severe-to-profound. It is associated with dilated vestibular aqueducts.

syndrome. It is important to make a syndrome diagnosis because: (i) it is important to monitor the individual and family for known complications and associations of the syndrome, such as renal or eye disease; (ii) inheritance may be clearly defined for many syndromic causes of deafness even if the gene is unknown; and (iii) molecular testing, which may confirm the diagnosis and aid genetic counselling, may be available for many of the commoner syndromes.

Although some syndromes may present in an obvious manner to the clinician, others require specialised investigation and a high index of suspicion in order to make the diagnosis. For these reasons, it is important to examine fully every individual with hearing impairment. Special attention should be paid to facial appearance, including the eyes, appearance of the external ears and neck, the skin (its pigmentation and its quality), and examination of the hands for unusual creases, extra or missing fingers and appearance of the digits. Those organs which cannot be easily seen, such as the eye and the kidney, with which syndromic associations are common, require additional investigations. Table 2 outlines the suggested clinical investigation of patients presenting with hearing impairment. The aim of this is to diagnose syndromic hearing loss, to exclude environmental causes and to build a picture of the phenotype of the hearing loss which may be valuable for directing molecular analysis. Table 3 gives examples of the genes underlying syndromic forms of hearing impairment.

In the remaining 70% of cases, hearing loss is not associated with additional clinical features and is termed 'non-syndromic'. Studies of marriages between the deaf have long indicated that a large number of genes are likely to be involved in human hearing impairment, and estimates have varied considerably[1]. More recent molecular analysis has borne out some of the higher estimates and indeed, to date, more than 40 genes for autosomal dominant deafness and more than 30 for autosomal recessive deafness mapped or cloned, although in some cases the same gene may be responsible for both dominant and recessive deafness[5]. Unsurprisingly, a wide variety of molecules has now been implicated in the causation of human hearing impairment, including transcription factors and activators, motor molecules, extracellular matrix components, cytoskeletal proteins, components of ion channels and gap junctions. These are summarized in Table 4.

For many years, this extreme heterogeneity hampered genetic studies because many different genetic forms of hearing loss give rise to similar clinical phenotypes, preventing the pooling of families in genetic linkage studies. Mapping strategies circumvented these problems by using single, large, dominant families, large consanguineous families and population isolates, where genetic homogeneity is far more likely. Although these approaches have been highly successful in mapping and identifying genes, they give no indication of molecular epidemiology of genetic deafness, *i.e.* how much a particular gene contributes to deafness world-wide or in a particular ethnically mixed country. Indeed, preliminary studies indicate that most recessively acting genes, with the exception of *GJB2* (*Connexin 26*), which encodes for the protein Connexin 26, are small contributors to hereditary deafness as a whole[6]. This means that genetic heterogeneity coupled with relative clinical homogeneity in presentation, require the clinician to use all available phenotypic clues in order to direct molecular testing and determine aetiology.

Autosomal recessive deafness

It is estimated that up to 75–80% of those with non-syndromic genetic hearing impairment have an autosomal recessive cause, 10–15% have an autosomal dominant cause, with the remainder being X-linked, mitochondrial or chromosomal. Autosomal dominant deafness loci are designated DFNA, autosomal recessive loci designated DFNB and X-linked loci, DFN. The loci are numbered according to the order in which they were mapped, DFNA1 being the first autosomal gene mapped in 1992[5].

Most of the recessively inherited forms of hearing impairment cause a phenotypically identical severe to profound, prelingual hearing loss[5], but mutations at a few loci – DFNB2 (MYO7A)[7], DFNB8/10 (*TMPRSS3*)[8] and DFNB16 (*STRC*)[9] – cause a delayed, childhood-onset hearing impairment. Also of note is that hearing loss caused by mutations at DFNB4 (*SLC26A4*) may be associated with dilated vestibular aqueducts and endolymphatic sacs[10], and there may be an associated auditory neuropathy with mutations in DFNB9 (*OTOF*)[11]. In addition, vestibular symptoms have been noted in DFNB2 (*MYO7A*), DFNB4 (*SLC26A4*) and DFNB12 (*CDH23*).

Hearing impairment caused by mutation in GJB2 (DFNB1) – a common cause of non-syndromic recessive and sporadic deafness

Epidemiological surveys of the deaf suggested that non-syndromic hearing loss was genetically heterogeneous, and that there was unlikely to be a single major gene involved. The discovery of *GJB2* and the subsequent realisation that it is a common cause of hearing impairment in many populations[12–18] was largely unexpected, although there was some previously published evidence of this in haplotype analysis of small families with non-syndromic deafness[19,20]. The gene *GJB2* encodes a gap junction protein known as Connexin 26. There is now good evidence that up to 50% of recessive non-syndromic hearing loss may be

Table 4 Cloned genes involved in non-syndromic hearing impairment

Locus	Name (gene)	Predicted functions	Phenotype of hearing loss (*denotes unusual phenotype)
DOMINANT GENES			
DFNA1 5q31	Diaphanous (*HDIA1*)	Cytokinesis and cell polarity	*Postlingual, low frequency. Onset 1st-2nd decade but rapidly progressive to involve all frequencies
DFNA2 1p34	Connexin 31 (*GJB3*)	Gap junction protein	Postlingual, high frequency. Onset 20–40 years. May cause deafness with auditory and peripheral neuropathy; also causes erythrokeratodermia variabilis (no deafness)
	KCNQ4 (*KCNQ4*)	Voltage gated potassium channel	Post-lingual, high frequency. Onset 10–30 years
DFNA3 13q12 (see also DFNB2)	Connexin 26 (*GJB2*)	Gap junction protein	See text. Prelingual, mainly high frequency, severe to profound or postlingual mild/moderate high frequency, onset 10–20 years. May also cause palmoplantar keratoderma, Vohwinkel's syndrome, or keratitis ichthyosis deafness (KID) syndrome
	Connexin 30 (*GJB6*)	Gap junction protein	Mid-high frequency (age of onset not stated)
DFNA5 7p15	ICERE-1 (*ICERE-1*)	Unknown	Postlingual high frequency onset age 5–15 years
DFNA6 4p16 (DFNA6/14/38 now confirmed to be same locus)	Wolframin (*WFS1*)	Unknown	See text. *Prelingual, low frequency. Onset 5–15 years with minimal progression except due to presbyacusis. No vestibular abnormalities, normal radiology
DFNA8/12 11q22-21	α-Tectorin (*TECTA*)	Structural component of tectorial membrane	See text. *Prelingual, mid-frequency. One family with high frequency progressive HI, and possibly delayed motor milestones[76]
DFNA9 14q12-13	Cochlin (*COCH*)	Extracellular matrix protein	See text. *Postlingual, high frequency, progressive with Menière-like symptoms
DFNA10 6q22-q23	EYA4 (*EYA4*)	Transcriptional activator	Postlingual, all frequencies, progressive. Onset 20–60 years
DFNA11 11q12-q21	Myosin 7A (*MYO7A*)	Motor molecule (unconventional myosin)	Postlingual, al frequencies, progressive. Onset 1st-2nd decade. Variable asymptomatic vestibular dysfunction.
DFNA12 11q 22-21 (see DNA8) DFNA13 6p21	Collagen 11A2 (*COL11A2*)	Structural molecule	See text. *Prelingual, mid/high frequency, progressive. 'Cookie bite' picture on audiogram
DFNA15 5q31	POU4F3 (*POU4F3*)	Transcription factor	Postlingual, all frequencies, progressive. Onset 20–40 years
DFNA17 22q12.2-13.3	MYH9 (*MYH9*)	Non-muscle myosin heavy chain	Postlingual, high-frequency. Onset by 10 years, moderate-to-severe by 30 years. Cochleosaccular degeneration
DFNA22 6q13	Myosin 6 (*MYO6*)	Motor molecule (unconventional myosin)	Postlingual, all frequencies, progressive. Onset 8–10 years
DFNA36 (see also DFNB7/11)	TMC1 (*TMC1*)	Transmembrane protein	Postlingual, initially high frequency, rapidly progressive across all frequencies. Onset in 1st decade. Or postlingual, slowly progressive. Onset 30–50 years
DFNA38 (see DFNA6)			

(Table 4 continued on next page)

Table 4 Cloned genes involved in non-syndromic hearing impairment (continued from previous page)

Locus	Name (gene)	Predicted functions	Phenotype of hearing loss (*denotes unusual phenotype)
RECESSIVE GENES			
DFNB1 13q12	Connexin 26 (GJB2)	Gap junction protein	See text. Prelingual, usually severe to profound (can be variable)
DFNB2 11q13.5	Myosin 7A (MYO7A)	Motor molecule (unconventional myosin)	Prelingual, severe-to-profound with reduced or absent vestibular function; *or variable age of onset (birth to 16 years) profound some with vertigo. Allelic with type 1B Usher
DFNB3 17p11.2	Myosin 15 (MYO15)	Motor molecule (unconventional myosin)	Prelingual, profound
DFNB4 7q13	Pendrin (SLC26A4)	Anion transporter	*Prelingual, sloping with profound high frequency hearing loss. May be progressive. Frequently associated with dilated vestibular aqueducts and endolymphatic ducts and sacs. Allelic with Pendred syndrome.
DFNB7/11 9q13-21 (see DFNA36)	TMC1 (TMC1)	Transmembrane protein	Prelingual, profound
DFNB8/10 21q22	TMPRSS3 (TMPRSS3)	Serine protease	Childhood onset (10–12 years) with profound losses across all frequencies within 4–5 years. Or prelingual profound
DFNB9 2p22	Otoferlin (OTOF)	Component of s synaptic vesicle	Prelingual, profound. *May be associated auditory neuropathy[11]
DFNB12 10q21	Otocadherin (CDH23)	Cell adhesion protein	Prelingual profound. Some families with atypical late onset retinitis pigmentosa and borderline vestibular dysfunction. Allelic with type 1D Usher
DFNB16 (possible second gene at 15q15)	Stereocilin (STRC)	Stereocilia protein	Early childhood onset (3–5 years), all frequencies moderate-to-severe (more severe in higher frequencies). Non-progressive. Or prelingual profound
DFNB18 11p15.5	Harmonin (USH1C)	PDZ domain protein	Prelingual profound (no vestibular pathology in non-syndromic cases). *Suspect if enteropathy (indicative of contiguous gene deletion). Allelic with type 1C Usher
DFNB21 11q22	α-tectorin (TECTA)	Structural component of tectorial membrane	Prelingual severe to profound
DFNB22 16p12.2	Otoancorin (OTOA)	Anchoring protein between acellular gels and non-sensory cells	Prelingual, moderate-to-severe
DFNB29 21q22	Claudin 14 (CLDN14)	Tight junction protein	Prelingual, profound
	Connexin 43 (GJA1)	Gap junction protein	Prelingual, profound

Note. The gene responsible for DFNB13 (uncloned at present) is reported to cause severe progressive sensorineural hearing loss.

Locus	Name (gene)	Predicted functions	Phenotype of hearing loss (*denotes unusual phenotype)
X-LINKED GENES			
DFN1 Xq22	Deafness dystonia protein (DDP)	Mitochondrial import protein	Postlingual but rapidly progressive in early childhood. Deafness is presenting symptom but may later be associated with dystonia, visual disability and mental impairment. *Suspect if X-linked agammaglobulinaemia (indicative of contiguous gene deletion)
DFN3 Xq13-21	POU3F4 (POU3F4)	POU domain transcription factor	Profound congenital deafness (mixed or pure sensorineural) with vestibular hypofunction. *Characteristic CT scan appearance[83]. Suspect if choroideremia and mental retardation (indicative of contiguous gene deletion)

Adapted from Van Camp and Smith[5].

accounted for by mutations in this gene in Caucasian and European populations[12,13]. In European, North American and Mediterranean populations, the most common mutation is a deletion of a single guanine nucleotide in a series of six guanines known as 35delG[18,20]. This mutation may account for 70% of mutant alleles of *GJB2* and the carrier frequency of this mutation alone is estimated at around 1 in 51 overall in Europe, but is considerably higher in some populations[12,13,21]. Originally, this mutation was thought to be a deletion hot-spot, but more recent evidence has suggested that it may be due to a founder effect, *i.e.* an ancient mutation which has become wide-spread possibly due to some undefined heterozygote advantage[22].

Study of other ethnic groups has shown that different mutations may be more common. For example, the 167delT mutation is the most prevalent mutation found in the Ashkenazi Jewish population with a probable carrier frequency of 3–4%, again possibly due to a founder effect[16,23]. In East Asian populations, the 235delC mutation is the most common mutation[17] and three mutations, W24X, W77X and Q124X, have been found commonly in families from different parts of the Indian subcontinent[24].

Not only is mutation in *GJB2* a common cause of non-syndromic recessive deafness, but mutations have been also been found in a significant number of sporadic cases – consistent with autosomal recessive inheritance[14,15]. Estimates vary, but between 10–30% of individuals with severe-to-profound non-syndromic hearing impairment of unknown cause have been shown to harbour mutations in this gene. Molecular analysis of *GJB2* in hearing-impaired individuals is simplified by the fact that this is a small gene consisting of two exons, only one of which codes for the protein, Connexin 26. Therefore, analysis of the gene in the diagnostic setting is relatively straightforward. This is a powerful argument for offering *GJB2* screening as part of the routine aetiological work-up in the diagnosis of all cases of non-syndromic deafness of unknown cause (Table 5). A further argument for offering *GJB2* testing on a wide-spread basis is the observation that the phenotype of hearing impairment caused by mutations in this gene is rather unremarkable, implying that one cannot select patients for analysis based on clinical phenotype[25]. There are no associated vestibular abnormalities or abnormality on the CT scan of the temporal bone. The deafness caused by mutations in *GJB2* is frequently severe or profound, but there can be considerable variation in severity even within families[23,26–28]. Deafness is usually stable, but progression has been reported[25,29]. Onset is nearly always pre-lingual, but not necessarily congenital, and it is possible that hearing may be normal at birth and progress rapidly during the first few months of life[30]. This implies that some babies with mutations in *GJB2* may pass new-born hearing screening but become profoundly deaf during infancy.

Table 5 Rationale of routine *GJB2 (Connexin 26)* mutation screening in all cases of non-syndromic hearing impairment where cause is unknown

	Common cause of hearing impairment
	Phenotype unremarkable and variable
	Small coding region
	Common mutations in some ethnic groups
	Enables accurate genetic information to be given to families
Disadvantages	
	Counselling difficulties with missense and heterozygous mutations

GJB2 may also be a rare cause of autosomal dominant deafness, both syndromic and non-syndromic (DFNA3)[31]. Phenotypes described include mild-to-profound hearing impairment, which is commonly progressive in nature, and may be associated with varying skin phenotypes including palmoplantar keratoderma (caused by the missense mutations G59A, R75W and DE42), Vohwinkel syndrome (associated with D66H), and keratitis-ichthyosis-deafness (KID, associated with D50N, G12R and S17F mutations)[32–36]. It would, therefore, seem sensible to screen the gene in individuals with deafness associated with epidermal defects. Interestingly, the R75W mutation appears to cause a variable skin phenotype since in some families it is reported to cause deafness with palmoplantar keratoderma, but in others the skin symptoms may be very mild or absent[33,37]. However, the missense mutations, W44C and C202F, definitely appear to cause non-syndromic deafness at the DFNA3 locus[5,31]. The role of the M34T allele in hearing loss is contentious since experimental studies show that there is a functional effect on the Connexin 26 molecule[38,39], but genetic studies now cast doubt on whether this is clinically significant[40,41].

Once *GJB2* analysis has been completed in the individual whose hearing loss is of unknown cause, there are very few further avenues for molecular investigation in small families or isolated cases at the present time. Recent data suggest that other recessive genes, with the exception of *SLC26A4*, contribute fairly equally to non-syndromic recessive deafness at least in Caucasian sibling pairs[6].

Hearing impairment caused by SLC26A4 (DFNB4/Pendred syndrome) – a significant cause of familial dilated vestibular aqueducts

Pendred syndrome describes the association of congenital deafness and goitre inherited in an autosomal recessive manner. Decades ago, Fraser estimated that mutations in this gene, giving rise to classical Pendred syndrome, may account for 5–10% of those with prelingual hearing impairment[42]. More recently, it has become apparent that the clinical presentation of individuals with mutations in this gene is highly variable. Features may range from those with classical Pendred syndrome presenting with goitre and prelingual profound sensorineural hearing loss, to those with absence of goitre, normal biochemical thyroid function and normal organification of iodine as demonstrated on a perchlorate discharge test, in whom the hearing impairment presents as non-syndromic. The most frequent presentation of the hearing loss is sensorineural, profound and prelingual but there may be a history of fluctuating progressive hearing loss that affects mainly the high frequencies[43]. Vestibular dysfunction has been demonstrated in a high proportion of individuals although not all are symptomatic. The major clue to diagnosis in an individual without overt goitre is, however, neuro-imaging. Enlargement of the vestibular aqueduct is the commonest abnormality which may be present in up to 80% of those with the disorder and in some cases there may also be a Mondini cochlea (1.5 cochlear turns instead of the normal 2.5)[44,45]. Dilatation or enlargement of the vestibular aqueducts is by no means diagnostic of Pendred syndrome, since these have been demonstrated in other genetic forms of hearing impairment including branchio-oto-renal syndrome and renal tubular acidosis with deafness[46,47]. However, in the absence of these syndromes where dilatation of the vestibular aqueduct and deafness is familial, there is a high chance of finding a mutation in the *SLC26A4* gene but a rather lower mutation pick-up rate in isolated cases[44].

PDS, the protein product of *SLC26A4*, is an anion transporter[48–50], expressed in the endolymphatic duct and sac from embryonic day 13 onwards and in non-sensory parts of the utricle, saccule and cochlea where it may be involved regulation and resorption of endolymph[51,52]. This is an attractive hypothesis since a protein involved in inner-ear fluid homeostasis might account for fluctuating hearing loss observed in individuals with mutations in the gene and for enlargement of the vestibular aqueduct and endolymphatic duct contained within it.

Many mutations have been described throughout the coding region of the gene including some which appear to be common[53,54]. Initial reports described a genotype–phenotype correlation based on functional study of chloride and iodide uptake by PDS transfected *Xenopus* oocytes[49,55]. Data suggested that mutations associated with full-blown Pendred syndrome cause a complete loss of transport whereas variants reported in those with non-syndromic deafness showed residual transport function. However, more recent assays of iodide efflux using transiently transfected mammalian cells, failed to show any correlation of mutation type with transport function and phenotype[56]. This is in keeping with the situation seen in human families in which there maybe clear phenotypic variation between siblings with the same mutation.

Autosomal dominant non-syndromic deafness

Most forms of autosomal dominant non-syndromic deafness are difficult to distinguish phenotypically. The majority of autosomal dominant genes are associated with hearing impairment that is post-lingual in onset, often beginning before the age of 20 years. Some forms, however, notably DFNA4, DNFA9 and DFNA10 are associated with hearing impairment starting somewhat later during the third and fourth decades. Mutations at the DFNA6/14/38 locus as well as those associated with the DFNA9 locus tend to have distinguishable clinical phenotypes, and DFNA12, DFNA13 and DFNA21 are characterised by mid-frequency hearing impairment.

WFS1 gene mutations (DFNA6/14/38) – a common cause of familial low frequency hearing loss

Mutations at only two loci are known to cause low-frequency sensorineural hearing loss; individuals from a single large Costa-Rican family with mutations at the DFNA1 locus have a rapidly progressive, fully penetrant form of hearing impairment in which affected individuals become profoundly deaf across all frequencies by the fourth decade of life[57].

In contrast to the DFNA1 phenotype, mutations at DFNA6/14/38 (caused by mutations in the gene WFS1) show overall mild progression consistent with presbyacusis[58–60]. Affected individuals show fully penetrant, early-onset, low-frequency hearing impairment which is bilateral and symmetrical. There is good speech discrimination and sometimes the hearing impairment may be asymptomatic as hearing at and below 2 kHz is predominantly affected. With the onset of presbyacusis, there is some flattening of the audiogram or even down-sloping configuration in older people. In a family from Newfoundland, the age of onset of hearing impairment was reported as the second decade although affected children could be identified before school age by an 'S-shaped' pure tone audiogram[59]. By the age of 40 years, hearing impairment was moderate-to-severe across all frequencies with males appearing to be more severely affected than females.

Mutation analysis studies of the WFS1 gene have shown that it is a common cause of dominantly inherited low frequency hearing loss[60], but not of sporadic, low-frequency hearing impairment[61]. The lower mutation pick-up rate in simplex cases suggests that there may be other non-genetic causes as well as genetic causes. It should be noted that mutations in the same gene cause Wolfram syndrome or DIDMOAD (diabetes insipidus, diabetes mellitus, optic atrophy and deafness inherited in an autosomal recessive manner)[62]. Mutations which cause Wolfram syndrome appear to be, in the most part, inactivating and tend to be spread throughout the gene. In contrast, the heterozygous missense mutations associated with low-frequency sensorineural hearing impairment tend to be non-inactivating and cluster at the C-terminal protein domain, an observation which may simplify mutation analysis of the 8 exons of the gene[61]. In summary, it is probably worthwhile screening the WFS1 gene in cases of low-frequency sensorineural hearing impairment where there is a positive family history.

Hearing impairment caused by mutations in the COCH gene (DFNA9) – familial progressive vestibulocochlear dysfunction with 'Menière-like' symptoms

The clinical presentation of mutations in this gene is remarkable in its consistency. Most families have presented at 40–60 years of age with a progressive autosomal dominant sensorineural hearing loss[63]. The exception to this is the family reported by Robertson et al in which the age of onset was somewhat younger, at 20–40 years of age[64]. Initially, high frequencies are affected but progression ultimately involves all frequencies so that severe-to-profound loss is seen by 60–80 years. However, the most notable feature is that of the vestibular symptoms, which may be present in some or all affected family members. Many individuals report a feeling of unsteadiness, difficulty walking in the dark, on uneven ground or up and down steps and vertigo has been reported in some individuals although it is not present in all. In some families, vestibular dysfunction has shown complete penetrance[63] but reduced penetrance in others[64-66]. The episodes of vertigo, tinnitus, aural fullness and progressive hearing impairment are reminiscent of symptoms of Menière's disease.

Endolymphatic hydrops, a characteristic of Menière's disease, has been confirmed in one patient histopathologically. Histopathological examination in the original DFNA9 families is said to have a unique appearance[67] with degeneration and acellularity of the spiral ligament, spiral limbus and stroma of the cristae and maculae, and replacement by eosinophilic acellular material. The actual function of the COCH gene product is, however, unknown, although it is likely to be a secreted protein[64].

The clinical presentation of this disorder does differ from classical Menière's disease in which the hearing loss usually begins as low-frequency as opposed to high-frequency in DFNA9. Meticulous clinical characterisation of this disorder has been described by Bom et al in a large Dutch family[68]. The progression of vestibular involvement was clearly documented and vestibular areflexia was found from the age of

47 years onwards, whereas younger individuals showed either severe hyporeflexia or unilateral caloric areflexia. In summary, it would appear that familial progressive hearing loss associated with progressive vestibular dysfunction is a good indication for mutation screening of the *COCH* gene.

Mid-frequency hearing loss (mutations at DFNA12, DFNA13 and DFNA21)

COL11A2 (DFNA12)

Mutations at three deafness loci (DFNA12, DFNA13 and DFNA21) are characterised by hearing impairment that affects the mid-frequencies.

Mutations at the locus DFNA13, in the *COL11A2* gene, give rise to a mid-frequency, or U-shaped ('cookie-bite') hearing loss with no significant progression beyond presbyacusis[69,70], which eventually produces a flattened audiogram[71]. Most individuals noted hearing problems 20–40 years of age, although actual age of onset may have been prelingual in some families. Study of a Dutch family revealed that about half of the mutation carriers also had caloric abnormalities[71]. It should be noted that mutations in the same gene, COL11A2, may cause Stickler syndrome without eye involvement. However, detailed clinical evaluation of the families described above confirms that their hearing impairment is non-syndromic.

Detailed clinical evaluation of a family with hearing impairment linked to DFNA13, but without a known mutation, again showed mid-frequency hearing impairment which became apparent at about the age of 30 years, but there was no evidence for congenital or prelingual onset. Speech had developed normally in all cases. Vestibular function as assessed by bithermal calorics was intact in most cases[72].

Studies of the hearing impaired *Col11a2*[−/−] mouse have shown that the tectorial membrane appeared to be thicker and less compacted than normal, due to disorganization of the type 2 collagen fibrils, which were not arranged in their usual parallel, evenly spaced manner[70]. It has been hypothesized that the type XI collagen is needed in the tectorial membrane for even spacing between type 2 collagen fibrils, the major collagen in the tectorial membrane. *Col11a2* mRNA was observed in vestibular sensory areas, compatible with the vestibular findings in some of the human families. Thus structural disorganization of the tectorial membrane appears to cause congenital, permanent hearing impairment, which is stable and affects the mid-frequencies predominantly.

Although the phenotype of mid-frequency hearing loss caused by mutations in this gene is more distinctive than many other autosomal dominant non-syndromic forms of hearing loss, the gene is large, consisting of 67 exons; therefore, prior linkage probably needs to be established in a family before mutation screening can be offered.

TECTA (DFNA8/12)

It is interesting to note that another component of the tectorial membrane, tectorin, causes a form of autosomal dominant deafness with a similar phenotype. Mutations in the zona pellucida domain of the *TECTA* gene, which encodes α-tectorin, also cause prelingual non-progressive, mid-frequency hearing impairment[73–75]. However, mutations in a different domain, the zonadhesin-like domain, cause autosomal dominant progressive high frequency hearing impairment which may be prelingual or postlingual in onset[76,77]. Homozygous loss of function mutation of *TECTA* may also result in the phenotype of severe-to-profound non-syndromic autosomal recessive hearing loss[78], DFNB21.

DFNA21

Mutation at the DFNA21 locus, mapped to 6p21-22, also may give rise to progressive non-syndromic mid-frequency sensorineural hearing impairment, with an age of onset estimated at around 3–4 years[79]. The gene responsible has not yet been identified.

Maternally inherited hearing impairment

The importance of maternally inherited hearing impairment, due to mutations in the mitochondrial genome, has only come to light in the last decade or so[80,81]. Mitochondria are intracellular organelles which are responsible for the generation of energy through oxidative phosphorylation. They contain their own DNA (mtDNA), which encodes 13 mRNAs (components of five enzymatic complexes necessary for oxidative phosphorylation), two rRNAs and twenty-two tRNAs. At fertilization, only the ovum contributes mitochondria to the zygote and; therefore, mutations in the mitochondrial genome are only inherited through the maternal line and are never transmitted by the father. Usually all the mitochondrial chromosomes in a cell carry identical copies of mtDNA (homoplasmy), but some mutations may be heteroplasmic (wild-type and mutant mitochondria in the same cell). Random distribution of mutations between cells following cell division may lead to differences in mutational loads between different cells and tissues.

Estimates of the contribution made by mitochondrial genes to inherited deafness vary between populations. Mitochondrial genes appear to be a rare cause of prelingual hearing loss[83], although data suggest that a considerable proportion of post-lingual hearing loss may be maternally inherited (T Hutchin, personal communication)[82,84].

A comprehensive description of the biology and phenotypes associated with mitochondrial hearing impairment is beyond the scope of this review and is available elsewhere[82,83], but suffice it to say that hearing impairment may be non-syndromic or syndromic and varies greatly in severity and age of onset even within families. Other systems which may be involved tend to include organs and tissues with a high energy requirement such as muscle, central nervous system, retina, heart, and gut, besides the ear. Symptoms such as ataxia, seizures, hypotonia, myopathy, ophthalmoplegia, optic atrophy, cardiomyopathy, retinopathy and endocrinopathies often occur in mitochondrial diseases (*e.g.* MERRF, MELAS, Pearson syndrome, Kearns-Sayre syndrome and maternally inherited diabetes and deafness). The hearing loss associated with these conditions tends to be of childhood or early adult onset, to involve high frequencies and is often progressive[81]. The hearing impairment appears to be cochlear in origin due to loss of outer hair cell function, and successful cochlear implantation indicates that the cochlear nerve is unaffected.

A number of mitochondrial mutations have been described which give rise to non-syndromic hearing impairment. The most important of these is the A1555G mutation in the 12SrRNA gene, which was originally described in a large Arab-Israeli family demonstrating maternally inherited deafness[80,81]. Most of the affected individuals had early onset severe to profound hearing loss in infancy, although other family members had adult onset hearing loss and some had normal hearing. It has subsequently been shown that the deafness phenotype in this family is probably modified by an unknown autosomal gene on chromosome 8[87]. In other cases, this mutation has been reported in families where there is deafness following exposure to aminoglycosides[84,88,89] in which case the age of onset of deafness in exposed individuals is younger[84]. Aminoglycoside-induced hearing impairment appears to be particularly common in some countries. For example, in one region of China, 25% of deaf mutes associated their hearing loss with aminoglycoside exposure, and where deafness was familial, transmission was compatible with maternal inheritance[90]. The A1555G mutation appears to be highly prevalent among Spanish deaf individuals where it is found in 27% of multigeneration families (with and without aminoglycoside exposure)[84], and also in Japanese where 10% of profoundly deaf individuals without aminoglycoside exposure carry the mutation[91]. A second mutation, 961delT, has also been associated with aminoglycoside induced deafness[92].

Other mutations, A7445G, 7472insC, T7510C and T7511C, in the tRNA[Ser(UCN)] gene, have been reported to cause non-syndromic hearing impairment, although A7445G has also been reported with palmoplantar keratoderma[93], and 7472insC with ataxia and myoclonus[94].

In summary, non-syndromic mitochondrial deafness should be considered in all multigeneration families, with and without exposure to aminoglycoside antibiotics, unless there is reliable documentation of transmission of deafness from a male. Syndromic mitochondrial deafness may underlie symptoms in multiple organ systems.

Conclusions

Thorough investigation of the aetiology of hearing loss is necessary for accurate genetic counselling and for the implementation and assessment of any future gene therapy. Investigation of non-syndromic deafness should include analysis of *GJB2* since it is the most common cause of inherited hearing loss and its clinical presentation is unremarkable. However, genetic heterogeneity underlying syndromic and non-syndromic deafness greatly complicates further genetic testing and diagnosis in small families and sporadic cases of deafness. Until genetic testing for large numbers of genes becomes cheaper, faster and less labour-intensive, clinicians must rely on the few audiological, vestibular and radiological clues that may suggest mutation at a particular locus. Detailed clinical description of the effects of gene mutations is an important part in realising the full potential.

Key points for clinical practice

- Characterize the hearing loss (audiology, vestibular tests and radiology)

- Rigorously exclude syndromic causes of hearing impairment, by history, examination and specialised investigation (ophthalmology, renal ultrasound, neuro-imaging)

- Consider *GJB2* mutation screen in all non-syndromic cases with unknown aetiology (common cause of hearing loss with few clinical pointers)

- Always consider mitochondrial inheritance in multigeneration families unless there is clear evidence of transmission from a male

References

1   Morton NE. Genetic epidemiology of hearing impairment. *Ann NY Acad Sci* 1991; **630**: 16–31
2   Green GE, Scott DA, McDonald JM *et al.* Performance of cochlear implant recipients with GJB2-related deafness. *Am J Med Genet* 2002; **109**: 167–70
3   Fortnum HM, Summerfield AQ, Marshall DH. Prevalence of childhood hearing impairment in the United Kingdom and implications for universal neonatal hearing screening: questionnaire based ascertainment study. *BMJ* 2001; **323**: 536–40
4   Davis AC. *Hearing in Adults*. London: Whurr, 1995
5   Van Camp G, Smith RJH. *Hereditary Hearing Loss*. Homepage at <http://www.uia.ac.be/dnalab/hhh>
6   Navarro-Coy N, Hutchin TP, Conlon HE *et al.* The relative contribution of mutations in the DFNB loci to congenital/early childhood non-syndromal hearing impairment/deafness. *J Med Genet* 2001; **38**: S38
7   Liu XZ, Walsh J, Mburu P *et al.* Mutations in the myosin VIIA gene cause non-syndromic recessive deafness. *Nat Genet* 1997; **16**: 188–90

8   Veske A, Oehlmann R, Younnus F et al. Autosomal recessive non-syndromic deafness locus (DFNB8) maps on chromosome 21q22 in a large consanguineous kindred from Pakistan. Hum Mol Genet 1996; 5: 165–8

9   Verpy E, Masmoudi S, Zwaenepohl I et al. Mutations in a new gene encoding a protein of the hair bundle cause non-syndromic deafness at the DFNB16 locus. Nat Genet 2001; 29: 345–9

10 Phelps PD, Coffey RA, Trembath RC et al. Radiological malformations of the ear in Pendred syndrome. Clin Radiol 1998; 53: 268–73

11 Rogers RJ, Kelley P, Keats BJB et al. Otoferlin mutations in non-syndromic recessive auditory neuropathy families. Molecular Biology of Hearing and Deafness Meeting. Bethesda, MD, 2001 (abstract 67)

12 Denoyelle F, Weil D, Maw MA et al. Prelingual deafness: high prevalence of a 30delG mutation in the connexin 26 gene. Hum Mol Genet 1997; 6: 2173–7

13 Zelante L, Gasparini P, Estivill X et al. Connexin 26 mutations associated with the most common form of non-syndromic neurosensory autosomal recessive deafness (DFNB1) in Mediterraneans. Hum Mol Genet 1997; 6: 1605–9

14 Estivill X, Fortina P, Surrey S et al. Connexin-26 mutations in sporadic and inherited sensorineural deafness. Lancet 1998; 351: 394–8

15 Lench N, Houseman M, Newton V et al. Connexin-26 mutations in sporadic non-syndromal sensorineural deafness. Lancet 1998; 351: 415

16 Morell RJ, Kim HJ, Hood LJ et al. Mutations in the connexin 26 gene (GJB2) among Ashkenazi Jews with non-syndromic recessive deafness. N Engl J Med 1998; 339: 1500–5

17 Abe S, Usami S, Shinkawa H et al. Prevalent connexin 26 gene (GJB2) mutations in Japanese. J Med Genet 2000; 37: 41–3

18 Green GE, Scott DA, McDonald JM et al. Carrier rates in the Midwestern United States for GJB2 mutations causing inherited deafness. JAMA 1999; 281: 2211–6

19 Maw MA, Allen-Powell DR, Goodey RJ et al. The contribution of the DFNB1 locus to neurosensory deafness in a Caucasian population. Am J Hum Genet 1995; 57: 629–35

20 Gasparini P, Estivill X, Volpini V et al. Linkage of DFNB1 to non-syndromic neurosensory autosomal recessive deafness in Mediterranean families. Eur J Hum Genet 1997; 5: 83–8

21 Gasparini P, Rabionet R, Barbujani G et al. High carrier frequency of the 35delG deafness mutation in European populations. Genetic Analysis Consortium of GJB2 35delG. Eur J Hum Genet 2000; 8: 19–23

22 Van Laer L, Coucke P, Mueller RF et al. A common founder for the 35delG GJB2 gene mutation in connexin 26 hearing impairment. J Med Genet 2001; 38: 515–8

23 Lerer I, Sagi M, Malamud E et al. Contribution of connexin 26 mutations to non-syndromic deafness in Ashkenazi patients and the variable phenotypic effect of the mutation 167delT. Am J Med Genet 2000; 95: 53–6

24 Rickard S, Kelsell DP, Sirimana T et al. Recurrent mutations in the deafness gene GJB2 (connexin 26) in British Asian families. J Med Genet 2001; 38: 530–3

25 Denoyelle F, Marlin S, Weil D et al. Clinical features of the prevalent form of childhood deafness, DFNB1, due to a connexin-26 gene defect: implications for genetic counselling. Lancet 1999; 353: 1298–303

26 Mueller RF, Nehammer A, Middleton A et al. Congenital non-syndromal sensorineural hearing impairment due to connexin 26 gene mutations – molecular and audiological findings. Int J Pediatr Otorhinolaryngol 1999; 50: 3–13

27 Cohn ES, Kelley PM, Fowler TW et al. Clinical studies of families with hearing loss attributable to mutations in the connexin 26 gene (GJB2/DFNB1). Pediatrics 1999; 103: 546–50

28 Wilcox SA, Saunders K, Osborn AH et al. High frequency hearing loss correlated with mutations in the GJB2 gene. Hum Genet 2000; 106: 399–405

29 Cohn ES, Kelley PM. Clinical phenotype and mutations in connexin 26 (DFNB1/GJB2), the most common cause of childhood hearing loss. Am J Med Genet 1999; 89: 130–6

30 Green GE, Smith RJ, Bent JP et al. Genetic testing to identify deaf newborns. JAMA 2000; 284: 1245

31 Denoyelle F, Lina-Grande G, Plauchu H et al. Connexin 26 linked to dominant deafness Nature 1998; 393: 319–20

32 Heathcote K, Syrris P, Carter ND *et al*. A connexin 26 mutation causes a syndrome of sensorineural hearing loss and palmoplantar hyperkeratosis (MIM 148350). *J Med Genet* 2000; **37**: 50–1

33 Richard G, White TW, Smith LE *et al*. Functional defects of Cx26 resulting from a heterozygous missense mutation in a family with dominant deaf-mutism and palmoplantar keratoderma. *Hum Genet* 1998; **103**: 393–9

34 Rouan F, White TW, Brown N *et al*. Trans-dominant inhibition of connexin-43 by mutant connexin-26: implications for dominant connexin disorders affecting epidermal differentiation. *J Cell Sci* 2001; **114**: 2105–13

35 Maestrini E, Korge BP, Ocana-Sierra J *et al*. A missense mutation in connexin 26, D66H, causes mutilating keratoderma with sensorineural deafness (Vohwinkel's syndrome) in three unrelated families. *Hum Mol Genet* 1999; **8**: 1237–43

36 Richard G, Rouan F, Willoughby CE *et al*. Missense mutations in GJB2 encoding *Connexin-26* cause the ectodermal dysplasia keratitis-ichthyosis-deafness syndrome. *Am J Hum Genet* 2002: **70**: 1341–8

37 Loffeld A, Kelsell DP, Moss C. Palmoplantar keratoderma and sensorineural deafness in an 8-year-old boy: a case report. *Br J Dermatol* 2000; **143**: 38

38 White TW, Deans MR, Kelsell DP *et al*. Connexin mutations in deafness. *Nature* 1998; **394**: 630–1

39 Martin PE, Coleman SL, Casalotti SO *et al*. Properties of connexin 26 gap junctional proteins derived from mutations associated with non-syndromal hereditary deafness. *Hum Mol Genet* 1999; **8**: 2369–76

40 Griffith AJ, Chowdhry AA, Kurima K *et al*. Autosomal recessive non-syndromic neurosensory deafness at DFNB1 not associated with the compound-heterozygous GJB2 (connexin 26) genotype M34T/167delT. *Am J Hum Genet* 2000; **67**: 745–9

41 Marlin S, Garabedian FN, Roger G *et al*. Connexin 26 gene mutations in congenitally deaf children: pitfalls for genetic counseling. *Arch Otolaryngol Head Neck Surg* 2001; **127**: 927–33

42 Fraser GR. Association of congenital deafness with goitre (Pendred's syndrome): a study of 207 families. *Ann Hum Genet* 1965; **28**: 201–49

43 Luxon LM, Cohen M, Coffey R *et al*. Neuro-otological abnormalities in Pendred syndrome. *Int J Audiol* 2002; In press

44 Reardon W, O'Mahoney CF, Trembath R *et al*. Enlarged vestibular aqueduct: a radiological marker of Pendred syndrome, and mutation of the PDS gene. *Q J Med* 2000; **93**: 99–104

45 Cremers CW, Admiraal RJ, Huygen PL *et al*. Progressive hearing loss, hypoplasia of the cochlea and widened vestibular aqueducts are very common features in Pendred's syndrome. *Int J Pediatr Otorhinolaryngol* 1998; **45**: 113–23

46 Chen A, Francis M, Ni L *et al* Phenotypic manifestations of branchio-oto-renal syndrome. *Am J Med Genet* 1995; **58**: 365–70

47 Berettini S, Forli F, Franceschini SS, Ravecca F, Massimetti M, Neri E. Distal renal tubular acidosis associated with isolated large vestibular aqueduct and sensorineural hearing loss. *Ann Otol Rhinol Laryngol* 2002; **115**: 385–91

48 Everett LA, Glaser B, Beck JC *et al*. Pendred syndrome is caused by mutations in a putative sulphate transporter gene (PDS). *Nat Genet* 1997; **17**: 411–22

49 Scott DA, Wang R, Kreman TM, Sheffield V, Karniski LP. The Pendred syndrome gene encodes a chloride iodide transporter. *Nat Genet* 1999; **21**: 440–3

50 Royaux IE, Wall SM, Karniski LP *et al*. Pendrin, encoded by the Pendred syndrome gene, resides in the apical region of renal intercalated cells and mediates bicarbonate secretion. *Proc Natl Acad Sci USA* 2001; **98**: 4221–6

51 Everett LA, Morsli H, Wu DK *et al*. Expression pattern of the mouse ortholog of the Pendred's syndrome gene (PDS) suggests a key role for pendrin in the inner ear. *Proc Natl Acad Sci USA* 1999; **96**: 9727–32

52 Everett LA, Belyantseva IA, Noben-Trauth K *et al*. Targeted disruption of mouse PDS provides insight about the inner-ear defects encountered in Pendred syndrome. *Hum Mol Genet* 2001; **10**: 153–61

53 Coyle B, Reardon W, Herbrick JA *et al*. Molecular analysis of the PDS gene in Pendred syndrome. *Hum Mol Genet* 1998; **7**: 1105–12

54 Campbell C, Cucci RA, Prasad S et al. Pendred syndrome, DFNB4, and PDS/SLC26A4 identification of eight novel mutations and possible genotype-phenotype correlations. *Hum Mutat* 2001; **17**: 403–11

55 Scott DA, Wang R, Kreman TM et al. Functional differences of the PDS gene product are associated with phenotypic variation in patients with Pendred syndrome and non-syndromic hearing loss (DFNB4). *Hum Mol Genet* 2000; **9**: 1709–15

56 Taylor JP, Metcalfe RA, Watson PF et al. Mutations of the PDS gene, encoding pendrin, are associated with protein mislocalization and loss of iodide efflux: implications for thyroid dysfunction in Pendred syndrome. *J Clin Endocrinol Metab* 2002; **87**: 1778–84

57 Lynch ED, Leon PE. Non-syndromic dominant DFNA1. *Adv Otorhinolaryngol* 2000; **56**: 60–7

58 McGuirt WT, Lesperance MM, Wilcox ER, Chen AH, Van Camp G, Smith RJH. Characterization of autosomal dominant non-syndromic hearing loss loci: DFNA4,6,10 and 13. *Adv Otorhinolaryngol* 2000; **56**: 84–96

59 Young TL, Ives E, Lynch E et al. Non-syndromic progressive hearing loss DFNA38 is caused by heterozygous missense mutation in the Wolfram syndrome gene WFS1. *Hum Mol Genet* 2001; **10**: 2509–14

60 Bespalova IN, Van Camp G, Bom SJ et al. Mutations in the Wolfram syndrome 1 gene (WFS1) are a common cause of low frequency sensorineural hearing loss. *Hum Mol Genet* 2001; **10**: 2501–8

61 Cryns K, Pfister M, Pennings RJ et al. Mutations in the WFS1 gene that cause low frequency sensorineural hearing loss are small non-inactivating mutations. *Hum Genet* 2002; **110**: 389–94

62 Barrett TG, Bundey SE, Macleod AF. Neurodegeneration and diabetes: UK nationwide study of Wolfram (DIDMOAD) syndrome. *Lancet* 1995; **346**: 1458–63

63 Kamarinos M, McGill J, Lynch M, Dahl H. Identification of a novel COCH mutation, I109N, highlights the similar clinical features observed in DFNA9 families. *Hum Mutat* 2001; **17**: 351

64 Robertson NG, Lu L, Heller S et al. Mutations in a novel cochlear gene cause DFNA9, a human non-syndromic sensorineural deafness with vestibular dysfunction. *Nat Genet* 1998; **20**: 229–303

65 Fransen E, Verstreken M, Verhagen WI et al. High prevalence of symptoms of Ménière's disease in three families with a mutation in the COCH gene. *Hum Mol Genet* 1999; **8**: 1425–9

66 de Kok YJ, Bom SJ, Brunt TM et al. A Pro51Ser mutation in the COCH gene is associated with late onset autosomal dominant progressive sensorineural hearing loss with vestibular defects. *Hum Mol Genet* 1999; **8**: 361–6

67 Merchant SN, Linthicum FH, Nadol JB. Histopathology of the inner ear in DFNA9. *Adv Otorhinolaryngol* 2000; **56**: 212–7

68 Bom SJ, Kemperman MH, De Kok YJ et al. Progressive cochleovestibular impairment caused by a point mutation in the COCH gene at DFNA9. *Laryngoscope* 1999; **109**: 1525–30

69 De Leenheer EM, Kunst HH, McGuirt WT et al. Autosomal dominant inherited hearing impairment caused by a missense mutation in COL11A2 (DFNA13). *Arch Otolaryngol Head Neck Surg* 2001; **127**: 13–7

70 McGuirt WT, Prasad SD, Griffith AJ et al. Mutations in COL11A2 cause non-syndromic hearing loss (DFNA13). *Nat Genet* 1999; **23**: 413–9

71 Kunst H, Huybrechts C, Marres H et al. The phenotype of DFNA13/COL11A2: non-syndromic autosomal dominant mid-frequency and high-frequency sensorineural hearing impairment. *Am J Otol* 2000; **21**: 181–7

72 Ensink RJ, Huygen PL, Snoeckx RL, Caethoven G, Van Camp G, Cremers CW. A Dutch family with progressive autosomal dominant non-syndromic sensorineural hearing impairment linked to DFNA13. *Clin Otolaryngol* 2001; **26**: 310–6

73 Verhoeven K, Van Laer L, Kirschhofer K et al. Mutations in the human alpha-tectorin gene cause autosomal dominant non-syndromic hearing impairment. *Nat Genet* 1998; **19**: 60–2

74 Kirschhofer K, Kenyon JB, Hoover DM et al. Autosomal-dominant, prelingual, non-progressive sensorineural hearing loss: localization of the gene (DFNA8) to chromosome 11q by linkage in an Austrian family. *Cytogenet Cell Genet* 1998; **82**: 126–30

75 Govaerts PJ, De Ceulaer G, Daemers K et al. A new autosomal-dominant locus (DFNA12) is responsible for a non-syndromic, midfrequency, prelingual and non-progressive sensorineural hearing loss. *Am J Otol* 1998; **19**: 718–23

76 Alloisio N, Morle L, Bozon M et al. Mutation in the zonadhesin-like domain of alpha-tectorin

associated with autosomal dominant non-syndromic hearing loss. *Eur J Hum Genet* 1999; **7**: 255–8

77 Balciuniene J, Dahl N, Jalonen P *et al*. Alpha-tectorin involvement in hearing disabilities: one gene – two phenotypes. *Hum Genet* 1999; **105**: 211–6

78 Mustapha M, Weil D, Chardenoux S *et al*. An alpha-tectorin gene defect causes a newly identified autosomal recessive form of sensorineural pre-lingual non-syndromic deafness, DFNB21. *Hum Mol Genet* 1999; **8**: 409–12

79 Kunst H, Marres H, Huygen *et al*. Non-syndromic autosomal dominant progressive non-specific mid-frequency hearing impairment with childhood to late adolescence onset (DFNA21). *Clin Otolaryngol* 2000; **25**: 45–54

80 Prezant TR, Agapian JV, Bohlman H *et al*. Mitochondrial ribosomal RNA mutation associated with both antibiotic-induced and non-syndromic deafness. *Nat Genet* 1993; **4**: 289–94

81 Hutchin TP, Haworth I, Higashi K *et al*. A molecular basis for human hypersensitivity to aminoglycoside antibiotics. *Nucleic Acids Res* 1993; **21**: 4174–9

82 Hutchin TP, Thompson KR, Parker M, Newton V, Bitner-Glindzicz M, Mueller RF. Prevalence of mitochondrial DNA mutations in childhood/congenital onset non-syndromal sensorineural hearing impairment. *J Med Genet* 2001; **38**: 229–31

83 Hutchin TP, Cortopassi GA. Mitochondrial defects and hearing loss. *Cell Mol Life Sci* 2000; **57**: 1927–37

84 Estivill X, Govea N, Barcelo E *et al*. Familial progressive sensorineural deafness is mainly due to the mtDNA A1555G mutation and is enhanced by treatment of aminoglycosides. *Am J Hum Genet* 1998; **62**: 27–35

85 Van Camp G, Smith RJ. Maternally inherited hearing impairment. *Clin Genet* 2000; **57**: 409–14

86 Tono T, Ushisako Y, Kiyomizu K *et al*. Cochlear implantation in a patient with profound hearing loss with the A1555G mitochondrial mutation. *Am J Otol* 1998; **19**: 754–7

87 Bykhovskaya Y, Estivill X, Taylor K *et al*. Candidate locus for a nuclear modifier gene for maternally inherited deafness. *Am J Hum Genet* 2000; **66**: 1905–10

88 Fischel-Ghodsian N, Prezant TR, Bu X, Oztas S. Mitochondrial ribosomal RNA gene mutation in a patient with sporadic aminoglycoside toxicity. *Am J Otolaryngol* 1993; **14**: 399–403

89 Usami S, Abe S, Kasai M *et al*. Genetic and clinical features of sensorineural hearing loss with the 1,555 mitochondrial mutation. *Laryngoscope* 1997; **107**: 483–90

90 Hu DN, Qiu WQ, Wu BT *et al*. Genetic aspects of antibiotic induced deafness: mitochondrial inheritance. *J Med Genet* 1991; **28**: 79–83

91 Usami S, Abe S, Akita J *et al*. Prevalence of mitochondrial gene mutations among hearing impaired patients. *J Med Genet* 2000; **37**: 38–40

92 Casano RA, Johnson DF, Bykhovskaya Y *et al*. Inherited susceptibility to aminoglycoside ototoxicity: genetic heterogeneity and clinical implications. *Am J Otolaryngol* 1999; **20**: 151–6

93 Sevior KB, Hatamochi A, Stewart IA *et al*. Mitochondrial A7445G mutation in two pedigrees with palmoplantar keratoderma and deafness. *Am J Med Genet* 1998; **75**: 179–85

94 Tiranti V, Chariot P, Carella F *et al*. Maternally inherited hearing loss, ataxia and myoclonus associated with a novel point mutation in mitochondrial tRNA$^{Ser(UCN)}$ gene. *Hum Mol Genet* 1995; **4**: 1421–7

95 Bilous RW, Murty G, Parkinson DB *et al*. Autosomal dominant familial hypoparathyroidism, sensorineural deafness, and renal dysplasia. *N Engl J Med* 1992; **327**: 1069–74

96 Van Esch H, Groenen P, Nesbit MA *et al*. GATA3 haplo-insufficiency causes human HDR syndrome. *Nature* 2000; **406**: 419–22

97 Muroya K, Hasegawa T, Ito Y *et al*. GATA3 abnormalities and the phenotypic spectrum of HDR syndrome. *J Med Genet* 2001; **38**: 374–80

98 Phelps PD, Reardon W, Pembrey M, Bellman S, Luxon L. X-linked deafness, stapes gushers and a distinctive defect of the inner ear. *Neuroradiology* 1991; **33**: 326–30

99 Bamiou DE, Phelps P, Sirimanna T. Temporal bone computed tomography findings in bilateral sensorineural hearing loss. *Arch Dis Child* 2000; **82**: 257–60

Microelectrode and neuroimaging studies of central auditory function

Alan R Palmer and **A Quentin Summerfield**

MRC Institute of Hearing Research, University of Nottingham, Nottingham NG7 2RD, UK

Imaging studies in humans are revealing parallels with the functional organisation of the auditory brain discovered in microelectrode studies in animals: the rate of amplitude modulation generating the strongest response declines systematically from the lower brain stem to the cortex; an increase in sound level induces a higher level and a greater extent of activity; spectra are represented tonotopically in multiple cortical areas. There are also differences: evidence of organisation reflecting the sound level of the stimulus is absent in animals, but has been found in humans. Additionally, imaging has revealed functional specialisations which have not (yet) been located in animals: areas that respond more strongly to sounds with stronger pitches and to sounds that move in space. Microelectrode studies suggest that vocalisations are represented by spatially distributed populations of neurones in secondary auditory areas. In humans, likewise, activation progressively more specific to speech is found as the search moves from primary to secondary to accessory areas.

Physiological and imaging methodologies to investigate central auditory function

Microelectrodes capable of recording from a single neurone or a small cluster of neurones have been the primary tools for investigating brain function for the last half century. For many purposes, they still provide unique information, although the information can be enhanced and extended by coupling microelectrode recordings with other techniques. For example, recorded cells can be filled with dyes to reconstruct their structure and connections. Neurotransmitters and their agonists can be injected locally to determine the nature of a cell's synaptic connections. Single ion channels can be studied to reveal biophysical mechanisms at the cell membrane. These combinations of techniques have allowed progressively finer resolution of the spatial and temporal properties of single neurone responses.

In the last two decades, a new set of weapons has been added to the research arsenal that has the potential for powerful complementarity with microelectrode techniques. These are imaging methodologies that allow the

Correspondence to:
Prof. Alan R Palmer, MRC Institute of Hearing Research, University Park, Nottingham NG7 2RD, UK

responses of large ensembles of neurones to be measured in awake human subjects. The oldest of these techniques, electroencephalography (EEG), measures electrical signals at the surface of the head that reflect activation of remote populations of neurones. By making up to 128 simultaneous spatially separated measurements, it is possible to calculate the location of one or more dipole sources within the brain that could have given rise to the voltages at the different electrodes. In this way, the location of the neural activity is inferred. A variant of the method, magnetoencephalo-graphy (MEG), detects not the voltage, but the magnetic field generated by the current flows that result from neural activity. MEG also requires multiple sensors to allow the location of a dipole source to be inferred. Both EEG and MEG achieve very high temporal resolution (of the order of milliseconds, but poor spatial accuracy due to the dispersion of the signals within the head before they reach the scalp.

Two other widely used imaging methods do not depend on the neural activity directly, but on the metabolic demands that neural activity imposes. To meet the requirement for oxygen by active neural tissue, the blood supply to the active regions in the brain is increased. The increase in blood flow is measured directly in positron emission tomography (PET) by monitoring the concentration within the brain of radioactive oxygen injected into the subject just before the start of the experiment. Functional magnetic resonance imaging (fMRI) also relies on the metabolic response to neural activity by detecting changes in the ratio of oxy- to deoxyhaemoglobin in blood. PET and fMRI provide good spatial resolution (down to millimetres), but their temporal resolution is generally poor, because they rely on cardiovascular changes which take place over several seconds. Recent developments in fMRI such as single-event paradigms are bringing this limit nearer to fractions of a second.

In the sections that follow we relate data from electrophysiological studies in animals are related to data from imaging studies in humans.

Frequency, tonotopicity, and pitch

Microelectrode studies have revealed that the most striking organising principle of all auditory nuclei, in all animal species, is tonotopicity. From the point at which the auditory nerve enters the brain in the cochlear nucleus up through the diverse nuclei of the auditory brain stem, mid-brain and thalamus to the multiple fields in the auditory cortex, each nucleus has a tonotopic organisation, replicating the logarithmic increase in frequency that occurs with distance from the apex along the cochlear epithelium[1]. The restricted place representation of any one frequency in the cochlea expands to become a slab of cells in the cortex, all responsive to the same frequency range, and so providing the substrate for parallel processing of various aspects of sound. The mere fact of tonotopicity, however, does not imply that the tuning curves of central neurones are simple 'V' shapes like those of auditory nerve fibre responses. Instead, convergence of excitatory and inhibitory inputs results in increasingly complicated response areas at higher levels of the system (*e.g.* Phillips *et al*[2]). Nonetheless, at the level of the primary auditory cortex, the topographical organisation of response types is systematic, with neurones at the centre of the region having the lowest thresholds, shortest latencies, and the narrowest and most symmetrical frequency response areas[3].

Electrophysiology in humans has provided a direct demonstration of tonotopicity along Heschl's gyrus – the site of the primary auditory cortex. Using electrodes implanted to detect the foci of seizures in epileptic patients[4], a lateral progression in frequency sensitivity from high frequency (3360 Hz) to lower frequency (1480 Hz) was found. A similar progression has been found using MEG: the source of the response in Heschl's gyrus again moves more laterally as frequency decreases[5]. This experiment also located an orthogonal tonotopic gradient in the secondary auditory cortex in planum temporale running from high to low frequency in a posterior direction.

Similar results have been obtained by using high resolution MRI to image the response to narrow-band noise stimuli[6]. By using high (above 2490 Hz) and low (below 600 Hz) bands, it was possible to identify regions on the supratemporal plane that were more responsive to one or other of the sounds. Eight regions were found (four that were activated more strongly by the low-frequency sound and four by the high-frequency sound) widely dispersed across the auditory cortex including Heschl's gyrus and planum temporale, suggesting the existence of multiple functionally distinct regions each with its own tonotopic axis. At least some of these regions coincided with anatomical divisions of the cortex, including the primary area on Heschl's gyrus.

Potentially, primary auditory cortex could be organised spatially with respect to pitch rather than frequency. Pitch is the subjective attribute of sounds such that they may be ordered on a musical scale: it is related to the repetition rate of the waveform of a sound. Early studies in monkey favoured frequency[7], although recent studies in the gerbil have indicated that pitch could be an additional organising principle[8]. This result awaits replication in other species. Whatever the outcome, a distinct cortical region responsive to the strength of pitch in sounds has been located in humans. It is possible to create stimuli whose spectral structure is not resolvable by the human auditory system and whose pitch is determined by their temporal structure alone. PET has been used with such stimuli to reveal bilateral areas of auditory cortex where the response magnitude increased parametrically with the temporal regularity, and hence the pitch strength, of the stimulus[9]. On the right, the region appeared to be in primary auditory cortex, while on the left the activation was more lateral extending onto the surface of the superior temporal gyrus. When the stimuli were presented in sequences forming melodies, additional regions more anterior (anterior temporal lobes) and posterior (superior temporal gyrus) to the primary auditory cortex showed activation dependent on the pitch strength. Temporal integration on a scale of ten's of milliseconds is required to detect pitch, and on a scale of seconds to detect melody. Given the limited temporal resolution of cortical neurones, it is likely that the primary areas were responding to evidence passed up from sub-cortical neurones which have the temporal resolution required to extract pitch, while the anterior and posterior areas themselves may be responsible for extracting the melody. Indeed, the nuclei of the brain stem show parametric increases in MRI activation as the temporal regularity of the stimulus increases[10].

Intensity and loudness

The perception of loudness, spatial position, and distance depend on sound level. How loud a sound appears is largely a reflection of its intensity, but also of its spectral content. In general, the higher the level of a sound or the greater the extent of its components in frequency, the louder it appears and the greater the magnitude and spread of the neural activation that it produces. In the auditory nerve, increases in the intensity of a single tone first cause an increase in the discharge rate of fibres tuned to that frequency and second a spread of activity to fibres tuned to adjacent frequencies. Eventually, at moderate levels of 70–80 dB SPL, virtually the whole nerve may be active to some extent[11]. Progressing centrally, the typically monotonic sigmoid function for discharge rate with sound level seen in auditory nerve fibres becomes less common, as inhibition shapes the range of sound levels to which neurones respond. By the level of the cortex, sharply non-monotonic rate-level functions can be found with each neurone responding only over very narrow ranges of sound levels[12], but in most mammals there is little evidence that the neurones are organised spatially by best or most effective sound level (referred to as an ampliotopic organisation).

In humans, in contrast, imaging studies have found some evidence of ampliotopy. MEG has revealed that the depth of the dipole source in response to 1000 Hz tones decreases monotonically with level from 30–80 dB HL (dB above hearing threshold at 1000 Hz)[13]. PET has also shown evidence of ampliotopic organisation: in the right temporal lobe, the location of the maximal response varied with the intensity, but not with the frequency of the stimuli[14]. More commonly, however, both with speech stimuli and with tones, an increase in the magnitude of activation[15] or in the volume of activated cortex[16,17] or both[14] have been found to accompany increases in sound level. These increases, even with simple tonal stimulation, are not restricted to the primary auditory areas and do not appear to saturate at high sound levels. For example, in medial geniculate and auditory cortex, activation by 4 kHz tones continued to increase between the high sound levels of 80 and 90 dB HL[14]. Increases in cortical activation at high sound levels have also been shown[18] with different growth functions for high and low frequency tones that were reminiscent of the growth functions for single neurones shown electrophysiologically[19].

Spatial position and movement

The spatial position of a sound source is computed from three types of cue: monaural spectral cues generated by the pinna and concha, and binaural differences in the timing of low-frequency sounds and the level of sounds, at the two ears, that result from longer transmission paths and head shadowing respectively[20]. Moving sound sources generate dynamic spatial cues which, when quite slow (2–6 Hz), lead human listeners to perceive a moving source. Lesion studies show that the auditory pathway up to the cortex is necessary for the perception of sound source position and motion[21,22], although the initial processing takes place in the brain stem.

The dorsal division of the cochlear nucleus has been implicated in the processing of pinna spectral cues, which are particularly important in determining sound source elevation. Somatosensory input to the dorsal cochlear nucleus may allow the position of head, neck, and pinna to be taken into account in evaluating the spectral cues[23]. To account for sensitivity to interaural timing, a network of coincidence detectors linked by delay lines was proposed originally by Jeffress[24]. Subsequent physiological studies[25] have shown that precisely timed action potentials from the auditory nerve are conducted via large high-fidelity synapses through the ventral cochlear nucleus to the binaural comparators in the superior olive. In the medial superior, olive cells receiving input from both ears act as coincidence detectors, firing when the inputs arrive simultaneously. Since the transmission paths to the two ears are not equal, coincidences occur only when the internal transmission delay exactly compensates for the interaural delay due to the sound source position: in the simplest form, the cells may be thought to be tuned for a particular direction in the horizontal plane. A pathway to the lateral superior olive subserves processing of interaural level differences. In this case, the path from the contralateral cochlear nucleus contains an extra synapse onto an inhibitory interneurone in the medial nucleus of the trapezoid body. The net result is that cells in the lateral superior olive are fed by inhibition from one ear and excitation from the other and are exquisitely sensitive to the exact balance of their inputs and hence to the interaural level difference. Microelectrode studies have shown sensitivity to interaural time and level differences throughout the auditory pathway up to the cortex, but sensitivity to the direction of auditory motion only appears beyond the auditory mid-brain[25].

The inferior parietal lobes, particularly on the right side, display greater MRI activation during localisation tasks than during other auditory discrimination tasks[26]. Selective activation of the parietal cortex by moving auditory sources has also been shown using PET and MRI[27]. In these studies, brain activations were compared under conditions in which the dynamic interaural time and level cues were complementary, resulting in perceived motion, or opposing resulting in little motion perception. A region of right parietal cortex was active only when the subject perceived motion not when the same dynamic cues were presented in opposition, nearly cancelling the motion percept. In contrast, primary auditory cortex displayed bilateral activation to both versions of the stimulus, and was not differentially activated when the subject perceived motion.

A movement sensitive area on the right supratemporal plane located on the planum temporale lateral to Heschl's gyrus has been identified with fMRI[28]. A complex broad-band stimulus was amplitude modulated either in phase at the two ears (stationary condition) or 90° out of phase at the ears (moving condition) relying on interaural level differences alone to generate the sound movement. Both moving and stationary signals activated different fields of the auditory cortex bilaterally compared to silence, but only the area in right planum temporale showed stronger activation to the moving stimulus.

Complex sounds and speech

Natural sounds, including speech, contain time-varying changes in spectral content and amplitude. Relatively simple temporally varying sounds have often been used to investigate the neural representation of complex sounds as a means of probing the basis for the analysis of speech sounds.

Responses to amplitude and frequency modulation have been studied at every level of the auditory pathway. Auditory nerve fibres discharge in synchrony with the modulation envelope up to frequencies determined by their tuning and phase locking capabilities, forming a low-pass transfer function[29]. From the cochlear nucleus upwards, neurones tend to be tuned to particular modulation rates, with progressively lower rates being favoured at higher processing stages such that at the cortex preferred rates are only a few tens of Hz. Remarkable parallels are found using MRI with humans[30,31] as shown in Figure 1: optimal rates of 32–256 Hz in the cochlear nucleus and lower brain stem decrease to 2–4 Hz in secondary auditory cortex.

At the mid-brain and cortex, maps of best modulation frequency that might serve pitch perception have been reported[8,32,33]. The existence and significance of these maps is controversial, however[34]. Similarly, only one imaging study, using MEG[35], has provided evidence of a map of modulation sensitivity in human cortex, and the results are equivocal. Other imaging studies show a postero-lateral region of the superior temporal gyrus to be activated selectively by frequency and amplitude modulated sounds[36–38]. Within the auditory region responsive to modulated signals, there appears to be a clustering of responsiveness to different modulation frequencies, but no systematic topographic organisation[30].

The number of neurophysiological studies of responses in auditory cortex to species-specific vocalisations peaked in the 1970s. Interest has revived recently with the development of techniques for studying awake behaving primates. The decline occurred because early expectations of populations of cortical feature-detector neurones were not sustained. Clearly, in primary auditory cortex, large numbers of cells are not

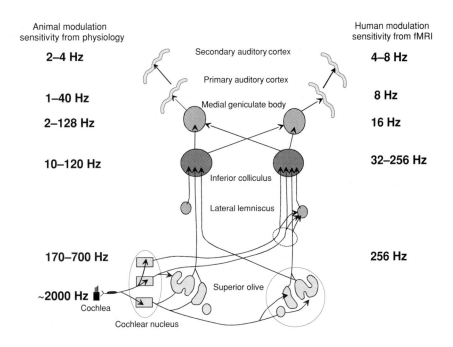

Fig. 1 Sensitivity to different rates of amplitude modulation at different nuclei along the auditory pathway. The animal data are taken from a variety of different studies using pure tone carriers and represent the range of best modulation frequencies. The human data are from an fMRI study[30] using broad-band noise and represent the modulation frequencies that best activated those regions.

specialised for vocalisations. Various alternatives have been proposed involving representations based on the collective response of populations of neurones whose individual responses reflect variations in frequency, tuning width, tuning asymmetry, *etc* (for example[39]). Neurones selective for vocalisations do exist, but are more common in secondary cortical areas[40–43]. Recently, evidence has been presented from neurophysiological and imaging studies that such stimuli can activate separate pathways originating in primary auditory cortex that determine 'what' sound has been produced and 'where' its source is located[43–46].

In imaging studies, speech generates wide-spread activation in auditory cortex including primary and non-primary areas in both hemispheres. Here we focus on speech-specific activation within and adjacent to the human auditory cortex.

Temporal analysis, which is a particular requirement in the encoding of acoustic cues for speech perception, is enhanced in areas of the left auditory cortex. Differential responses to voiced and voiceless stop consonants in primary and secondary auditory areas on the left, but not right, have been recorded from electrodes implanted along the supratemporal plane of epilepsy patients[47]. The auditory cortex on both sides responded strongly to the syllables, but responses were time-locked to the different components of the syllable only on the left. The asymmetries in the temporal processing in these areas were also found for simplified acoustical models of the stimuli, that were not perceived as speech.

MRI and PET, possibly because of their relatively poor temporal resolution, often fail to show hemispheric asymmetries between speech and non-speech sounds, but have provided evidence of an anterior/ventral network involved in processing speech. Activation has been measured to a range of stimuli that included sequences of words and tones, white noise, reversed speech, and pseudowords[48]. No difference was found in the strength of activation in primary or secondary cortex, in either hemisphere, between sequences of words and sequences of pure tones of different frequencies. Activation by the words spread ventrally towards the superior temporal sulcus, to a greater extent on the left side. Primary auditory cortex responded equally to all of the stimuli. In contrast, surrounding non-primary auditory areas, responded more strongly to tone sequences than to white noise, suggesting a preference for sound sequences of changing frequency. The lateral surface of the superior temporal gyrus responded to words more than tones suggesting the emergence of some degree of speech specificity. Ventrolateral areas, primarily in left superior temporal sulcus, were unresponsive to noise, weakly responsive to the tones, but strongly responsive to the words, pseudowords and reversed speech. It remains to be determined whether this result originates in differences in acoustical, phonetic, or lexical processing. Other findings also suggest that, as analysis moves from

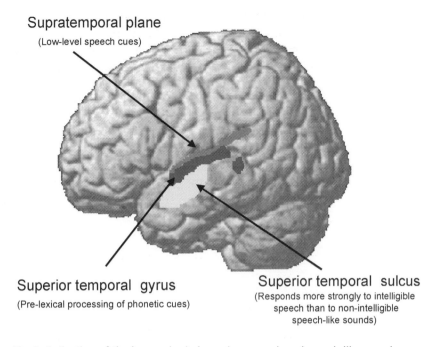

Supratemporal plane
(Low-level speech cues)

Superior temporal gyrus
(Pre-lexical processing of phonetic cues)

Superior temporal sulcus
(Responds more strongly to intelligible speech than to non-intelligible speech-like sounds)

Fig. 2 Activation of the human brain by various speech and speech-like sounds as determined by fMRI in a variety of studies. The primary auditory cortex in humans is on the transverse gyrus located on the supratemporal plane in the Sylvian fissure (from Palmer and Hall[50], with permission).

primary cortex across the superior temporal gyrus to the superior temporal sulcus, processing becomes more specific for speech[49]. Activation differences were measured with a variety of speech and speech-like sounds configured to have equivalent spectral and temporal complexity, but to vary in phonetic information and intelligibility. While the lateral surface of the superior temporal gyrus and posterior superior temporal sulcus were activated by all stimuli that contained perceptible phonetic features, regardless of intelligibility, the anterior part of the superior temporal sulcus was specifically activated only by intelligible stimuli.

A possible synthesis of these results is shown in Figure 2: speech processing involves distinct subsystems in the left temporal lobe that form a dorsal-ventral-anterior pathway. Low-level auditory cues are processed in primary and surrounding secondary auditory areas, while prelexical processing of phonetic cues and their sequencing may take place on the lateral surface of superior temporal gyrus. Activation by intelligible speech occurs in the anterior superior temporal sulcus which projects widely to other brain areas including the prefrontal cortex and medial temporal lobe.

References

1 Merzenich MM, Roth GL, Andersen RA, Knight PL, Colwell SA. Some basic features of organisation of the central auditory nervous system. In: Evans EF, Wilson JP. (eds) *Psychophysics and Physiology of Hearing*. London: Academic Press, 1977; 485–97

2 Phillips DP, Orman SS, Musicant AD, Wilson GF. Neurons in the cat's primary auditory-cortex distinguished by their responses to tones and wide-spectrum noise. *Hear Res* 1985; **18**: 73–86

3 Ehret G. The auditory cortex. *J Comp Physiol A-Sens Neural Behav Physiol* 1997; **181**: 547–57

4 Howard MA, Volkov IO, Abbas PJ, Damasio H, Ollendieck MC, Granner MA. A chronic microelectrode investigation of the tonotopic organization of human auditory cortex. *Brain Res* 1996; **724**: 260–4

5 Lutkenhoner B, Steinstrater O. High-precision neuromagnetic study of the functional organization of the human auditory cortex. *Audiol Neuro-Otol* 1998; **3**: 191–213

6 Talavage TM, Ledden PJ, Benson RR, Rosen BR, Melcher JR. Frequency-dependent responses exhibited by multiple regions in human auditory cortex. *Hear Res* 2000; **150**: 225–44

7 Schwarz DWF, Tomlinson RWW. Spectral response patterns of auditory-cortex neurons to harmonic complex tones in alert monkey (*Macaca mulatta*). *J Neurophysiol* 1990; **64**: 282–98

8 Schulze H, Langner G. Auditory cortical responses to amplitude modulations with spectra above frequency receptive fields: evidence for wide spectral integration. *J Comp Physiol A-Sens Neural Behav Physiol* 1999; **185**: 493–508

9 Griffiths TD, Buchel C, Frackowiak RSJ, Patterson RD. Analysis of temporal structure in sound by the human brain. *Nat Neurosci* 1998; **1**: 422–7

10 Griffiths TD, Uppenkamp S, Johnsrude I, Josephs O. Encoding of the temporal regularity of sound in the human brainstem. *Nat Neurosci* 2001; **4**: 633–7

11 Palmer AR. Neural signal processing. In: Moore BCJ. (ed) *Hearing*. San Diego: Academic Press, 1995; 75 121

12 Pfingst BE, O'Connor TA. Characteristics of neurons in auditory-cortex of monkeys performing a simple auditory task. *J Neurophysiol* 1981; **45**: 16–34

13 Pantev C, Hoke M, Lehnertz K, Lutkenhoner B. Neuromagnetic evidence of an amplitopic organization of the human auditory-cortex. *Electroencephalogr Clin Neurophysiol* 1989; **72**: 225–31

14 Lockwood AH, Salvi RJ, Coad ML *et al*. The functional anatomy of the normal human auditory system: Responses to 0.5 and 4.0 kHz tones at varied intensities. *Cereb Cortex* 1999; **9**: 65–76

15 Mohr CM, King WM, Freeman AJ, Briggs RW, Leonard CM. Influence of speech stimuli intensity on the activation of auditory cortex investigated with functional magnetic resonance imaging. *J Acoust Soc Am* 1999; **105**: 2738–45

16 Strainer JC, Ulmer JL, Yetkin FZ, Haughton VM, Daniels DL, Millen SJ. Functional MR of the primary auditory cortex: An analysis of pure tone activation and tone discrimination. *Am J Neuroradiol* 1997; **18**: 601–10

17 Jänke L, Shah NJ, Posse S, Grosse-Ryuken M, Müller-Gärtner H-W. Intensity coding of auditory stimuli: an fMRI study. *Neuropsychologica* 1998; **36**: 875–83

18 Hart HC, Hall D, Palmer AR. Growth of activation in Heschl's gyrus with increasing level of low and high frequency tones. *25th Midwinter Meeting of the Association for Research in Otolaryngology*. St Petersburgh Beach, FL: 2002; S1238

19 Phillips DP, Semple MN, Calford MB, Kitzes LM. Level-dependent representation of stimulus frequency in cat primary auditory-cortex. *Exp Brain Res* 1994; **102**: 210–26

20 Rayleigh L. On our perception of sound direction. *Philos Mag* 1907; **13**: 214–32

21 Jenkins WM, Merzenich MM. Role of cat primary auditory-cortex for sound-localization behavior. *J Neurophysiol* 1984; **52**: 819–47

22 Zatorre RJ, Penhune VB. Spatial localization after excision of human auditory cortex. *J Neurosci* 2001; **21**: 6321–8

23 Young ED. Circuitry and function of the dorsal cochlear nucleus. In: Oertel D, Popper AN, Fay RR. (eds) *Integrative Functions in the Mammalian Auditory Pathway*. New York: Springer, 2001

24 Jeffress LA. A place theory of sound localization. *J Comp Physiol Psychol* 1948; **61**: 468–86

25 Spitzer MW, Semple MN. Transformation of binaural response properties in the ascending auditory pathway: Influence of time-varying interaural phase disparity. *J Neurophysiol* 1998; **80**: 3062–76

26 Weeks RA, Aziz-Sultan A, Bushara KO *et al*. A PET study of human auditory spatial processing. *Neurosci Lett* 1999; **262**: 155–8

27 Griffiths TD, Rees G, Rees A *et al*. Right parietal cortex is involved in the perception of sound movement in humans. *Nat Neurosci* 1998; **1**: 74–9

28 Baumgart F, Gaschler-Markefski B, Woldorff MG, Heinze HJ, Scheich H. A movement-sensitive area in auditory cortex. *Nature* 1999; **400**: 724–6

29 Joris PX, Yin TCT. Responses to amplitude-modulated tones in the auditory nerve of the cat. *J Acoust Soc Am* 1992; **91**: 215–32

30 Giraud AL, Lorenzi C, Ashburner J *et al*. Representation of the temporal envelope of sounds in the human brain. *J Neurophysiol* 2000; **84**: 1588–98

31 Harms M, Melcher J. Time courses of fMRI signals in the inferior colliculus, medial geniculate body, and auditory cortex show different dependencies on noise burst rate. *Neuroimage* 1999; **7**: S847

32 Schreiner CE, Langner G. Periodicity coding in the inferior colliculus of the cat. 2. Topographical organization. *J Neurophysiol* 1988; **60**: 1823–40

33 Schulze H, Langner G. Periodicity coding in the primary auditory cortex of the Mongolian gerbil (*Meriones unguiculatus*): two different coding strategies for pitch and rhythm? *J Comp Physiol A-Sens Neural Behav Physiol* 1997; **181**: 651–63

34 Krishna BS, Semple MN. Auditory temporal processing: responses to sinusoidally amplitude-modulated tones in the inferior colliculus. *J Neurophysiol* 2000; **84**: 255–73

35 Langner G, Sams M, Heil P, Schulze H. Frequency and periodicity are represented in orthogonal maps in the human auditory cortex: evidence from magnetoencephalography. *J Comp Physiol A-Sens Neural Behav Physiol* 1997; **181**: 665–76

36 Thivard L, Belin P, Zilbovicius M, Poline JB, Samson Y. A cortical region sensitive to auditory spectral motion. *Neuroreport* 2000; **11**: 2969–72

37 Hall DA, Johnsrude IS, Haggard MP, Palmer AR, Akeroyd MA, Summerfield AQ. Spectral and temporal processing in human auditory cortex. *Cereb Cortex* 2002; **12**: 140–9

38 Mirz F, Ovesen T, Ishizu K *et al*. Stimulus-dependent central processing of auditory stimuli – a PET study. *Scand Audiol* 1999; **28**: 161–9

39 Versnel H, Shamma SA. Spectral-ripple representation of steady-state vowels in primary auditory cortex. *J Acoust Soc Am* 1998; **103**: 2502–14

40 Wang XQ. On cortical coding of vocal communication sounds in primates. *Proc Natl Acad Sci USA* 2000; **97**: 11843–9

41 Rauschecker JP. Parallel processing in the auditory cortex of primates. *Audiol Neuro-Otol* 1998; **3**: 86–103

42 Rauschecker JP. Parallel processing in the auditory cortex of human and nonhuman primates. *Eur J Neurosci* 2000; **12**: 450–

43 Rauschecker JP, Tian B. Mechanisms and streams for processing of 'what' and 'where' in auditory cortex. *Proc Natl Acad Sci USA* 2000; **97**: 11800–6

44 Clarke S, Maeder P, Meuli R *et al*. What and where in human audition: distinct cortical processing pathways revealed by fMRI. *Eur J Neurosci* 2000; **12**: 129–

45 Bellmann A, Clarke S, Adriani M *et al*. What and where in audition: selective deficits following circumscribed hemispheric lesion. *Eur J Neurosci* 2000; **12**: 495–

46 Belin P, Zatorre RJ. 'What', 'where' and 'how' in auditory cortex. *Nat Neurosci* 2000; **3**: 965–6

47 Liégeois-Chauvel C, de Graaf JB, Laguitton V, Chauvel P. Specialization of left auditory cortex for speech perception in man depends on temporal coding. *Cereb Cortex* 1999; **9**: 484–96

48 Binder JR, Frost JA, Hammeke TA, Rao SM, Cox RW. Function of the left planum temporale in auditory and linguistic processing. *Brain* 1996; **119**: 1239–47

49 Scott SK, Blank CC, Rosen S, Wise RJS. Identification of a pathway for intelligible speech in the left temporal lobe. *Brain* 2000; **123**: 2400–6

50 Palmer AR, Hall D. *Open University Reader*, 2002; In press

Central auditory pathologies

Timothy D Griffiths

Newcastle University Medical School, Newcastle-upon-Tyne, UK

This chapter considers specific deficits in auditory processing ('negative' disorders) due to neurological conditions and 'positive' disorders of central auditory processing caused by abnormal activity in central auditory mechanisms. Recent work focuses on the assessment of auditory processing in disorders that are not specifically auditory. In this case, auditory measurement may provide a 'window' into the condition.

This chapter considers disorders of central auditory processing. These are disorders in the processing of sound after the transduction of the sound into neural activity in the cochlea. Such processing involves the characterisation of auditory patterns in frequency or time that are used to identify and localise sound objects. I restrict the term central auditory disorder to deficits in the processing of auditory pattern before the patterns acquire labels or schemata[1]. The attribution of labels after central auditory processing constitutes semantic processing.

The definition of disorders of central auditory processing is broad and can involve a number of brain mechanisms in the ascending auditory pathway and cortex. The initial processing of spectral and temporal patterns occurs in the cochlear nuclei at the ponto-medullary junction, whilst the initial processing of binaural cues for spatial analysis occurs in the superior olives in the pons. On the other hand, processing mechanisms for higher-order patterns in sound occur well beyond the primary auditory cortex located in medial Heschl's gyrus in the superior temporal plane[2]. Such widely distributed processing mechanisms can be affected by a number of brain processes.

In this chapter, I will describe a clinical approach to the identification of central auditory pathology and describe types of pathology that can be identified using such an approach. The aim is to describe approaches that help diagnosis in typical clinical settings, rather than detailed assessments that are most appropriate for the cognitive neuropsychological studies in the case literature. The initial consideration of methodology concentrates on techniques that are widely available and appropriate for a routine clinical setting. Some research techniques that might in future prove useful in routine clinical practice are also highlighted. This methodological description will also allow readers to consider the thoroughness of assessments used in the case literature.

Correspondence to:
Dr Timothy D. Griffiths,
Reader in Cognitive
Neurology, Newcastle
University Medical
School, Framlington
Place, Newcastle-upon-
Tyne NE2 4HH, UK

Clinical assessment of central auditory disorders

The various techniques used in the clinical assessment of central auditory disorders are summarised an Table 1.

History and examination

As with any neurological disorder, the most important aspect of the assessment of central auditory pathologies is a careful history to determine the nature of the disorder. This allows further assessment to be 'tailored' to an individual patient, which is important in view of the extensive battery of tests that would be needed to 'screen' patients blindly for these disorders. The suggestions here are based on an intuitive approach, and might in future be systematised into structured questionnaires for which the predictive value of different questions could be formally assessed. This would have the added advantage of standardising the clinical approach to a group of disorders that are seen in a number of different specialties (neurology, otolaryngology, speech and language therapy, and audiology). An important aspect of the history is the assessment of any features that might be associated with cochlear or vestibular disorder: difficulty hearing, tinnitus, vertigo, or features of recruitment. Specific deficits in hearing particular classes of sound (speech, music, and environmental sounds) or particular sound attributes (such as location) should also be sought and can often be helpful in pointing towards a particular psycho-acoustic deficit. For example, one subject with particular difficulty in recognising tunes

Table 1 Clinical assessment of central auditory disorders

History/clinical examination	Essential to guide appropriate investigation
Audiometry	Pure tone audiometry essential
EEG	May be helpful in children to exclude Landau Kleffner syndrome (when sleep EEG needed): not routinely indicated in adults
Evoked potentials	Brain stem responses to click helpful to define lesions in ascending auditory pathway. Mismatched negativity responses and modulation responses not routinely indicated
Psycho-acoustic assessment	Should be guided by history and clinical examination. There is no standard form of assessment appropriate to all central auditory disorders
Structural imaging	High quality structural imaging essential for the adequate characterisation of central disorders
Functional imaging	No routine indication at present

where these had a high tempo was demonstrated to have a deficit in the perception of sound sequences with a high tempo[3]. He had a posterior right hemisphere lesion. Another patient with a pontine vascular lesion[4] reported particular difficulty in sound localisation. That patient was found to have a deficit in the detection of interaural phase and intensity cues. This is consistent with the lesion involving the trapezoid body, preventing comparison of the input to the two ears at the superior olives. In both of these examples, the appropriate psychophysical tests were suggested by the history. Neurological examination is also essential in patients with central neurological disorder. This is the case even if high-resolution structural scanning is available, as this might miss small vascular or inflammatory lesions.

Audiometry

Audiometry is a critical part of the assessment of patients with suspected central auditory pathology. Pure-tone audiometry is essential. In subjects with hearing disorders, the presence of normal pure-tone audiometry makes the diagnosis of a central auditory disorder more likely. However, abnormal audiometry is not an exclusion criterion for central auditory pathology, and normal audiometry alone is not a guarantee that a subtle cochlear deficit is not present. Firstly, it is possible for a degree of cochlear or central deafness to co-exist with other disorders, such as auditory agnosia[5]. Secondly, deafness can be a feature of central auditory disorder in its own right (see below). A number of reports describe evolution of central deafness into auditory agnosia[5]. Finally, normal audiometry does not guarantee that there is no cochlear deficit, as it is theoretically possible to have an outer hair cell disorder that could produce deficits in frequency discrimination in the presence of normal pure-tone audiometry. The detection of such deficits requires psychophysical assessment of auditory filter width using a method such as notched noise[6,7]. Such techniques have been used in research studies of clinical populations[8], but are not routinely used in most audiology departments.

EEG and evoked potentials

EEG recording is important in the evaluation of children with acquired disorders of complex sound perception and language to exclude the rare condition of Landau Kleffner syndrome (acquired epileptic aphasia)[9]. EEG abnormalities in this condition may be subtle, in that they may be present only during sleep, when continuous spike and slow wave activity can occur. In general, however, there is no specific indication for EEG in the routine evaluation of central auditory disorders in adults. EEG-evoked potentials in response to sound[10] are useful for the evaluation of the level of the system at which the abnormality occurs. Auditory brain stem responses to clicks can provide a measure to corroborate the presence or absence of cochlear hearing loss, when there will be an alteration in waves I–V. The amplitude of wave V can be used as a measure of threshold in cases of cochlear hearing loss. Dissociation between the early brain stem responses and the middle latency responses to clicks can allow identification of the site of central pathology. The earliest middle latency responses arise from primary auditory cortex in the medial part of Heschl's gyrus[11,12]. This response may be absent in patients with central deafness, when the brain stem responses will be preserved. Pre-attentive and attentive responses to acoustic 'oddball' stimuli (the mismatched negativity or MMN, and P300 responses, respectively) have also been extensively investigated in clinical conditions. These responses may in future prove to be useful indicators of specific brain activity at and beyond the auditory cortex. The pre-attentive component may in future prove to be the most useful as this does not require the subject to carry out any task. For example, recent studies suggest that the presence of the MMN predicts a better functional outcome from coma[13,14]. However, the MMN response can be difficult to obtain even in normal, conscious individuals; the general usefulness of this technique remains to be proven if consistent results are only obtainable in laboratories with specific expertise. Other measures of central auditory processing that may prove to be useful are responses to modulated sound. Stefanatos et al[15] described a specific deficit in responses to frequency-modulated sound in children with receptive language disorder.

Psycho-acoustic assessment

Psycho-acoustic evaluation of subjects with central auditory disorders can allow demonstration of deficits that may be related to the symptoms from which the patients suffer. The presence of deficits in acoustic processing in patients with acquired aphasia due to left hemisphere lesions was first suggested nearly 40 years ago[16]. That work assessed judgements of the temporal order of two tones at different rates of presentation. Subsequent work has assessed temporal order judgement in developmental disorders including dyslexia and specific language impairment (see Bishop[17] for a review). Recent work has addressed the presence of deficits in modulation processing in developmental and acquired disorders[18,19].

There are a number of practical and theoretical problems with the psycho-acoustic evaluation of subjects with central neurological conditions. The major practical limitation in clinical practice, more than in a research setting, is the amount of time available for testing. Many psycho-acoustic procedures require hundreds of responses to achieve reliable parameters, and were developed using paid volunteers or undergraduates. This will not be appropriate for, say, a 50-year-old subject who has recently had a stroke. This also raises the issue of the appropriate control data to use. Published data based on highly trained young observers may not be appropriate and the use of control data from age-matched controls who are have undergone a similar amount of training are ideal. The other important issue with respect to psychophysical measures is whether deficits that are demonstrated correspond to perceptual deficits or attentional deficits. This is a particular issue in subjects with lesions of the auditory cortices and beyond. With the now widely used and efficient adaptive tracking procedures, it is not possible to say as they yield a single measure for a given task – the threshold. An alternative approach is to use full psychometric functions where the performance at different stimulus levels is estimated. This allows determination of both threshold and whether the subject reaches ceiling performance at **any** stimulus level; this does not occur if the subject shows an attentional deficit. The measurement of full psychometric functions allows a measure of attentional lapses (reflected by the slope[20,21]). However, this technique is very time-consuming and, therefore, limited for realistic studies of neurological patients.

A battery of psycho-acoustic tasks for the evaluation of neurological patients has been released recently[22]. The principal purpose of this battery is to provide a tool for research studies of clinical populations where a psycho-acoustic deficit is predicted, but some of the measures may in future prove to be useful in more routine clinical settings. Full psychometric functions are used for all of the tests. The battery systematically assesses temporal processing by measuring thresholds for the perception of the pitch of regular interval sound[23], amplitude and frequency modulation processing at different rates, and gap detection[24]. Binaural processing is also assessed by the measurement of thresholds for the detection of fixed and dynamic interaural amplitude and phase change of a narrow band carrier.

Structural imaging

Structural imaging is essential in the assessment of subjects with suspected disorders of central auditory processing. The history, clinical evaluation and acoustic tests will yield a description of the phenomenology and hypotheses about its cause that can be tested by the use of structural imaging. Vascular and inflammatory lesions are best demonstrated by specific magnetic resonance images (high resolution T2 and proton density weighted) and the sensitivity may be further increased by the use of gadolinium contrast. Such imaging may be particularly helpful in the evaluation of brain stem lesions to which computerised tomography radiographs are not sensitive. Even the most sensitive MRI may miss small lesions, however.

Functional imaging

Since the first auditory studies in the late 1980s using positron emission tomography (PET), and in the early 1990s using functional MRI (fMRI), there has been a huge increase in our knowledge and understanding of normal human central sound processing. These techniques measure responses related to the brain blood flow following acoustic stimulation. Studies of patients with certain central auditory disorders have been carried out for research purposes to characterise better the conditions[25-27]. At the present time, these techniques are not suitable for the routine investigation of central auditory disorders.

Types of specific central auditory disorder

Various types of specific central auditory disorder are summarised in Table 2.

Brain stem disorders

Specific disorders of auditory processing (*i.e.* deficits that occur in the absence of other perceptual or cognitive disorders) are unusual. This is

Table 2 Various types of specific central auditory disorder

Brainstem disorders (unusual)	
Deafness	Very unusual result of brain stem lesion
Temporal-cue detection deficit	Can occur in multiple sclerosis
Binaural-cue detection deficit	Can occur in multiple sclerosis and vascular conditions
Higher-level disorders	
Central deafness	Requires bilateral lesions of cerebrum. The older term 'cortical deafness' may be incorrect as the causative lesion may be in auditory radiation. May evolve into auditory agnosia
Auditory agnosia	Abnormal perception of complex sound in the presence of preserved hearing. Often, but not always, associated with bilateral lesions in region of superior temporal lobe
Auditory agnosia 1: (pure) word deafness	Inability to perceive oral words
Auditory agnosia 2: amusia	Deficit in musical perception
Auditory agnosia 3: environmental sound agnosia	Deficit in the perception of environmental sounds

particularly so in the case of conditions affecting the brain stem. Here, the auditory pathway is closely related to key motor and sensory tracts and nuclei, and the incomplete decussation of the auditory pathway means that the ascending auditory tracts (the lateral lemnisci) transmit information from both ears. It follows from this that many hearing disorders can only be produced by bilateral lesions of the brain stem, which would usually be expected to produce striking neurological features in addition.

Deafness due to disorders of the brain stem is unusual, but has been described due to a vascular lesion[28] and is described as occurring in multiple sclerosis (MS). Most neurologists, however, would be very reluctant to ascribe deafness to MS, and would search hard for another cause in patients with this disorder.

The brain stem is the first point of convergence of the input from the two ears, with important points of convergence occurring at the superior olives (in the pons) and between the two inferior colliculi (in the midbrain). These points of convergence allow binaural processing, the comparison of the phase and intensity of sounds presented to the two ears. A derangement of such processing can occur in MS[29–31] and vascular lesions[4]. In the case of MS, the lesions demonstrated by MRI in these patients and associated deficits in brain stem-evoked potentials make it likely that the disease in the brain stem is causal. Many of these patients had psychophysical deficits that were not symptomatic.

Temporal processing deficits are described in MS as well. Early studies suggested deficits in the perception of frequency modulation and formant frequency changes in synthetic speech[32,33]. It would seem plausible that such deficits might occur as a result of involvement of mechanisms for modulation processing in the ascending pathway in brain stem. Such mechanisms are well described in animal models (see, for example, Rees and Moller[34]). Other studies have demonstrated deficits in the detection of temporal gaps in noise in MS[35,36]. The gap detection studies cannot be interpreted unequivocally in terms of brain stem versus cerebral involvement.

Higher-level disorders

Deafness can also occur in lesions of the cerebrum[37–41] and there is a long-standing debate as to whether should be called 'cortical deafness' to parallel the better-established cortical blindness. The disorder is always associated with bilateral lesions (usually vascular, see Griffiths *et al*[5] for detailed description of individual cases in terms of hearing loss, evoked potentials, and lesion). The idea has been controversial, firstly because of debate as to whether the disorder might represent a disorder of auditory perception or attention. Many of the patients show an initial profound hearing loss with recovery, which parallels the effect of cortical lesions in the macaque[42] but not lower mammals[43]. For human subjects, variability in the audiograms of affected individuals[40] is consistent with a variable attentional component to the condition, but there is always a degree of deafness after this is taken into account. A second source of controversy has been whether the condition is a truly cortical disorder. Tanaka *et al*[40] described two cases with partial sparing of Heschl's gyrus (containing the primary auditory cortex in its medial part) on one or both sides. This suggests the possible importance of projections to the auditory cortex rather than lesions of the cortex itself. For this reason, I have proposed the term central deafness for this condition[5].

Auditory agnosia is a condition where there is impaired perception of complex sounds with preservation of the pure tone audiogram[3,25,39,44–66]. The disorder can evolve from central deafness, and is also associated with bilateral lesions of the superior temporal lobes, although cases in association with unilateral lesions are described. Three different forms of auditory agnosia have been described: for words (word deafness), music (amusia) and environmental sounds (environmental-sound agnosia). There is often overlap between the three forms, and I have argued on the basis of this that the disorder can be characterised as an apperceptive disorder[5]. This term is used in the sense of an inability to perceive particular patterns in sound, in distinction to the attribution of meaning to those sounds after initial pattern processing. Common deficits in the analysis of particular stimulus features might on this basis be manifest with a number of different sorts of sound. For example, the slow changes in pitch, intensity and timing of musical sounds have a parallel in prosody or the 'melody of language'[67]. There is a well-established association between amusia and deficits in prosodic perception, even in cases where language function is otherwise spared. This is consistent with a common deficit in the perception these two sound patterns characterised by features that change at similar rate. Consistent with this, psycho-acoustic studies of one subject with amusia[19] demonstrated a profound deficit in amplitude and frequency modulation perception, that was particularly marked at low modulation rates, corresponding to slow temporal changes. Interestingly, the same subject was still able to detect the emotion in music despite an almost total loss of musical recognition[60,68]. It is important to stress that this account of apperceptive agnosia does not exclude the existence of associative forms of auditory agnosia, where the spectrotemporal patterns corresponding to an acoustic object are analysed normally but the association of those patterns with semantic labels or schema[1] is lost. Recent functional imaging work[69] suggests the possibility that the planum temporale, the part of the superior temporal plane behind Heschl's gyrus, may be an important locus for such association.

Recent studies of congenital auditory agnosia

There are reports of subjects with 'tune deafness' or 'tone deafness' going back a century in the absence of any known neurological insult. This disorder may represent a developmental form of amusia, although there are clear differences, such as the absence of any associated deficit in the detection of prosody in speech. The disorder has just been just been systematically described for the first time[70–72]. Striking deficits in the perception of music were demonstrated in subjects otherwise considered 'normal' using the battery of tasks originally developed by Peretz for the characterisation of acquired amusia. Further studies are needed to show how common this disorder is in the population, at what level the deficit lies, and what brain structural and functional brain deficits can be demonstrated. The striking pitch difference limens found (greater than four semitones in one subject[72]) suggests that this is a central rather than a cochlear disorder. In the converse situation, where subjects have good musical skills, interesting brain correlates have been described such as greater structural asymmetry in the planum temporale associated with absolute pitch[73]. It will be interesting to see if anatomical and functional correlates exist at this level.

'Positive' disorders of central auditory processing

Tinnitus may be associated with abnormal activity in the ascending auditory system or auditory cortex. Using PET, Lockwood and colleagues studied patients with tinnitus evoked by facial or eye movements[27,74], a condition that allows subjects to 'switch' the tinnitus on and off to allow demonstration of activity associated with the percept. Gaze-evoked tinnitus was originally thought to be rare, even amongst patients with eighth nerve section for acoustic neuroma, but turned out to be common in this particular group. Unilateral activation of the auditory cortex or auditory pons without auditory input was been demonstrated in these subjects. This pattern would not be seen with actual auditory input even to one ear, due to the incomplete decussation of the auditory pathway. Lockwood has argued that central tinnitus associated with abnormal activity of the auditory cortex or pons might be likened to the phenomenon of alien limb in amputees. A recent fMRI study[75] has examined the basis for tinnitus in more typical tinnitus patients who had not undergone surgery. The use of subjects with normal hearing and lateralised tinnitus simplified the interpretation. Indirect inference about abnormal activity in the inferior colliculus was made on the basis of less increase in activity with sound stimulation. This effect might be due either to masking of abnormal central activity by external sound or saturation effects when the effect of central activity and external stimulation is combined. In either case, the results support abnormal activity in the central pathway in this more common form of tinnitus.

Musical hallucinations need to be distinguished from tinnitus, but also appear to be due to abnormal central auditory activity[26]. This disorder may occur in subjects who are in middle-to-later life with moderate-to-profound hearing loss. More rarely, the condition can also occur due to central lesions, epilepsy or psychosis. In the common form, subjects typically experience melodies that were previously familiar and it can be argued on the basis of the phenomenology that the condition is due to the inappropriate activity of a normal mechanism for musical perception and imagery. Supporting this, functional imaging demonstrated a network of brain areas where activation increased with severity of the hallucination. This network was similar to that shown in normal hearing subjects actually listening to sound sequences. This bilateral network includes the planum temporale and frontal operculum.

Auditory processing in disorders that are not specific auditory disorders

Many of the specific disorders with localised pathologies, as described above, are rare. There has been considerable recent interest in assessing central auditory processing in neurological conditions that are not restricted to audition, as a 'window' into the condition. In coma due to a variety of causes, EEG-evoked potential studies suggest that the early brain stem responses to click are often preserved, but that their absence correlates with poor survival[76-79]. Recent studies mentioned above have shown that the presence of MMN can correlate with a good prognosis at the level of functional outcome. Whilst any conclusion about unique predictive power for auditory tests would be premature, the results to date (and reasoning based on the distributed nature of many auditory cortical processes) suggests a useful application of auditory testing in the intensive care ward.

A PET study of five patients in vegetative state due to diffuse hypoxia has shown activation in primary auditory cortex in the region of Heschl's gyrus and in the planum temporale in response to click stimuli, despite decreases in resting metabolism[80]. These activations occur in a similar region to that demonstrated in normal controls in the same experiment, and in MEG studies of normal click response[11]. Less activation in response to clicks was observed in more posterior cortex in the temporoparietal junction in patients compared to controls, and an analysis of functional connectivity showed a functional disconnection between the posterior superior temporal lobe and the inferior parietal lobule, anterior cingulate and hippocampus. This suggests a deficit in connections beyond the auditory cortices in these patients.

Conclusions

Increasingly, systematic assessment of specific deficits in central auditory processing has led to greater understanding of their psycho-acoustic and anatomical basis. Recent work has characterised a developmental form of auditory agnosia, and re-organisation and aberrant activity within the central auditory system is becoming increasingly recognised as a cause of pathology. The use of sound stimuli to probe the unconscious brain is a developing area, with the potential to define distributed brain mechanisms relevant to functional outcome from coma and vegetative state. Auditory stimuli have the potential to probe the integrative function of the brain needed for normal conscious functioning and a challenge for the future is to develop auditory stimuli and techniques that can probe this integrative function in routine clinical settings.

References

1 Bregman AS. *Auditory Scene Analysis*. Cambridge, MA: MIT Press, 1990

2 Morosan P, Rademacher J, Schleicher A, Amunts K, Schormann T, Zilles K. Human primary auditory cortex: cytoarchitechtonic subdivisions and mapping into a spatial reference system. *Neuroimage* 2001; **13**: 684–701

3 Griffiths TD, Rees A, Witton C, Cross PM, Shakir RA, Green GGR. Spatial and temporal auditory processing deficits following right hemisphere infarction. A psychophysical study. *Brain* 1997; **120**: 785–94

4 Griffiths TD, Bates D, Rees A, Witton C, Gholkar A, Green GGR. Sound movement detection deficit due to a brainstem lesion. *J Neurol Neurosurg Psychiatry* 1997; **62**: 522–6

5 Griffiths TD, Rees A, Green GGR. Disorders of human complex sound processing. *Neurocase* 1999; **5**: 365–78

6 Patterson RD, Moore BCJ. Auditory filters and excitation patterns as representations of frequency resolution. In: Moore BCJ. (ed) *Frequency Selectivity in Hearing*. London: Academic Press, 1986

7 Hartmann WM. *Signals, Sound, and Sensation*. New York, NY: AIP Press, 1997

8 Chinnery PF, Elliott C, Green GR *et al*. The spectrum of hearing loss due to mitochondrial DNA defects. *Brain* 2000; **123**: 82–92

9 Landau WM, Kleffner FR. Syndrome of acquired aphasia with convulsive disorder in children. *Neurology* 1957; **7**: 523–30

10 Abramovich SJ. *Electric Response Audiometry in Clinical Practice*. Edinburgh: Churchill Livingstone, 1990

11 Yvert B, Crouzeix A, Bertrand O, Seither-Preisler A, Pantev C. Multiple supratemporal sources of magnetic and electric auditory evoked middle latency components in humans. *Cereb Cortex* 2001; **11**: 411–23

12 Liegeois-Chauvel C, Musolino A, Chauvel P. Localisation to the primary auditory area in man. *Brain* 1991; **114**: 139–53

13 Kane NM, Butler SR, Simpson T. Coma outcome prediction using event related potentials: P3 and mismatch negativity. *Audiol Neuro-otol* 2000; **5**: 186–91

14 Fischer C, Morlet D, Giard M-H. Mismatch negativity and N100 in comatose patients. *Audiol Neuro-otol* 2000; **5**: 192–7

15 Stefanatos GA, Green GGR, Ratcliff GG. Neurophysiological evidence of auditory channel anomalies in developmental dysphasia. *Arch Neurol* 1989; **46**: 871–5

16 Efron R. Temporal perception, aphasia, and *deja vu*. *Brain* 1963; **86**: 403–24

17 Bishop DVM. *Uncommon Understanding*. Hove: Psychology Press, 1997

18 Talcott JB, Witton C, McLean MF *et al.* Dynamic sensory sensitivity and children's word decoding skills. *Proc Natl Acad Sci USA* 2000; **97**: 2952–7

19 Griffiths TD, Penhune V, Peretz I, Dean JL, Patterson RD, Green GGR. Frontal processing and auditory perception. *Neuroreport* 2000; **11**: 919-22

20 Wichmann FA, Hill NJ. The psychometric function: I. Fitting, sampling, and goodness of fit. *Percept Psychophys* 2001; **63**: 1293–313

21 Wichmann FA, Hill NJ. The psychometric function: II. Bootstrap-based confidence intervals and sampling. *Percept Psychophys* 2001; **63**: 1314–29

22 Griffiths TD, Dean JL, Woods W, Rees A, Green GGR. The Newcastle Auditory Battery (NAB): a temporal and spatial test battery for use on individual naïve subjects. *Hear Res* 2001; **154**: 165–9

23 Yost WA, Patterson R, Sheft S. A time domain description for the pitch strength of iterated rippled noise. *J Acoust Soc Am* 1996; **99**: 1066–78

24 Phillips DP, Taylor TL, Hall SE, Carr MM, Mossop JE. Detection of silent intervals between noises activating different perceptual channels: some properties of 'central' auditory gap detection. *J Acoust Soc Am* 1997; **101**: 3694–705

25 Engelien A, Silbersweig D, Stern E *et al.* The functional anatomy of recovery from auditory agnosia. A PET study of sound categorisation in a neurological patient and normal controls. *Brain* 1995; **118**: 1395–409

26 Griffiths TD. Musical hallucinosis in acquired deafness. Phenomenology and brain substrate. *Brain* 2000; **123**: 2065–76

27 Lockwood AH, Wack DS, Burkard RF *et al.* The functional anatomy of gaze-evoked tinnitus and sustained lateral gaze. *Neurology* 2001; **56**: 472–80

28 Egan CA, Davies L, Halmagyi GM. Bilateral total deafness due to pontine haematoma. *J Neurol Neurosurg Psychiatry* 1996; **61**: 628–31

29 Van der Poel JC, Jones SJ, Miller DH. Sound lateralisation, brainstem auditory evoked potentials and magnetic resonance imaging in multiple sclerosis. *Brain* 1988; **111**: 1453–74

30 Furst M, Levine RA, Korczyn AD, Fullerton BC, Tadmore R, Algom D. Brainstem lesions and click lateralisation in patients with multiple sclerosis. *Hear Res* 1995; **82**: 109–24

31 Griffiths TD, Elliott C, Coulthard A, Cartlidge NEF, Green GGR. A distinct low-level mechanism for interaural timing analysis in human hearing. *Neuroreport* 1998; **9**: 3383–6

32 Quine DB, Regan D, Murray TJ. Degraded discrimination between speech-like sounds by patient's with multiple sclerosis and Friedreich's ataxia. *Brain* 1984; **107**: 1113–22

33 Quine DB, Regan D, Beverly KI, Murray TJ. Patients with multiple sclerosis experience hearing loss for shifts of tone frequency. *Arch Neurol* 1984; **41**: 506–7

34 Rees A, Moller AR. Responses of neurons in the inferior colliculus of the rat to AM and FM tones. *Hear Res* 1983; **10**: 301–30

35 Hendler T, Squires WK, Emmerich DS. Psychophysical measures of central auditory dysfunction in multiple sclerosis: neurophysiological and neuroanatomical correlates. *Ear Hear* 1990; **11**: 403–16

36 Rappaport JM, Gulliver JM, Phillips DP, Van Dorpe RA, Maxner CE, Bhan V. Auditory temporal resolution in multiple sclerosis. *J Otolaryngol* 1994; **23**: 307–24

37 Bahls FH, Chatrian GE, Mesher RA, Sumi SM, Ruff RL. A case of persistent cortical deafness: clinical , neurophysiological and neuropathologic observations. *Neurology* 1988; **38**: 1490–3

38 Leicester J. Central deafness and subcortical motor aphasia. *Brain Lang* 1980; **10**: 224–42

39 Mendez MF, Geehan GR. Cortical auditory disorders: clinical and psychoacoustic features. *J Neurol Neurosurg Psychiatry* 1988; **51**: 1–9

40 Tanaka Y, Kamo T, Yoshida M, Yamadori A. 'So-called' cortical deafness. Clinical, neurophysiological and radiological observations. *Brain* 1991; **114**: 2385–401

41 Woods DL, Knight RT, Neville HJ. Bitemporal lesions dissociate auditory evoked potentials and perception. *EEG Clin Neurophysiol* 1984; **57**: 208–20

42 Heffner HE, Heffner RS. Effect of unilateral and bilateral auditory cortex lesions on the discrimination of vocalisations by Japanese macaques. *J Neurophysiol* 1986; **56**: 683–701

43 Neff WD, Diamond IT, Casseday JH. Behavioural studies of auditory discrimination: central nervous system. In: Keidel WD, Neff WD. (eds) *Handbook of Sensory Physiology*, vol 5. Berlin: Springer, 1975; 307–400

44 Auerbach SH, Allard T, Naeser M, Alexander MP, Albert ML. Pure word deafness. Analysis of a case with bilateral lesions at the prephonemic level. *Brain* 1982; **105**: 271–300

45 Buchman AS, Garron DC, Trost-Cardamone JE, Wichter MD, Schwartz M. Word deafness: a hundred years later. *J Neurol Neurosurg Psychiatry* 1986; **49**: 489–99

46 Buchtel HA, Stewart JD. Auditory agnosia: apperceptive or associative disorder? *Brain Lang* 1989; **37**: 12–25

47 Caramazza A, Berndt RS. The selective impairment of phonological processing: a case study. *Brain Lang* 1983; **18**: 128–74

48 Coslett HB, Brashear HR, Heilman KM. Pure word deafness after bilateral auditory cortex infarcts. *Neurology* 1984; **34**: 347–52

49 Eustache F, Lechevalier B, Viader F, Lambert J. Identification and discrimination disorders in auditory perception: a report on two cases. *Neuropsychologia* 1990; **28**: 257–70

50 Fujii T, Fukatsu R, Watabe S *et al*. Auditory sound agnosia without aphasia following a right temporal lobe lesion. *Cortex* 1990; **26**: 263–8

51 Godefroy O, Leys D, Furby A *et al*. Psychoacoustical deficits related to bilateral subcortical haemorrhages. A case with auditory agnosia. *Cortex* 1995; **31**: 149–59

52 Habib M, Daquin G, Milandre L *et al*. Mutism and auditory agnosia due to bilateral insular damage – role of the insula in human communication. *Neuropsychologia* 1995; **33**: 327–39

53 Lambert J, Eustache F, Lechevalier B, Rossa Y, Viader F. Auditory agnosia with relative sparing of speech perception. *Cortex* 1989; **25**: 71–82

54 Metz-Lutz M-N, Dahl E. Analysis of word comprehension in a case of pure word deafness. *Brain Lang* 1984; **23**: 13–25

55 Miceli G. The processing of speech sounds in a patient with cortical auditory disorder. *Neuropsychologia* 1982; **20**: 5–20

56 Motomura N, Yamadori A, Mori E. Auditory agnosia: analysis of a case with bilateral subcortical lesions. *Brain* 1986; **109**: 379–91

57 Oppenheimer DR, Newcombe F. Clinical and anatomical findings in a case of auditory agnosia. *Arch Neurol* 1978; **35**: 712–9

58 Peretz I, Kolinsky R, Tramo M *et al*. Functional dissociations following bilateral lesions of auditory cortex. *Brain* 1994; **117**: 1283–301

59 Peretz I, Belleville S, Fontaine F. Dissociations entre musique et langage apres atteint cerebrale; un nouveau cas d'amusie sans aphasie. *J Can Psychol Exp* 1997; **51**: 354–68

60 Peretz I, Gagnon L. Dissociation between recognition and emotion for melodies. *Neurocase* 1999; **5**: 21–30

61 Praamstra P, Hagoort P, Maassen B, Crul T. Word deafness and auditory cortical function. *Brain* 1991; **114**: 1197–225

62 Takahashi N, Kawamura M, Shinotou H, Hirayama K, Kaga K, Shindo M. Pure word deafness due to left hemisphere damage. *Cortex* 1992; **28**: 295–303

63 Tanaka Y, Yamadori A, Mori E. Pure word deafness following bilateral lesions. *Brain* 1987; **110**: 381–403

64 von Stockert TR. On the structure of word deafness and mechanisms underlying the fluctuations of disturbances of higher cortical functions. *Brain Lang* 1982; **16**: 133–46

65 Yaqub BA, Gascon GG, Al-Nosha M, Whitaker H. Pure word deafness (acquired verbal auditory agnosia) in an Arabic speaking patient. *Brain* 1988; **111**: 457–66

66 Gold M, Rojiani A, Murtaugh R. A 66-year-old woman with a rapidly progressing dementia and basal ganglia involvement. *J Neuroimaging* 1997; 7: 171–5

67 Monrad-Krohn GH. Dysprosody or altered 'melody of language'. *Brain* 1947; **70**: 405–15

68 Peretz I, Blood AJ, Penhune V, Zatorre R. Cortical deafness to dissonance. *Brain* 2001; **124**: 928–40

69 Griffiths TD, Warren JD. The planum temporale as a computational hub. *Trends Neurosci* 2002; **25**: 348-353

70 Peretz I. Brain specialization for music. New evidence from congenital amusia. *Ann NY Acad Sci* 2001; **930**: 153–65

71 Ayotte J, Peretz I, Hyde K. Congenital amusia. A group study of adults afflicted with a music-specific disorder. *Brain* 2002; **125**: 238–51

72 Peretz I, Ayotte J, Zatorre RJ *et al*. Congenital amusia: a disorder of fine-grained pitch discrimination. *Neuron* 2002; **33**: 185–91

73 Zatorre RJ, Perry DW, Beckett CA, Westbury CF, Evans AC. Functional anatomy of musical processing in listeners with absolute pitch and relative pitch. *Proc Natl Acad Sci USA* 1998; **95**: 3172–7

74 Lockwood AH, Salvi RJ, Coad ML, Towsley ML, Wack DS, Murphy BW. The functional neuroanatomy of tinnitus: evidence for limbic system links and neural plasticity. *Neurology* 1998; **50**: 114–20

75 Melcher JR, Sigalovsky IS, Guinan JJJ, Levine RA. Lateralized tinnitus studied with functional magnetic resonance imaging: abnormal inferior colliculus activation. *J Neurophysiol* 2000; **83**: 1058–72

76 Ganji S, Peters G, Frazier E. Somatosensory and brainstem auditory evoked potential studies in nontraumatic coma. *Clin Electroencephalogr* 1988; **19**: 55–67

77 Lutschg J, Pfenninger J, Ludin HP, Vassella F. Brain-stem auditory evoked potentials and early somatosensory evoked potentials in neurointensively treated comatose children. *Am J Dis Child* 1983; **137**: 421–6

78 Tsubokawa T, Nishimoto H, Yamamoto T, Kitamura M, Katayama Y, Moriyasu N. Assessment of brainstem damage by the auditory brainstem response in acute severe head injury. *J Neurol Neurosurg Psychiatry* 1980; **43**: 1005–11

79 Rosenberg C, Wogensen K, Starr A. Auditory brain-stem and middle- and long-latency evoked potentials in coma. *Arch Neurol* 1984; **41**: 835–8

80 Laureys S, Faymonville ME, Degueldre C *et al*. Auditory processing in the vegetative state. *Brain* 2000; **123**: 1589–601

Psychoacoustics of normal and impaired hearing

Brian C J Moore

Department of Experimental Psychology, University of Cambridge, Cambridge, UK

Recent developments in the field of psychoacoustics are presented, focusing on areas which have application in the diagnosis and understanding of impaired hearing. Cochlear hearing loss often results in a loss of the compressive non-linearity that operates in normal ears; this loss is probably the main cause of loudness recruitment. Forward masking can be used as a tool to assess the strength of cochlear compression in human listeners. Hearing impairment can sometimes be associated with complete loss of function of inner hair cells over a certain region of the cochlea, resulting in a 'dead region'. Two psychoacoustic methods for detecting dead regions and defining their limits are described. The implications of the results for fitting hearing aids are discussed. Finally, the effect of cochlear hearing loss on the perception of rapid sequences of sounds (stream segregation) is described.

This chapter presents a selective review of recent developments in the field of psychoacoustics. It focuses on areas which have application in the diagnosis and understanding of impaired hearing. It does not repeat topics covered in my earlier *British Medical Bulletin* review[1]. For more comprehensive coverage of the psychoacoustics of impaired hearing, the reader is referred to reviews elsewhere[2,3].

Using forward masking to assess cochlear compression

Recent physiological studies of the mechanics of the basilar membrane within the cochlea indicate that the response to sinusoidal tones can be highly compressive[4,5]. The compression can be quantified by plotting the magnitude of the response as a function of the magnitude of the input, giving an input–output function. A schematic example is given in Figure 1. The solid line shows what would be observed for a tone at the characteristic frequency (CF) of the place being studied (the CF is the frequency giving maximal response at that place for a low-level input). For mid-range sound levels, the output grows by only 2.5 dB for each 10-dB increase in input level, indicating compression. The function becomes

Correspondence to:
Prof. Brian C J Moore,
Department of
Experimental Psychology,
University of Cambridge,
Downing Street,
Cambridge CB2 3EB, UK

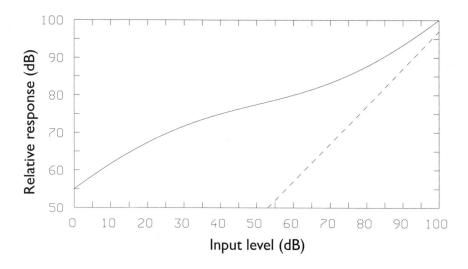

Fig. 1 The solid line shows a schematic illustration of an input–output function on the basilar membrane for a tone with frequency close to CF. The dashed line shows a linear input-output function. This is typical of what might be observed for a tone with frequency well below CF.

more linear (steeper) for very low and very high sound levels. The long-dashed line shows the type of function that would be observed for a tone with frequency well below CF. In this case, the response grows in a linear manner; each 10-dB increase in input level gives rise to a 10-dB increase in response.

The compression on the basilar membrane is believed to arise from the operation of an 'active' physiological mechanism which depends on the motile behaviour of the outer hair cells (see chapters by Ashmore and by Kemp in this volume). The compression is very fast-acting[6] and it allows the normal auditory system to operate over a wide range of sound levels, *i.e.* it provides the large dynamic range of about 120 dB. It also plays a role in many other aspects of auditory perception, including intensity discrimination, masking, loudness, and timbre perception[7]. Hearing loss is often caused by loss of function of the outer hair cells (see chapters by Forge & Wright and by Raphael in this volume). This leads to the loss of compression, which is probably the main cause of the reduced dynamic range and loudness recruitment that are typically associated with cochlear hearing loss[3,8].

Compression in the cochlea can be quantified in human listeners using forward masking. The listener is required to detect a brief signal presented just after the end of a masker that typically lasts 100–300 ms. It is assumed that the threshold for detecting the signal is monotonically related to the 'internal' effect produced by the masker at the place in the cochlea where the signal is detected. This place will have a CF close to the signal frequency. The advantage of forward masking is that the signal and the masker are separated in time, so the masker and the signal are processed independently on the basilar membrane, and non-linear interactions between them are minimal.

In forward masking, a given increment in masker level often does not produce an equal increment in amount of forward masking. For example, if the masker level is increased by 10 dB, the masked threshold may only increase by 3 dB[9,10]. This effect can be quantified by plotting the signal threshold (in dB) as a function of the masker level (in dB). The resulting function is called a growth-of-masking function. In simultaneous masking, such functions often have slopes close to one, when a broad-band noise masker is used. In forward masking, the slopes are usually less than one.

Oxenham and Moore[11] have suggested that the shallow slopes of the growth-of-masking functions can be explained in terms of the compressive input–output function of the basilar membrane. Such an input–output function is shown schematically in Figure 2. It has a shallow slope for medium input levels, but a steeper slope at very low input levels. Assume that, for a given time delay of the signal relative to the masker, the response evoked by the signal at threshold is directly proportional to the response evoked by the masker. Assume, as an example, that a masker with a level of 50 dB produces a signal threshold of 12 dB. Consider now what happens when the masker level is increased by 20 dB. The increase in masker level, denoted by ΔM in Figure 2, produces a relatively small

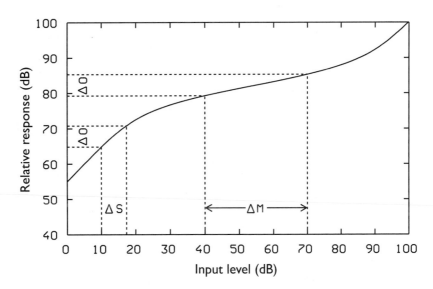

Fig. 2 The curve shows a schematic input-output function on the basilar membrane. When the masker is increased in level by ΔM, this produces an increase in response of ΔO. To restore signal threshold, the response to the signal also has to be increased by ΔO. This requires an increase in signal level, ΔS, which is markedly smaller than ΔM.

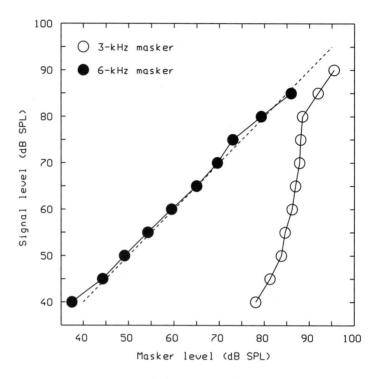

Fig. 3 Data from Oxenham and Plack[12] for normally hearing subjects. Thresholds for detecting a 6-kHz signal following a 3-kHz or 6-kHz masker are shown. The signal level was fixed, and the masker level was varied to determine the threshold. Symbols represent the mean thresholds of three normally hearing subjects. Error bars represent ± 1 SEM. They are omitted where they would be smaller than the relevant data point.

increase in response, ΔO. To restore the signal to threshold, the signal has to be increased in level so that the response to it increases by ΔO. However, this requires a relatively small increase in signal level, ΔS, as the signal level falls in the range where the input–output function is relatively steep. Thus, the growth-of-masking function has a shallow slope.

Oxenham and Plack[12] have investigated forward masking for a 6-kHz sinusoidal masker and a signal of the same frequency. They showed that if the signal is made very brief and the time delay between the masker and signal is very short, the level of the signal at threshold is approximately equal to the masker level. Under these conditions, the signal and the masker are compressed by a similar amount on the basilar membrane, and the growth-of-masking function has a slope of unity. This is illustrated in Figure 3 (filled symbols). When a masker frequency well **below** the signal frequency was used (3 kHz instead of 6 kHz), the growth-of-masking function had a slope much **greater** than unity; a 10-dB increase in masker level was accompanied by a 40-dB increase in signal level, as shown by the open symbols in Figure 3. This can be explained as follows: the signal

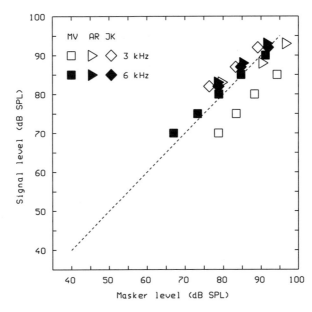

Fig. 4 Data from Oxenham and Plack[12] for three subjects with cochlear hearing loss. Individual data from subjects MV, AR and JK are plotted.

threshold depends on the response evoked by the masker at the place with CF close to the signal frequency. The growth of response on the basilar membrane for tones with frequency well below CF is linear (see the long-dashed line in Fig. 1). Thus, the signal is subject to compression while the masker is not (essentially the opposite of the situation illustrated in Fig. 2). This gives rise to the steep growth-of-masking function.

If the compression on the basilar membrane is lost as a consequence of cochlear hearing loss, then the growth-of-masking functions in forward masking (in dB per dB) should have slopes close to unity, except when the signal is very close to its absolute threshold. Furthermore, the slope should remain close to unity, regardless of the relative frequencies of the masker and signal, as all frequencies should be processed linearly. Empirical data have confirmed these predictions[11-13]. This is illustrated in Figure 4, which shows individual data from three subjects with moderate cochlear hearing loss in the same conditions as those used for the normally hearing subjects in Figure 3. In contrast to Figure 3, all three hearing-impaired subjects in Figure 4 show linear growth-of-masking functions for both the 6-kHz and the 3-kHz masker. This is consistent with the view that cochlear damage results in a loss of basilar membrane compression.

While forward masking is a useful laboratory tool for quantifying cochlear compression, it is probably not suitable as a clinical tool, because quite a lot of practice is required before stable results are obtained. However, a simple measure of frequency selectivity, based on the measurement of thresholds for detecting a sinusoidal signal in a noise with a spectral notch[14-16] gives results that are quite highly correlated with measures of cochlear compression obtained using forward masking[17]. This correlation probably occurs because both cochlear compression, and the sharpness of tuning (selectivity) of the cochlea are strongly dependent on the active mechanism. Thus, the strength of cochlear compression can be estimated indirectly from the detection threshold of a tone in a noise with a spectral notch.

Diagnosis of dead regions in the cochlea

Cochlear hearing loss is sometimes associated with complete destruction of the inner hair cells (IHCs)[18]. Sometimes the IHCs may still be present, but may be sufficiently abnormal that they no longer function. The IHCs are the transducers of the cochlea, responsible for converting the vibration patterns on the basilar membrane into action potentials in the auditory nerve[19]. When the IHCs are non-functioning over a certain region of the cochlea, no transduction will occur in that region. Hence, such a region is called a dead region[8,20,21].

A dead region can be defined in terms of the CFs of the IHCs and/or neurones immediately adjacent to the dead region[21]. For example, if there is a dead region at the basal end of the cochlea, and the CF of the IHCs/neurones immediately adjacent to the dead region is 2 kHz, this is described as a dead region extending from 2 kHz upwards. A tone with frequency falling in a dead region is detected via the apical or basal spread of the vibration pattern to places where there are surviving IHCs and neurones[22]. Thus, the 'true' hearing loss at a given frequency may be greater than suggested by the audiometric threshold at that frequency.

The audiogram cannot be used to determine whether or not a dead region is present in a given individual, although a large low-frequency loss or a loss that increases rapidly with increasing frequency is often associated with a dead region[21]. In the laboratory, dead regions have been diagnosed by using simultaneous masking to measure psychophysical tuning curves (PTCs)[22,23]. The signal is fixed in frequency and in level, usually at a level just above the absolute threshold. The masker is usually a narrow band of noise. For each of several masker centre frequencies, the level of the masker needed just to mask the signal is determined. For normally hearing subjects, the tip of the PTC (*i.e.* the frequency at which the masker level is lowest) always lies close to the signal frequency; the masker is most effective when its frequency is close to that of the signal.

When hearing-impaired listeners are tested, PTCs have sometimes been found whose tips are shifted well away from the signal frequency[20,23]. This happens when the signal frequency falls in a dead region. For example, when there is a low-frequency dead region, the detection of low-frequency tones is mediated by neurones with high CFs, so a high-frequency masker is more effective than a masker close to the signal frequency.

PTCs are rather time consuming to determine, and have rarely been used in clinical practice. Recently, Moore *et al*[20] described a test for the identification of dead regions which is intended to be short and simple enough for use in clinical practice. The test is based upon the detection of sinusoids in the presence of a broad-band noise, designed to produce almost equal masked thresholds (in dB SPL) over a wide frequency range, for normally hearing listeners and for listeners with hearing impairment but without dead regions. This noise is called threshold equalizing noise (TEN). The detection threshold is approximately equal to the level of the noise in a one-ERB wide band centred at 1 kHz; ERB stands for equivalent rectangular band-width of the auditory filter, and its normal value at 1000 Hz is about 132 Hz[15]. For example, a noise level of 70 dB/ERB usually leads to a masked threshold of about 70 dB SPL.

When a tone has a frequency that falls well within a dead region, the tone is detected using neurones with CFs remote from the signal frequency. The amplitude of basilar membrane vibration at the remote place will generally be less than the amplitude in the dead region. Therefore, the broad-band noise masks the tone much more effectively than would normally be the case, as the noise only has to mask the reduced response at the remote place. Thus, if the threshold for detecting a tone in the TEN is **markedly** higher than normal, this indicates a lack of functioning IHCs/neurones with CFs corresponding to the frequency of the tone (*i.e.* a dead region).

To validate the TEN test, Moore *et al*[20] measured PTCs and applied the TEN test in the same hearing-impaired listeners. The hypothesis tested was that higher-than-normal thresholds in the TEN would be associated with PTCs with shifted tips. Results for a hearing-impaired person who does not appear to have a dead region are shown in Figure 5. The lower panel shows results obtained with the TEN, except that filled squares indicate absolute thresholds (in dB SPL). Over the frequency range where the TEN produces masking, the masked thresholds are only slightly higher than normal, being around 71–75 dB for the TEN level of 70 dB/ERB. For frequencies of 3000 Hz and above, the TEN level of 70 dB/ERB is not sufficient to produce masking, so the masked thresholds are close to the absolute thresholds.

The upper panel of Figure 5 shows PTCs determined for three signal frequencies. In each case, the signal level and frequency are indicated by a filled symbol. The corresponding PTC is indicated by an open symbol of the same shape. For each PTC, the tip is close to the signal frequency. The PTCs are consistent with the results using the TEN, indicating that each signal was detected via IHCs/neurones with CFs close to the signal frequency.

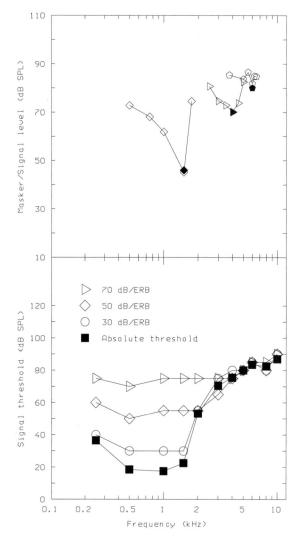

Fig. 5 Results for a hearing-impaired person who does not have a dead region. The lower panel shows results obtained with the TEN, except that filled squares indicate absolute thresholds. The upper panel shows PTCs determined for three signal frequencies. In each case, the signal level and frequency are indicated by a filled symbol. The corresponding PTCs are indicated by open symbols of the same shape.

Figure 6 shows results for a hearing-impaired person who probably does have a dead region. This person has near-normal hearing for frequencies up to 1000 Hz, but a severe-to-profound loss at higher frequencies. For signal frequencies of 1500 Hz and above, masked thresholds in the 70 dB/ERB noise were 10 dB or more higher than the mean normal value. For signal frequencies from 3000–5000 Hz, the masked thresholds in the 30 dB/ERB noise were elevated above the absolute thresholds and were at

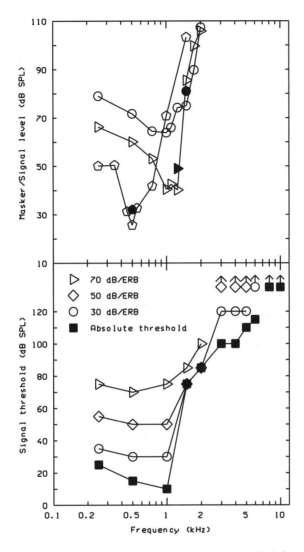

Fig. 6 Results for a person with a dead region at high frequencies. Otherwise, as Figure 5. Symbols with up-pointing arrows indicate cases where the threshold was too high to be measured; the highest measurable threshold (determined by equipment limitations) was 120 dB SPL. The specific symbol used with the arrow indicates the lowest TEN level for which a threshold could not be measured.

120 dB SPL, *i.e.* 90 dB higher than for normal-hearing subjects! This strongly suggests that tones with frequencies of 1500 Hz and above were being detected via IHCs/neurones with CFs below 1500 Hz.

The PTC for this subject for a signal frequency of 500 Hz has a tip at 500 Hz. However, the PTCs for signal frequencies of 1200 and 1500 Hz are shifted downwards to about 1000–1200 Hz. This suggests that the dead region starts at 1000–1200 Hz, and extends upwards from there, which is consistent with the finding that thresholds in the TEN were near normal for frequencies up to 1000 Hz, but were higher than normal for frequencies of 1500 Hz and above.

In total, Moore *et al*[20] tested 20 ears of 14 subjects with sensorineural hearing loss. Generally, there was a very good correspondence between the results obtained using the TEN and the PTCs; if, for a given signal frequency, the masked threshold in the TEN was 10 dB or more higher than normal **and** the TEN produced at least 10 dB of masking (*i.e.* the masked threshold was 10 dB or more above the absolute threshold), then the tip of the PTC determined using that signal frequency was shifted. If the masked threshold in the TEN was not 10 dB or more higher than normal, the tip of the PTC was not shifted. Hence, the following 'rule' was formulated: if the threshold in the TEN is 10 dB or more above the TEN level/ERB, and the TEN produces at least 10 dB of masking, this is indicative of a dead region at the signal frequency. It should be noted, however, that if the TEN does not produce at least 10 dB of masking, the result must be regarded as inconclusive; a dead region may or may not be present.

The presence or absence of dead regions can have important implications for the fitting of hearing aids. People with moderate-to-severe high-frequency hearing loss often do not benefit from amplification of high frequencies[24–26]. In several of these studies, it was suspected that there were dead regions at high frequencies, although there was little direct evidence to support this idea. Recently, Vickers *et al*[27] measured the identification of nonsense syllables by people with high-frequency hearing loss. One group of subjects was diagnosed as having high-frequency dead regions, using the tests described above. The other group did not have dead regions. For both groups, the stimuli were subjected to frequency-dependent linear amplification according to the 'Cambridge' formula[28], which is intended to restore the audibility of speech presented at a moderate level (about 65 dB SPL). Then, the stimuli were low-pass filtered with various cut-off frequencies. For subjects without dead regions, performance generally improved progressively with increasing cut-off frequency. For most subjects with dead regions, performance improved with increasing cut-off frequency until the cut-off frequency was somewhat above the estimated edge frequency of the dead region, but hardly changed with further increases. For a few subjects, performance initially improved with increasing cut-off frequency and then worsened with further increases. The cut-off frequency giving optimum performance was estimated to be 1.5–2 times the estimated edge frequency of the dead region. Baer *et al*[29] found similar results for speech presented in background noise.

The practical implications of these results are as follows. Firstly, for a person with an extensive high-frequency dead region, the ability to understand speech will probably be rather poor, and a hearing aid may be of limited benefit. However, as noted above, amplification should be applied for frequencies up to about 1 octave above the estimated edge frequency of the dead region. There may be several benefits of reducing the gain for frequencies above this. Firstly, this may actually lead to improved speech intelligibility, as described above. Secondly, it may reduce problems associated with acoustic feedback (whistling). Thirdly, it may reduce distortion in the hearing aid. Finally, it allows the dispenser to concentrate efforts on providing appropriate amplification over the frequency range where there is useful residual hearing.

Perceptual streaming

A rapid sequence of sounds may perceived as coming from a single source (called fusion), or as coming from more than one source (called fission or stream segregation)[30,31]. The term 'streaming' is used to denote the processes determining whether one stream or multiple streams are heard. Streaming has often been studied using sequences of the form ABA–ABA–..., where A and B represent brief sinusoidal tone bursts and – represents a silent interval[30]. When the frequency separation of A and B is large, two streams are heard, one (A tones) going twice as fast as the other (B tones). When the frequency separation is small, fusion occurs and a characteristic 'gallop' rhythm is heard. For intermediate frequency separations of A and B, the subject may either hear two streams or one. The frequency separation at which the subject cannot perceive two streams, but only hears the gallop rhythm, is called the fission boundary.

It has been proposed[32,33] that streaming depends primarily upon the filtering that takes place in the cochlea. For example, the computer model of Beauvois and Meddis[33] is based on the idea that streaming depends upon the overlap of the excitation patterns evoked by successive sounds in the cochlea; a large degree of overlap leads to fusion while a small degree leads to fission. People with cochlear hearing loss usually have reduced frequency selectivity, which leads to broader excitation patterns[3]. If the model of Beauvois and Meddis is correct, the fission boundary should be larger than normal in people with cochlear hearing loss.

This prediction was tested by Rose and Moore[34]. They measured fission boundaries for the ABA–ABA– sequence described above, using both normally hearing subjects and subjects with unilateral and bilateral cochlear hearing loss. For the unilaterally hearing-impaired listeners, there was no consistent difference in the fission boundary across ears. The bilaterally hearing-impaired listeners sometimes showed fission boundaries within the normal range, and sometimes showed larger than normal fission boundaries. These results indicate that factors other than overlap of excitation patterns must influence streaming for sequences of pure tones. It may be that the pitches of successive tones need to be clearly different for fission to be heard. If the pitches of the tones are unclear, this may lead to larger-than-normal fission boundaries. It is known that the frequency discrimination of sinusoids is worse than normal in people with cochlear hearing loss[2], and this may indicate that the pitch sensation is less clear.

Grimault et al[35] studied streaming for sequences of harmonic complex tones, comparing the results for young, normally hearing subjects and elderly subjects having either impaired or normal hearing for their age. They used the ABA–ABA– sequence. The tones A and B differed in fundamental frequency (F0), but were band-pass filtered so as to contain harmonics in the same frequency region (1375–1875 Hz). When the F0s of the A and B tones were low (around 88 Hz), the harmonics would not have been resolved by the auditory system[36], and excitation patterns would have been very similar for the A and B tones. In this condition, performance was similar for the young and for the elderly hearing-impaired subjects. Thus, consistent with earlier results using similar stimuli, the results indicate that streaming can occur in the absence of differences in the excitation patterns[37–39]. Presumably, the streaming depends on differences in the time pattern (F0) of the successive tones.

When the F0s of the tones were higher (around 250 Hz), some of the harmonics would have been resolved in the auditory periphery of the normally hearing subjects, but the harmonics probably were not resolved by the elderly subjects, owing to their reduced frequency selectivity. In this condition, the former showed significantly more stream segregation than the latter.

The results of Rose and Moore[34] and of Grimault et al[35] suggest that the stream segregation of both pure and complex tones can be adversely affected by cochlear hearing loss. This may contribute to the difficulties experienced by hearing-impaired people in understanding speech in situations where there are competing sounds such as other speakers and music.

Key points for clinical practice

- Cochlear hearing loss is usually associated with damage to the active mechanism in the cochlea. This results in reduced frequency selectivity, which contributes to difficulty in understanding speech in noise, and reduced cochlear compression, which is probably the main cause of loudness recruitment. Cochlear compression can be assessed in the laboratory using forward masking, but in the clinic it can be more easily measured by an indirect method, based on the detection of a tone in notched noise.

- Cochlear hearing loss is sometimes associated with complete loss of function of inner hair cells over a certain region of the cochlea, called a dead region. People with extensive dead regions often do not benefit much from a hearing aid, although there can be some benefit of amplifying frequencies up to an octave above the edge frequency of a high-frequency (basal) dead region.

- Dead regions can be diagnosed in the laboratory using psychophysical tuning curves. A method suitable for clinical use involves measuring detection thresholds for tones in quiet and in threshold-equalising noise (TEN).

- Cochlear hearing loss is often associated with abnormalities in the perception of rapid sequences of sounds (stream segregation). This may be a side-effect of reduced frequency selectivity, and it may contribute to the difficulties experienced by hearing-impaired people in understanding speech in situations where there are competing sounds such as other speakers and music.

References

1 Moore BCJ. Psychophysics of normal and impaired hearing. *Br Med Bull* 1987; **43**: 887–908
2 Moore BCJ. *Perceptual Consequences of Cochlear Damage*. Oxford: Oxford University Press, 1995
3 Moore BCJ. *Cochlear Hearing Loss*. London: Whurr, 1998
4 Rhode WS. Observations of the vibration of the basilar membrane in squirrel monkeys using the Mössbauer technique. *J Acoust Soc Am* 1971; **49**: 1218–31
5 Ruggero MA, Rich NC, Recio A, Narayan SS, Robles L. Basilar-membrane responses to tones at the base of the chinchilla cochlea. *J Acoust Soc Am* 1997; **101**: 2151–63
6 Recio A, Rich NC, Narayan SS, Ruggero MA. Basilar-membrane responses to clicks at the base of the chinchilla cochlea. *J Acoust Soc Am* 1998; **103**: 1972–89
7 Moore BCJ, Oxenham AJ. Psychoacoustic consequences of compression in the peripheral auditory system. *Psychol Rev* 1998; **105**: 108–24
8 Moore BCJ, Glasberg BR. A model of loudness perception applied to cochlear hearing loss. *Auditory Neurosci* 1997; **3**: 289–311
9 Jesteadt W, Bacon SP, Lehman JR. Forward masking as a function of frequency, masker level, and signal delay. *J Acoust Soc Am* 1982; **71**: 950–62
10 Moore BCJ, Glasberg BR. Growth of forward masking for sinusoidal and noise maskers as a function of signal delay: implications for suppression in noise. *J Acoust Soc Am* 1983; **73**: 1249–59
11 Oxenham AJ, Moore BCJ. Additivity of masking in normally hearing and hearing-impaired subjects. *J Acoust Soc Am* 1995; **98**: 1921–34
12 Oxenham AJ, Plack CJ. A behavioral measure of basilar-membrane nonlinearity in listeners with normal and impaired hearing. *J Acoust Soc Am* 1997; **101**: 3666–75
13 Oxenham AJ, Moore BCJ. Modeling the effects of peripheral nonlinearity in listeners with normal and impaired hearing. In: Jesteadt W. (ed) *Modeling Sensorineural Hearing Loss*. New Jersey: Erlbaum, 1997; 273–88
14 Patterson RD. Auditory filter shapes derived with noise stimuli. *J Acoust Soc Am* 1976; **59**: 640–54
15 Glasberg BR, Moore BCJ. Derivation of auditory filter shapes from notched-noise data. *Hear Res* 1990; **47**: 103–38

16   Stone MA, Glasberg BR, Moore BCJ. Simplified measurement of impaired auditory filter shapes using the notched-noise method. *Br J Audiol* 1992; **26**: 329–34

17   Moore BCJ, Vickers DA, Plack CJ, Oxenham AJ. Inter-relationship between different psychoacoustic measures assumed to be related to the cochlear active mechanism. *J Acoust Soc Am* 1999; **106**: 2761–78

18   Schuknecht HF. *Pathology of the Ear*. Cambridge, MA: Harvard University Press, 1974

19   Yates GK. Cochlear structure and function. In: Moore BCJ. (ed) *Hearing*. San Diego, CA: Academic Press, 1995; 41–73

20   Moore BCJ, Huss M, Vickers DA, Glasberg BR, Alcántara JI. A test for the diagnosis of dead regions in the cochlea. *Br J Audiol* 2000; **34**: 205–24

21   Moore BCJ. Dead regions in the cochlea: diagnosis, perceptual consequences, and implications for the fitting of hearing aids. *Trends Amplif* 2001; **5**: 1–34

22   Thornton AR, Abbas PJ. Low-frequency hearing loss: perception of filtered speech, psychophysical tuning curves, and masking. *J Acoust Soc Am* 1980; **67**: 638–43

23   Moore BCJ, Alcántara JI. The use of psychophysical tuning curves to explore dead regions in the cochlea. *Ear Hear* 2001; **22**: 268-78

24   Murray N, Byrne D. Performance of hearing-impaired and normal hearing listeners with various high-frequency cut-offs in hearing aids. *Aust J Audiol* 1986; **8**: 21–8

25   Hogan CA, Turner CW. High-frequency audibility: benefits for hearing-impaired listeners. *J Acoust Soc Am* 1998; **104**: 432–41

26   Ching T, Dillon H, Byrne D. Speech recognition of hearing-impaired listeners: predictions from audibility and the limited role of high-frequency amplification. *J Acoust Soc Am* 1998; **103**: 1128–40

27   Vickers DA, Moore BCJ, Baer T. Effects of lowpass filtering on the intelligibility of speech in quiet for people with and without dead regions at high frequencies. *J Acoust Soc Am* 2001; **110**: 1164–75

28   Moore BCJ, Glasberg BR. Use of a loudness model for hearing aid fitting. I. Linear hearing aids. *Br J Audiol* 1998; **32**: 317–35

29   Baer T, Moore BCJ, Kluk K. Effects of lowpass filtering on the intelligibility of speech in noise for listeners with and without dead regions at high frequencies. *J Acoust Soc Am* 2002; In press

30   van Noorden LPAS. *Temporal Coherence in the Perception of Tone Sequences*. PhD Thesis, Eindhoven University of Technology, 1975

31   Bregman AS. *Auditory Scene Analysis: The Perceptual Organization of Sound*. Cambridge, MA: Bradford Books/MIT Press, 1990

32   Hartmann WM, Johnson D. Stream segregation and peripheral channeling. *Music Percept* 1991; **9**: 155–84

33   Beauvois MW, Meddis R. Computer simulation of auditory stream segregation in alternating-tone sequences. *J Acoust Soc Am* 1996; **99**: 2270–80

34   Rose MM, Moore BCJ. Perceptual grouping of tone sequences by normally hearing and hearing-impaired listeners. *J Acoust Soc Am* 1997; **102**: 1768–78

35   Grimault N, Micheyl C, Carlyon RP, Arthaud P, Collet L. Perceptual auditory stream segregation of sequences of complex sounds in subjects with normal and impaired hearing. *Br J Audiol* 2001; **35**: 173–82

36   Plomp R. The ear as a frequency analyzer. *J Acoust Soc Am* 1964; **36**: 1628–36

37   Vliegen J, Oxenham AJ. Sequential stream segregation in the absence of spectral cues. *J Acoust Soc Am* 1999; **105**: 339–46

38   Vliegen J, Moore BCJ, Oxenham AJ. The role of spectral and periodicity cues in auditory stream segregation, measured using a temporal discrimination task. *J Acoust Soc Am* 1999; **106**: 938–45

39   Moore BCJ, Gockel H. Factors influencing sequential stream segregation. *Acta Acustica* 2002; **88**: 320–32

Auditory processing and the development of language and literacy

Peter J Bailey and **Margaret J Snowling**

Department of Psychology, University of York, York, UK

This paper considers evidence for basic auditory processing impairments associated with dyslexia and specific language impairment, against a back-drop of findings from studies of the normal development of auditory and phonological processing. A broad range of auditory impairments have been implicated in the aetiology of these language-learning disorders, including deficits in discriminating the temporal order of rapid sequences of auditory signals, elevated thresholds for frequency discrimination and for detection of amplitude and frequency modulation, impaired binaural processing and increased susceptibility to backward masking. Current evidence is inconsistent, but suggests that not all children with language difficulties have non-verbal auditory processing impairments, and for those that do, the impact on language development is poorly understood. Some implications for clinical practice are discussed.

Although children make use of visual cues when learning language, audition is of primary importance for language acquisition. The fact that language development can be severely compromised as a consequence of audiometrically-defined hearing impairment is *prima facie* evidence for the role of auditory processing in language development. Here we review claims that a range of more subtle impairments of auditory processing may be associated with, and possibly causally linked to, specific deficiencies in language and literacy. Space limitations prohibit discussion of claims concerning co-occurring subtle sensory impairments in vision and touch[1].

The language learning impairments that have received most attention in this context are dyslexia and specific language impairment (SLI). A commonly accepted definition of dyslexia is that it is a specific learning difficulty, primarily affecting the acquisition of reading and spelling, such that these skills are below the level to be expected for a given age and general cognitive ability. Some dyslexic children have concomitant language problems, but in 'discrepancy defined' samples of children with at least average IQ, oral language deficits are not wide-spread. In contrast, the term specific language impairment is applied typically when the non-verbal IQ score is at least 80, and performance on at least

Correspondence to:
Dr Peter Bailey,
Depart. of Psychology,
University of York,
Heslington,
York YO10 5DD, UK

two oral language tasks is significantly below the level predicted from IQ. However, it is important to note that there is no consensus about the IQ criterion that should be applied, and there is considerable heterogeneity within language-impaired samples[2].

Some investigators have assumed a common substrate for dyslexia and SLI (in effect that dyslexia is a mild form of SLI), but this assumption is likely only to be justified for children whose SLI is characterised by expressive language difficulties and phonological processing problems, rather than for those who exhibit pragmatic language abnormalities, involving difficulties with use of language in interaction. The distinctions between different forms of language difficulty have sometimes been obscured by the use of the term 'language learning impaired', but it is important to note that SLI children have more extensive language problems than dyslexic children, encompassing poor vocabulary, grammatical deficits and problems with the comprehension and production of sentence structure.

Normal development of auditory processing in relation to speech perception

The perception of speech requires a capacity to determine spectral shape, to detect and discriminate amplitude modulation and modulation of fundamental and spectral frequency, and to do so with temporal resolution that encompasses both the relatively slow changes that extend over an entire utterance and the relatively fast changes that occur as a result of rapid consonantal articulations. Moreover, given that speech is rarely heard in isolation from other sounds, the listener must segregate the signal of interest from background sounds (including other speech sounds), and attend appropriately to the auditory patterns in the segregated speech.

At least some of these capabilities are present *in utero*. The cardiac orienting reflex has been used to demonstrate that late gestational age fetuses respond more to pulsed than continuous sounds[3], suggesting a sensitivity to amplitude modulation, and have a limited ability to discriminate complex tones differing in pitch[4]. It is presumably capabilities of these kinds that make it possible for neonates to discriminate low-pass filtered maternal from non-maternal speech[5].

The auditory capabilities of normally-developing children are probably sufficient early in infancy to support discrimination of the linguistically-relevant contrasts in speech. By 6 months of age, infants' frequency selectivity is similar to that of adults[6], which suggests an ability to extract information about spectral shape, and temporal resolution is adequate for extraction of phonetically-relevant details in the amplitude envelope of speech[7]. However, there are some indications that infants do not have adult-like attentional capabilities[8]; limitations on selective listening may constrain their ability to extract information from speech heard against a background of noise, particularly the speech of other talkers.

Sensitivity to the acoustic cues that carry supra-segmental information in speech has been demonstrated in neonates using habituation–dishabituation procedures; a change in language (from Dutch to Japanese) was detected, but only for speech waveforms played forwards, and not when the waveforms were reversed[9]. A corresponding pattern of performance found for monkeys suggests that this language discrimination may depend on processes common to mammalian auditory systems generally. The extent to which similarities between the speech discrimination capabilities of humans and non-humans should be taken to argue against specialisation of human brains for speech perception remains controversial[10].

An influential view for many years has been that neonates are pre-programmed to perceive speech categorically, but sufficiently generally to afford the potential for learning any of the world's languages. Sensitivity to phonetically relevant acoustic variation is then gradually shaped during the first year of life to home in on those phonetic contrasts that are relevant in the native language[11]. However, Nittrouer[12], using a visually-reinforced conditioned head-turning procedure, reported that, of her 6–14-month-old participants, only 65% reached the criterion for discrimination of a vowel contrast and only 35% for a consonantal voicing contrast. It seems, therefore, that the speech perception capabilities of young infants may have been overstated. Nittrouer concluded that if lack of conditioning to the criterion in these procedures is due to a failure of discrimination, rather than due to infant temperament as has often been assumed, then the performance of young listeners is unreliable, but not randomly so.

According to Nittrouer and her colleagues, a child's experience with their native language affects the perceptual weight assigned to individual acoustic properties of speech[13]. They argue that children begin by relying on dynamic spectral properties, useful for recognising syllabic structure, whereas older children and adults tend to give more weight to steady-state acoustic properties, on which the development of fine-grained phonological representations depends. These developmental changes have only been demonstrated so far for a relatively limited set of phonetic contrasts, and it has been suggested that young children simply use the most acoustically salient cues[14]; however, Nittrouer and Crowder[15] found that 5- and 7-year-old children and adults did not differ in their relative sensitivity to steady state and dynamic acoustic cues, and argued that the developmental weighting shift is not the result of a change in sensitivity to the relevant acoustic parameters.

Thus the prevailing, but not settled, view on the normal development of speech perceptual abilities is that from birth, infants are sensitive to the acoustic cues that signal phonetic contrasts, but that the cues they use will change with age in response to environmental input. An important issue is how any auditory processing deficits present at this stage might influence the establishment of the fine-grained phonological represent- ations that underpin language development.

Auditory deficits associated with specific language impairment

According to one prominent theory[16], both oral and written language disorders in childhood can be traced to a non-verbal processing deficit that manifests itself when auditory information arrives at a rapid rate. This view was developed from an initial series of studies of children with SLI using a procedure often referred to as the Auditory Repetition Task (ART)[17,18]. In the ART, the child listens to two complex tones that differ clearly in pitch, separated by an inter-stimulus interval (ISI). Following training to the criterion on trials in which the tones are associated with different responses, the child has to copy the order of the tones in the order of their responses. Tallal and Piercy[18] reported that their sample of 12 SLI children found this task more difficult than controls only when there was a relatively short ISI (<150 ms). Temporal order judgement tasks like this have been used widely as an indicator of the general efficacy of auditory temporal processing.

This rapid auditory processing deficit found with non-speech sounds is assumed within the theory to have a critical impact on the perception of consonants distinguished by rapid spectrotemporal changes; a further key assumption is that the relationship between auditory processing and language skill is a causal one mediated by phonological processing. Both of these assumptions are contentious. It has been claimed recently that training rapid auditory processing improves language skills[19], providing potentially powerful support for the validity of a causal theory linking the two abilities. Thus, it is important for theoretical and practical reasons that this theory be properly evaluated.

There have been rather few studies of temporal auditory processing in SLI. One of these used a version of the ART to investigate the auditory processing skills of 55 SLI children selected from twin pairs, and 76 control twins with normal language skills[20]. The ART performance of the SLI group was significantly worse than that of controls but, contrary to Tallal and Piercy's original findings[18], group differences tended to be larger at slow than at fast rates of presentation. The primary focus of the study was the heritability of auditory processing (performance on the ART) and phonological processing skills, assessed by a test of non-word repetition. Although deficits on the non-word repetition task showed a significant degree of heritability, ART scores did not. These findings suggest that the relationship between non-verbal auditory processing and language skills is not mediated by phonological processing abilities. If ART deficits are principally determined by environmental factors, perhaps children with SLI experience difficulties in auditory processing tasks as a consequence of their language impairment.

Bishop and colleagues went on to explore in more detail the auditory processing capabilities of SLI and control children from the above sample[21]. Backward masking thresholds correlated with performance in the ART measured 2 years earlier, attesting to the consistency of these measures, but did not predict language impairment. Moreover, there were no group differences in absolute threshold, thresholds for frequency modulation detection or pitch discrimination, or thresholds under forward or backward masking. The absence of a group difference in backward-masked thresholds is inconsistent with a previous report that children with SLI had elevated backward-masked thresholds compared to controls[22]. A logical problem for the hypothesis that auditory processing deficits lead to language impairments is the finding that some control children had elevated backward masked thresholds and performed poorly on the ART but were not language impaired[21].

Auditory deficits associated with dyslexia

Many recent studies have investigated auditory processing skills in so-called 'well-compensated' dyslexic adults who may no longer have reading problems. There are grounds for caution in the interpretation of some of these studies. First, such participants are likely to differ from those in childhood samples that are recruited at the time they have reading problems. Second, a failure to find a difference between dyslexic adults and controls in an auditory processing task does not rule out the possibility that a deficit earlier in development compromised the development of phonological representations. Slow or delayed development of one process (albeit along normal lines) may alter the course of development of a related process in a sensitive period.

Auditory temporal order judgements

The auditory repetition task described above has been used in a variety of forms with reading-impaired participants. Tallal[23] reported that ART performance was poor relative to that of controls for 9 of the 20 reading-impaired children in her study, and that ART scores were correlated with performance on a phonological task, suggesting that impairments of reading, as well as impairments of oral language, can be the consequence of a reduced ability to process rapidly-occurring auditory stimuli. A recent report has suggested that a relationship between auditory temporal order judgements and phonological measures is also found for average and above-average readers[24].

Contrasting results were obtained by Nittrouer[25], who found that good and poor readers did not differ in performance of an ART-like task, nor did the poor readers show impairments in use of brief formant transitions to cue a phonemic contrast involving manner of articulation. Similarly, a study in our laboratory[26] found no differences between dyslexic and control children in mean ART performance, although there was a small subgroup of dyslexics (24%) whose ART performance was outside the normal range. Marshall et al[26] noted that children who were impaired on the ART also tended to take longer reaching the criterion in a tone identification and response mapping pre-test; this observation suggests that verbal labelling skill, rather than simply efficiency in rapid auditory processing, is important for ART performance. Indeed, the large individual differences in performance of ART-like tasks may be related to language skills, with low scores reported only for poor readers having concomitant weak language skills[27].

Despite its superficial simplicity, the ART requires a range of non-auditory capabilities, including attentional and verbal labelling skills, as well as tone segregation, pitch perception and judgements of the temporal order of auditory events. The effects of reading and language impairments on these diverse aspects of the task remain unclear, as does the nature of any relationship between rapid auditory processing and phonological representations. In view of this, pragmatic caution should be exercised before implementing remediation programmes designed to improve language and reading performance by training rapid auditory processing skills.

Frequency discrimination

There have been several reports that dyslexic adults are impaired in tasks involving pure tone frequency discrimination, relative to normal-reading controls[28-31]. McAnally and Stein[28] proposed that the dyslexic participants' elevated difference limens for frequency (DLF) could be understood in terms of an impairment in the ability to extract information about the temporal fine structure of auditory stimuli from the phase locking of auditory nerve firing patterns. This hypothesis predicts that any differences between dyslexic and control listeners should be more evident for tones at low frequencies, where phase locking information is available, than at frequencies above 4–5 kHz, where it is not. However, the demonstration by Hill *et al*[32] that DLFs were similar for dyslexic and control listeners for pure tones at both 1 kHz and 6 kHz is not consistent with the prediction.

The magnitude of threshold elevation for DLFs reported for dyslexic listeners across different studies shows considerable variation, possibly as a result of differences in the severity of dyslexia in the participant sample, and also of differences in aspects of the psychophysical procedures, such as the trial structure and the availability of feedback. A recent report has confirmed an influence of trial structure (2-interval *versus* 7-interval) on the magnitude of DLF differences between dyslexic and control listeners[33]. Such results question the extent to which differences between good and poor readers' psychophysical thresholds directly reflect fundamental limitations in low-level sensory processing. Even highly constrained psychophysical tasks require attentional and memory processes, and little is known yet about the impact of dyslexia on such processes in the context of threshold estimates. As with most measures of poor readers' performance, there are large individual differences in frequency discrimination[34], and DLF estimates for dyslexic and control listeners typically show considerable overlap.

Poor readers have been reported to have elevated thresholds for detection of frequency modulation (FM), but only at slow modulation rates (2 Hz); detection of FM at fast rates (240 Hz) – which is dependent on resolution of spectral side-bands rather than on detection of FM *per se* – was not impaired[35]. A modest, but significant, relationship between phonological skill and auditory sensitivity to low rates of FM has been demonstrated in a class of normal primary-school children[36]. Thresholds for amplitude modulation are also reported to be elevated for dyslexic listeners, and, in contrast to FM thresholds, across a relatively wide range of modulation frequencies (10–320 Hz)[37].

Given the importance of frequency and amplitude modulations in carrying information in speech, a reduction in sensitivity to frequency and amplitude variation, present when infants are refining their phonological representations on the basis of the speech they hear, might be expected to result in weak or inappropriate phonological representations that could affect subsequent language and literacy development. To be convincing, this position requires that the thresholds typically reported for dyslexic participants are high relative to the magnitude of modulations typically found in speech. Such comparisons are necessarily crude, but may be informative. For example, the stop consonants in the syllables [ba] and [ga] are differentiated primarily by the characteristics of the initial second-formant transitions, which typically differ in onset frequency by at least 500 Hz[38]. Although there are few normative data on which to base an estimate, 100 Hz is probably a reasonable rough approximation to the difference limen for formant frequency transition onset frequency[38]. The mean threshold for detection of slow FM reported by Witton *et al*[35] for dyslexic adults was approximately 50% larger than that of controls. If such estimates from dyslexic adults using tonal stimuli are indicative of the magnitude of threshold elevation for formant discrimination by infants at risk of dyslexia, it is not obvious why the threshold elevation alone would be sufficient to cause significant problems with speech perception.

Binaural processing

The binaural masking level difference provides an elegant approach to measuring the use dyslexic listeners can make of the fine-grain temporal structure of sounds. It has been reported that the masking level difference – in this case the difference between the masked thresholds for binaural tones that were in phase at the two ears and for binaural tones that were 180° out of phase at the two ears, presented in binaurally-identical noise – was significantly smaller for dyslexic than for control listeners[28] (although see Hill *et al*[32]). There is also evidence that dyslexic children were impaired in a dichotic pitch identification task, where pitch sensations depended on interaural timing mismatches[39].

Backward masking

If dyslexics are impaired in their processing of rapid sound sequences, this may be because they are particularly susceptible to masking of a sound by temporally adjacent sounds. In one study, masked thresholds for dyslexic children were normal under forward masking, but (for 5 of the 8 participants) elevated under backward masking[40]. In addition to this demonstration of abnormal backward **detection** masking, deficits have been reported in backward **recognition** masking, but only for poor readers with concomitant oral language problems[41].

The asymmetries in backward and forward masking led Rosen and Manganari[40] to hypothesise that the acoustic cues to initial consonants might be backward-masked by the energy in the following vowel. In fact the dyslexic children in their study were not impaired on discrimination of syllable-initial relative to syllable-final formant transitions. This was true for synthetic speech syllables and for non-speech sounds with analogous spectral properties (isolated second formants); dyslexic children's performance was slightly worse overall for synthetic speech syllables than for the non-speech isolated formants, but it is not clear whether this difference is attributable to the perceptual status of the sounds as speech or non-speech, or to the differences in acoustic complexity between synthetic syllables and isolated formants.

Tasks involving speech and non-speech sounds

In contrast to the proposal that impairments in basic auditory processes play a causal role in SLI and dyslexia[16], it has been suggested that the deficit is not a general auditory impairment but is specific to the processing of speech sounds. Consistent with this is the finding that poor readers, whose performance discriminating acoustically-similar speech syllables was impaired relative to that of control children, were not reliably impaired in discriminating non-speech 'sine-wave' analogues of the syllables, in which the formant frequency pattern was simulated with frequency-modulated pure tones[42].

Similar sine-wave analogues of consonant-vowel syllables have been used in an experiment comparing discrimination performance of dyslexic and control children in two conditions – first where the sounds were described to the listeners as electronic whistles, and second where the sounds were described as speech-like[43]. Discrimination performance did not differ significantly between participant groups when the stimuli were described as whistles, but when described as speech-like, dyslexic children's performance indicated a reduced tendency to categorise the sounds phonemically.

The extent to which any perceptual deficits in poor readers are speech-specific or associated with general auditory processing problems is the subject of continuing debate[44-46]. A hindrance to resolving the issue experimentally is the difficulty in designing appropriate non-speech auditory stimuli so that performance with speech and non-speech sounds can be meaningfully compared. Sine-wave speech has the virtue that it can be made to mimic some of the spectrotemporal properties of formant patterns, and is typically heard, initially at least, as whistles without phonemic value; however, for some listeners it can evoke phonemic percepts on first presentation, and it differs greatly from speech in its acoustic complexity.

Key points and conclusions

- Advances in the understanding of the role of auditory processing in the genesis of language difficulties have been hampered theoretically by a lack of agreement about the relationship between basic auditory skills, speech perception and phonological processing abilities, and also methodologically by frequent uncontrolled group differences in experimental studies.

- It should be clear from this review that by no means all children with language learning impairments demonstrate non-verbal auditory processing problems. It has been suggested that, where present, auditory processing deficits may be a 'synergistic risk factor' for language impairment[20], that exerts a moderating influence when children are already at genetic risk of language disorder, but they are neither necessary nor sufficient to explain language difficulties.

- Children with oral language impairments require comprehensive assessment of their cognitive strengths and difficulties to specify more accurately the nature of their difficulties. It is premature given the present state of knowledge to advocate training in auditory skills for these children[47,48]. While this might bring about some benefit for their auditory attention and listening skills, the large-scale adoption of such training programmes is counter-indicated until the causal relationships among auditory, phonological and language impairments are clarified.

- Children with oral language impairments beyond the pre-school years require intensive programmes of speech and language therapy and there is good evidence of the benefits of phonological awareness training for dyslexia[49].

Acknowledgements

Our work on auditory deficits associated with dyslexia, in collaboration with Nick Hill and Yvonne Griffiths, has been supported by the Wellcome Trust through project grant No. 55671. We thank Charles Hulme, Nick Hill, Yvonne Griffiths and Brian Moore for helpful comments.

References

1 Wright BA, Bowen RW, Zecker SG. Nonlinguistic perceptual deficits associated with reading and language disorders. *Curr Opin Neurobiol* 2000; **10**: 482–6
2 Bishop DVM. Cognitive neuropsychology and developmental disorders: Uncomfortable bedfellows. *Q J Exp Psychol A* 1997; **50**: 899–923
3 Groome LJ, Mooney DM, Holland SB *et al*. Temporal pattern and spectral complexity as stimulus parameters for eliciting a cardiac orienting reflex in human fetuses. *Percept Psychophys* 2000; **62**: 313–20
4 Lecanuet JP, Graniere-Deferre C, Jacquet AY, DeCasper AJ. Fetal discrimination of low-pitched musical notes. *Dev Psychobiol* 2000; **36**: 29–39
5 Spence MJ, Freeman MS. Newborn infants prefer the maternal low-pass filtered voice, but not the maternal whispered voice. *Inf Behav Dev* 1996; **19**: 199–212
6 Spetner NB, Olsho LW. Auditory frequency resolution in human infancy. *Child Dev* 1990; **61**: 632–52
7 Trainor LJ, Samuel SS, Desjardins RN, Sonnadara RR. Measuring temporal resolution in infants using mismatch negativity. *Neuroreport* 2001; **12**: 2443–8
8 Bargones JY, Werner LA. Adults listen selectively – infants do not. *Psychol Sci* 1994; **5**: 170–4
9 Ramus F, Hauser MD, Miller C, Morris D, Mehler J. Language discrimination by human newborns and by cotton-top tamarin monkeys. *Science* 2000; **288**: 349–51
10 Trout JD. The biological basis of speech: what to infer from talking to the animals. *Psychol Rev* 2001; **108**: 523–49
11 Jusczyk PW, Bertoncini J. Viewing the development of speech perception as an innately guided learning process. *Lang Speech* 1988; **31**: 217–38

12 Nittrouer S. Challenging the notion of innate phonetic boundaries. *J Acoust Soc Am* 2001; **110**: 1598–605

13 Nittrouer S, Miller ME. Predicting developmental shifts in perceptual weighting schemes. *J Acoust Soc Am* 1997; **101**: 2253–66

14 Sussman JE. Vowel perception by adults and children with normal language and specific language impairment: based on steady states or transitions? *J Acoust Soc Am* 2001; **109**: 1173–80

15 Nittrouer S, Crowther CS. Examining the role of auditory sensitivity in the developmental weighting shift. *J Speech Lang Hear Res* 1998; **41**: 809–18

16 Tallal P, Miller SL, Jenkins WM, Merzenich MM. The role of temporal processing in developmental language-based learning disorders: research and clinical implications. In: Blachman BA. (ed) *Foundations of Reading Acquisition and Dyslexia: Implications for Early Intervention.* Mahwah, NJ: Lawrence Erlbaum, 1997; 49–66

17 Tallal P, Piercy M. Defects of non-verbal auditory perception in children with developmental aphasia. *Nature* 1973; **241**: 468–9

18 Tallal P, Piercy M. Developmental aphasia: impaired rate of non-verbal processing as a function of sensory modality. *Neuropsychologia* 1973; **11**: 389–98

19 Tallal P, Miller SL, Bedi G *et al*. Language comprehension in language-learning impaired children improved with acoustically modified speech. *Science* 1996; **271**: 81–4

20 Bishop DVM, Bishop SJ, Bright P *et al*. Different origin of auditory and phonological processing problems in children with language impairment: Evidence from a twin study. *J Speech Lang Hear Res* 1999; **42**: 155–68

21 Bishop DVM, Carlyon RP, Deeks JM, Bishop SJ. Auditory temporal processing impairment: Neither necessary nor sufficient for causing language impairment in children. *J Speech Lang Hear Res* 1999; **42**: 1295–310

22 Wright BA, Lombardino LJ, King WM *et al*. Deficits in auditory temporal and spectral resolution in language-impaired children. *Nature* 1997; **387**: 176–8

23 Tallal P. Auditory temporal perception, phonics, and reading disabilities in children. *Brain Lang* 1980; **9**: 182–98

24 Au A, Lovegrove B. Temporal processing ability in above average and average readers. *Percept Psychophys* 2001; **63**: 148–55

25 Nittrouer S. Do temporal processing deficits cause phonological processing problems? *J Speech Lang Hear Res* 1999; **42**: 925–42

26 Marshall CM, Snowling MJ, Bailey PJ. Rapid auditory processing and phonological ability in normal readers and readers with dyslexia. *J Speech Lang Hear Res* 2001; **44**: 925–40

27 Heath SM, Hogben JH, Clark CD. Auditory temporal processing in disabled readers with and without oral language delay. *J Child Psychol Psychiatry* 1999; **40**: 637–47

28 McAnally KI, Stein JF. Auditory temporal coding in dyslexia. *Proc R Soc Lond B Biol Sci* 1996; **263**: 961–5

29 Hari R, Saaskilahti A, Helenius P, Uutela K. Non-impaired auditory phase locking in dyslexic adults. *Neuroreport* 1999; **10**: 2347–8

30 Baldeweg T, Richardson A, Watkins S, Foale C, Gruzelier J. Impaired auditory frequency discrimination in dyslexia detected with mismatch evoked potentials. *Ann Neurol* 1999; **45**: 495–503

31 Ahissar M, Protopapas A, Reid M, Merzenich MM. Auditory processing parallels reading abilities in adults. *Proc Natl Acad Sci USA* 2000; **97**: 6832–7

32 Hill NI, Bailey PJ, Griffiths YM, Snowling MJ. Frequency acuity and binaural masking release in dyslexic listeners. *J Acoust Soc Am* 1999; **106**: L53–8

33 France SJ, Rosner BS, Hansen PC *et al*. Auditory frequency discrimination in adult developmental dyslexics. *Percept Psychophys* 2002; **64**: 169–79

34 Amitay S, Ahissar M, Nelken I. Auditory processing deficits in reading disabled adults. *J Assoc Res Otolaryngol* 2002; <http://link.springer-ny.com/link/service/journals/10162/contents/00/10093/>

35 Witton C, Talcott JB, Hansen PC *et al*. Sensitivity to dynamic auditory and visual stimuli predicts nonword reading ability in both dyslexic and normal readers. *Curr Biol* 1998; **8**: 791–7

36 Talcott JB, Witton C, McLean MF *et al*. Dynamic sensory sensitivity and children's word decoding skills. *Proc Natl Acad Sci USA* 2000; **97**: 2952–7

37 Menell P, McAnally KI, Stein JF. Psychophysical sensitivity and physiological response to amplitude modulation in adult dyslexic listeners. *J Speech Lang Hear Res* 1999; **42**: 797–803

38 Stevens KN. *Acoustic Phonetics*. Cambridge, MA: MIT Press, 1998

39 Dougherty RF, Cynader MS, Bjornson BH, Edgell D, Giaschi DE. Dichotic pitch: a new stimulus distinguishes normal and dyslexic auditory function. *Neuroreport* 1998; **9**: 3001–5

40 Rosen S, Manganari E. Is there a relationship between speech and nonspeech auditory processing in children with dyslexia? *J Speech Lang Hear Res* 2001; **44**: 720—36

41 McArthur GM, Hogben JH. Auditory backward recognition masking in children with a specific language impairment and children with a specific reading disability. *J Acoust Soc Am* 2001; **109**: 1092–100

42 Mody M, Studdert-Kennedy M, Brady S. Speech perception deficits in poor readers: auditory processing or phonological coding? *J Exp Child Psychol* 1997; **64**: 199–231

43 Serniclaes W, Sprenger-Charolles L, Carre R, Demonet JF. Perceptual discrimination of speech sounds in developmental dyslexia. *J Speech Lang Hear Res* 2001; **44**: 384–99

44 Denenberg VH. A critique of Mody, Studdert-Kennedy, and Brady's 'Speech perception deficits in poor readers: auditory processing or phonological coding?' *J Learning Disabil* 1999; **32**: 379–83

45 Studdert-Kennedy M, Mody M, Brady S. Speech perception deficits in poor readers: a reply to Denenberg's critique. *J Learning Disabil* 2000; **33**: 317–21

46 Studdert-Kennedy M. Deficits in phoneme awareness do not arise from failures in rapid auditory processing. *Reading Writing* 2002; **15**: 5–14

47 Gillam RB, Crofford JA, Gale MA, Hoffman LM. Language change following computer-assisted language instruction with Fast ForWord or Laureate Learning Systems software. *Am J Speech-Lang Pathol* 2001; **10**: 231–47

48 Gillam RB, Loeb DF, Friel-Patti S. Looking back: a summary of five exploratory studies of Fast ForWord. *Am J Speech-Lang Pathol* 2001; **10**: 269–73

49 Snowling MJ. *Dyslexia*, 2nd edn. Oxford: Blackwell, 2000

Electronic aids to hearing

Stuart Gatehouse

MRC Institute of Hearing Research, Glasgow Royal Infirmary, Glasgow, UK

Despite many scientific developments in the biology of hearing, there remain no wide-spread medical or surgical interventions for listeners with sensorineural hearing impairments. In addition to describing technical advances, this chapter identifies important aspects of candidature for hearing aids and some issues of service delivery.

Despite many scientific advances in the biology of hearing, there remain no wide-spread medical or surgical interventions for listeners with sensorineural hearing impairments. The provision of amplification and associated rehabilitation remains the only effective intervention available for sensorineural hearing loss[1-6]. It is also effective for conductive hearing loss when surgical intervention to improve hearing (and medical intervention to eradicate pathology) is either not appropriate or not available. There is a danger when concentrating on 'advances and developments' to place too great a focus on advances in the technological content of amplification devices at the expense of the rehabilitative context within which those devices are embedded. In addition to describing technical advances, this chapter identifies important aspects of candidature for hearing aids and some issues of service delivery. Here 'electronic aids to hearing' includes assistive listening devices and communicators as well as head- or ear-worn personal amplifiers (hearing aids) whether they be of a conventional air-conduction, bone-conduction or implantable configuration. Cochlear implants are covered elsewhere (see Ramsden, this volume).

Hearing aids may overcome some, though not all, of the deficits associated with a hearing loss[2]. Some sounds are inaudible, while others can be detected because part of their spectrum is audible, but may not be correctly identified because other parts of their spectrum (typically the high-frequency parts) remain inaudible. The dynamic range between the weakest sound that can be heard and the threshold of discomfort is less for a person with sensorineural hearing loss than for a normal-hearing person. To compensate for this, a hearing aid would have to amplify quiet sounds more than intense sounds. In addition, sensorineural impairment diminishes the ability of a person to detect and analyze energy at one frequency in the presence of energy at other frequencies. A hearing-impaired person also has decreased ability to hear a signal that rapidly

Correspondence to:
Prof. Stuart Gatehouse,
MRC Institute of Hearing
Research, Glasgow Royal
Infirmary, Queen
Alexander Building, 16
Alexandra Parade,
Glasgow G31 2ER, UK

follows, or is rapidly followed by, a different signal. This decreased frequency and temporal resolution makes it more likely that speech understanding will be disrupted in adverse listening environments, and is discussed in detail elsewhere in this volume.

Hearing aids are often classified according to where they are worn. In order of decreasing size, these categories are: body, spectacle, behind-the-ear, in-the-ear, in-the-canal and completely-in-the-canal. Decreasing size has been a driving force during the history of the development of the hearing aid, but it is important to recognise that size and style are not exclusively related to cosmetic appearance. Some years ago, listeners who opted for smaller in-the-ear or in-the-canal devices paid a definite penalty in terms of processing capability, sound quality, and battery life. Technical advances in circuitry and battery technology have largely eradicated that penalty, although the choice or recommendation of a hearing aid style still does interact with the features in a hearing aid. For each style there are advantages relating to ease of insertion, ease of manipulation, visibility, amount of gain, sensitivity to wind noise, directivity, reliability, telephone compatibility, processing flexibility, ease of cleaning, and avoidance of occlusion and feed-back[1]. The need for specific features such as a volume control, tele-coil, direct audio input and directional microphone have to be determined on an individual basis and will influence professional recommendation and client choice, almost independent of cosmetic factors.

Much hearing aid research and promotional literature from manufacturers concentrates on the signal processing contained within a hearing aid. However, the first piece of technology encountered by a sound entering a hearing aid is the microphone, and there can still be occasions where the performance of a hearing aid is limited, not by the electronics, but by this component. Modern miniature electrical microphones provide high sound quality, with only minor imperfections associated with internal noise and sensitivity to vibration. Directional microphones, which have two entry ports, are more sensitive to frontal sound than to sound arriving from other directions[7]. The benefits of directionality are based on the ecologically reasonable assumption that listeners will orientate themselves to face a sound source of interest, and that interfering sound sources are likely to be at other locations in space. High directionality in hearing aids might compromise access to new sound sources of definite interest in those with the cognitive capacity to benefit. However, the trade-off between such a restriction and improved selectivity for wanted sound has yet to be quantified for a range of listeners. Directional microphones enable hearing aids to improve the signal-to-noise ratio by 3–5 dB relative to their omni-directional counterparts, and hence improve the intelligibility of speech in noise when speech and noise do not come from the same source angle. Dual-microphone hearing aids can be switched by the users to be either directional, or omni-directional, as required in different listening situations. Although dual microphone hearing aids impose stringent requirements regarding matching and stability on their constituent components, they do offer listeners the opportunity to select the microphone sensitivity mode most appropriate for any given listening circumstance. Hearing aids are now in the market-place which attempt to identify the location in space of an interfering noise source and to adapt their directional pattern to suppress optimally the interfering source (which is always assumed to be other than straight ahead from the listener). Data on the effectiveness of such schemes are only beginning to emerge.

The use of a remote microphone located near the source of sound is effective, but often socially unpractical. Apart from this, multi-microphone directional arrays (including directional microphones) are the most effective way to improve intelligibility in noisy environments. Until recently, directional microphones used in hearing aids have been fixed arrays, meaning that they have the same directional pattern (represented by their polar response) in all situations. These fixed arrays use processing in which the signals from two microphones, or the sounds entering the two inlet ports of a single microphone, are subtracted to form a difference signal. Although microphone arrays offer attractive theoretical possibilities and laboratory results can be encouraging[8–10], it is a formidable challenge to deliver such processing schemes in real products. The products have to give advantages to hearing-impaired listeners in circumstances amenable to the processing without complementary disadvantages in other circumstances. Single-microphone schemes for noise reduction are not very effective. They can improve sound comfort, and the overall signal-to-noise ratio, but as conventionally and simply measured they do not improve the crucial signal-to-noise ratio for the frequency bands carrying the important information over any short time period. Consequently, they do not significantly improve intelligibility, except for highly unusual background noises.

Hearing aids can be classified by their technology into analogue, digitally programmable analogue, and fully digital types. Digitally programmable hearing aids employ conventional analogue circuits for processing the sound, but use a digital control circuit to alter the characteristics of the analogue elements. This enables the circuit, and hence the sound, to be more flexibly altered than is possible with fully analogue devices. The digital programming circuit also enables the user to switch between listening programmes in different situations. Fully digital circuits may be constructed to perform any arithmetic operation, in which case the type of processing they do depends on the software that is loaded into them. They can thus process sounds in ways specific to each device. Some manipulations of sound are performed more efficiently with digital processing, and some complex operations are only feasible with digital processing. At the time of writing, the hearing-aid industry is in a transition period from reliance on analogue and digitally-controlled analogue technology to fully digital products, and the cost penalties of fully digital implementation relative to a similarly featured analogue counterpart (where that is possible) are gradually disappearing. The 'benefits of digital hearing aids' was always a misleading issue, but it will soon become totally irrelevant[11]. The scientifically valid issue of the benefits of different features that may be incorporated into a hearing aid rationale and fitting can then return to the fore.

The performance of hearing aids is most conveniently measured when the hearing aid is connected to an acoustic coupler. While test boxes provide a convenient way to get sound into the hearing aid in a controlled manner, they are an imperfect means to an end. That end is the performance of the hearing aid in an individual patient's ear. This performance can be directly measured using a soft, thin probe-tube inserted in the ear canal. A singular development in recent years has been the gradual incorporation of real-ear measures of hearing aid performance into both the fitting, fine-tuning and evaluation of hearing aids[12]. The increasing complexities of hearing aid processing have placed increasing demands upon the signals, equipment and procedures for such measures.

Feedback ('whistling') is a major problem in hearing aids. It occurs when the amplification from the microphone to the receiver is greater than the attenuation of sound leaking from the output back to the input. Feedback can be made less likely be several means. One simple technique is to decrease the gain only for those frequencies and input levels at which oscillation is likely. A second technique involves adding a controlled internal feedback path that has the gain and phase response needed to cancel the accidental leakage around the ear-mould or shell[13]. These techniques are already available in advanced hearing aids. Feedback has been one of the predominant problems with hearing aid fitting and a significant bar to acceptance both on the part of hearing-impaired listeners themselves, but also their family and significant others. The advent of flexible feedback management and suppression algorithms, though as yet by no means perfect, has led to significant advances in the degrees and forms of amplification provided and the overall acceptability of fittings. Even where a feedback suppression or management regimen leads to no overall change in the acoustical characteristics of the amplification delivered, but simply results in the ability to employ an ear-mould delivery system which leads to significantly less occlusion, there will be a material benefit to listeners. Such a fitting will result in increased use and comfort of the hearing aid, with a resultant increase in satisfaction.

The ear-mould is designed to fit an individual's ear and retains the hearing aid on the head[14]. It also provides the soundpath from the receiver to the ear canal. In many cases, the ear-mould provides a second sound path, referred to as a vent, between the air outside the head and the ear canal. One unwanted consequence of an ear-mould can be the occlusion effect, in which the aid wearer's own voice is excessively amplified by bone-conducted sound. At present, most occlusion management techniques are based around ear-mould alterations. The acoustical, as opposed to the discomfort, aspects of occlusion are still poorly understood, though preliminary experiments using acoustical cancelling techniques to offset, or at least alleviate, the acoustical elements of occlusion are underway.

Because of the non-linear elements of SNHL, many hearing aid rationales employ amplitude compression[15]. Compression's major role is to match the range of sound levels in the environment to the dynamic range of a hearing-impaired person better. The compressor may be most active at low, mid or high sound levels. Alternatively, it may vary its gain across a wide range of sound levels, in which case it is known as a wide dynamic range compressor. Compressors can react to a change in input levels within a few milliseconds, or they can take many tens of seconds to react fully. Simple compression systems can be classified as input controlled, where the compressor is controlled by a signal prior to the hearing aid's volume control, or as output controlled, where the compressor is controlled by a signal subsequent to the volume control. This classification is irrelevant for hearing aids with no volume control. Compression systems have been used to achieve various specific aims and different compression parameters are needed for each rationale. Output-controlled compression limiting can prevent the output from ever causing loudness discomfort[16,17]. Fast-acting compression with a low compression thresholds can be used to increase the audibility of the softer syllables of speech, whereas slow-acting compression will leave the relative intensities unchanged, but will alter the overall level of a speech signal. Compression applied with a medium compression threshold will make hearing aids more comfortable to wear in noisy places, without the advantages or disadvantages that occur when lower level sounds are compressed[18]. Multichannel compression can be used to enable a hearing-impaired person to hear sounds at the same loudness as a normal-hearing person listening to the same sounds. Alternatively, it can be used to maximize intelligibility, while making the overall loudness of sounds normal (rather than normalizing the loudness at each frequency)[19,20]. Compression can be used to decrease the disturbing effects of background noise by reducing gain at those frequencies where the signal-to-noise ratio is poorest. Gain reduction of this type increases listening comfort and, with some unusual noises, may also increase intelligibility. Finally, compression can be applied by using the combination of compression parameters that patients are believed to prefer, irrespective of whether there is a theoretical rationale guiding the application.

Despite some complexity, the benefits of compression demonstrated in clinical trials can be summarized as follows. Compression can make low-level speech more intelligible, by increasing gain, and hence audibility. Compression can make high-level sounds more comfortable and less distorted. In mid-level environments, compression offers little advantage relative to a well-fitted linear aid. Once the input level goes up, of course, the advantages of compression become evident. Major disadvantages of compression include greater likelihood of feedback oscillation, and excessive amplification of unwanted lower level background noises. These considerations of compression give some indications of how the choices might interact with aspects of candidature and rehabilitation[21,22]. Although the research base is still small, it does appear logical that those implementations of compression designed to function well across wide ranges of auditory environment are likely to be most beneficial to listeners who do experience those conditions[23]. On the other hand, compression regimens which are optimally configured to overcome the restrictions in dynamic range, masking and frequency and temporal resolution are more likely to be most beneficial to listeners who suffer most from those deficits.

The most complex forms of amplification, which are not yet widely available, involve enhancing speech in ways that vary from one speech sound to the next. These methods include exaggerating the peaks and troughs in the spectrum of a speech sound, lengthening and shortening the duration of particular sounds, and increasing the amount of amplification whenever a consonant occurs. On the evidence available so far, however, none of these techniques will produce a large increase in intelligibility compared to conventional amplification.

Many hearing-aid fittings need to be fine-tuned, either electronically or physically, after the patient has had sufficient listening experience[2,22]. In those cases where it is not clear which control should be adjusted, or by how much it should be adjusted, a systematic fine-tuning can be performed using one of two general methods. The first of these is paired comparisons, in which the patient is asked to choose between two amplification characteristics presented in quick succession. Multiple characteristics can be compared by arranging them in pairs. Paired comparisons can be used to adaptively fine-tune a hearing aid control if the settings compared in each trial are based on the patient's preference in the preceding trial. Such techniques can also be used as part of the initial fitting process[24]. The second general method for fine-tuning relies on the patient making an absolute rating of sound quality. The best amplification characteristic (out of those compared) is simply the characteristic that is given the highest rating by the patient. The absolute rating method can also be used to alter adaptively a chosen hearing aid control. This is achieved by deciding on a target rating (*e.g.* just right) and adjusting a control in the direction indicated by the patient's rating (*e.g.* too shrill, or too dull). The paired comparisons and absolute rating methods are best carried out while the patient listens to continuous discourse speech material. Depending on the complaint being investigated, this can be supplemented with recordings of commonly encountered background noises.

A notable development in audiological practice throughout the world is the increasing commitment to formalised outcome measures as part of both an evaluation and a patient centred optimisation process[25]. Because of time constraints, these are often by simple self-report rather than performance measurement. Systematic measurement of outcomes helps inform clinicians which of the practices, procedures and devices are achieving the intended aims[26]. Appropriate outcome measures can also help determine how the rehabilitation for individual patients should be structured and when they might be ended or delivered in some other way. Self-report measures that assess benefit can be grouped into various classes. First, patients can be asked to make a direct assessment of the benefit of rehabilitation. Alternatively, patients' views of their disability can be assessed both before and after the rehabilitation programme. The change in score provides a measure of the effects of rehabilitation. Measures obtained both before and after rehabilitation provide a more complete view of disability or handicap status and change. These difference measures probably assess change less accurately than those that directly assess benefit because they involve subtracting two scores. The second way in which self-report measures differ is the extent to which the items are the same for all patients or are determined individually for each patient. Results can more easily be compared across patients if a standard set of items is used for all patients. When the items are individually selected for each patient, however, the questionnaires become shorter and can more easily be incorporated within interviews with the patient. Self-report measures are the only viable way to assess hearing aid use and satisfaction. Some measures contain questions that address only one dimension (benefit, use, or satisfaction) whereas others address more than one dimension. While outcomes can be assessed any time after hearing aid fitting, the extent of benefit does not appear to stabilize until about 6 weeks after fitting. Hearing aid use is associated with general improvements in health-related and quality-of-life[27]. However, generic measures of health outcome are not all efficient means to assess the outcomes of rehabilitation, because they are sensitive to too many other variables.

Sensing sounds in two ears (binaural hearing) makes it possible for a person to locate the source of sound and increases speech intelligibility in noisy situations[28–30]. Wearing two hearing aids (a bilateral fitting) instead of one hearing aid (a unilateral fitting) increases the range of sound levels for which binaural hearing is possible. Bilateral fitting is thus increasingly important as hearing loss increases. Bilateral fitting of hearing aids has several other advantages[31-33]. These include improved sound quality, suppression of tinnitus in both ears, and greater convenience when one hearing aid breaks down. In addition, a unilateral fitting can lead to decreased speech processing ability in the unaided ear if this ear is deprived of auditory stimulation for too long. Although bilateral fitting of devices has long been held to be an appropriate goal to aim at (two aidable ears deserve two hearing aids), the evidence base for cost-effectiveness in providing the second aid has yet to be established. Particular processing strategies which specifically implement or enhance binaural processing capabilities have been investigated in laboratory settings though have yet to reach the commercial market.

Hitherto this section has discussed conventional air conduction hearing aids. Bone-conduction devices output a mechanical vibration instead of an air-borne sound wave. They are most suited to people who (usually for medical reasons) cannot wear a hearing aid that includes the ear in any way. For patients with sensorineural hearing loss, bone-conduction hearing aids do not stimulate the cochlea as effectively as air-conduction devices due to the relative inefficiency of the bone-conduction route, but can for patients with substantial conductive hearing losses. Bone-conduction hearing aids require mechanical coupling to the head usually via a head band, though occasionally via spectacles. Such devices have limited cosmetic appeal and patient acceptability. An established alternative form of bone-conduction aid is the bone-anchored hearing aid, in which the vibrations are transmitted to the skull via an embedded titanium screw[34-36]. Numerous clinical trials have demonstrated the effectiveness and acceptability of this implementation for specific patient groups. Benefits of bilateral provision are beginning to be developed[37]. At an experimental level, devices can also enable vibrations to be transmitted directly to the tympanic membrane, the ossicular chain or to the round window[38-40]. Clinical trials are under way concerning the effectiveness of and candidature for such devices, though at present the potential impact would appear to be limited to certain specific patient sub-groups.

Apart from directional microphones, success for signal processing schemes to improve actively the intelligibility of speech in noise remains elusive. The most effective way to make speech more intelligible is to locate the microphone nearer the person talking. This decreases interfering noise and reverberation, but does require a means of transmitting the signal from the microphone to the hearing aid at a remote distance. Methods currently include magnetic induction to a small telecoil inside the hearing aid, radio and infrared transmission, each of which has advantages and disadvantages. Although not the subject of dramatic technological improvements (with the possible exception of the miniaturisation of coupling systems to acceptable dimensions), there is an increasing realisation and use of such remote coupling particularly in circumstances where the orientation of speakers and listeners is relatively fixed, such as in classrooms, meeting rooms and residential care facilities. A broad approach to technical capabilities can deliver significant benefits to patients.

Finally the term 'electronic aids to hearing' does not have to be hearing aids that are worn entirely or on the head or body of the hearing impaired person. These are usually classified as assistive listening devices[41] and include the remote transmission systems described above, as well as devices that are specific to particular pieces of instrumentation (such as television or telephone amplifiers) and those that convert signals into another modality (such as smoke detectors or doorbells that cause a light to flash or provide a vibratory sensation). Technological advances in this domain are relatively limited, though all benefits of miniaturisation that have accompanied developments in the electronic industry do flow almost automatically. A major step forward in services for hearing impaired people is the growing realisation that a sensible and coherent coupling of the technical capabilities and features in the acoustical processing features of personal hearing aids with the listening and life-style demands of patients in the context of remote and assistive listening devices when delivered as part of a comprehensive rehabilitation programme is the optimal way of delivering new developments to the benefit of patients.

References

1 Byrne D. Hearing aid selection for the 1990s: Where to? *J Am Acad Audiol* 1996; 7: 377–95

2. Dillon H. *Hearing Aids*. New York: Thieme, 2001

3 Kricos P, Holmes A, Doyle D. Efficacy of a communication training program for hearing-impaired elderly adults. *J Acad Rehabil Audiol* 1992; **25**: 69–80

4 Kricos PB, Holmes efficacy of audiologic rehabilitation for older adults. *J Am Acad Audiol* 1996; 7: 219–29

5 Ross M. A retrospective look at the future of aural rehabilitation. *J Acad Rehabil Audiol* 1997; **30**: 11–28

6 Sweetow RW. *Counselling for Hearing Aid Fittings*. San Diego, CA: Singular, 1999

7 Leeuw A, Dreschler W. Advantages of directional hearing aid microphones related to room acoustics. *Audiology* 1991; **30**: 330–44

8 Greenfield DG, Zurek P. Evaluation of an adaptive beam-forming method for hearing aids. *J Acoust Soc Am* 1992; **91**: 1662–76

9 Schweitzer CKG. Binaural beamforming and related digital processing for enhancement of signal-to-noise ratio in hearing aids. *Curr Opin Otolaryngol Head Neck Surg* 1996; **4**: 335–9

10 Stadler RW, Rabinowitz WM. On the potential of fixed arrays for hearing aids. *J Acoust Soc Am* 1993; **94**: 1332–42

11 Taylor RS, Paisley S, Davis A. Systematic review of the clinical and cost effectiveness of digital hearing aids. *Br J Audiol* 2001; **35**: 271–88

12 Mueller HG, Hawkins DB, Northern JL. *Probe Microphone Measurements: Hearing Aid Selection and Assessment*. San Diego, CA: Singular, 1992.

13 Engebretson AM, St French M, O'Connell B *et al*. Adaptive feedback stabilization of hearing aids. *Scand Audiol* 1993; **38**: 56–64

14 Morgan R. The art of making a good impression. *Hear Rev* 1994; **1**: 60–5

15 Moore BCJ, Peters RW, Stone MA. A comparison of four methods of implementing automatic gain control (AGC) in hearing aids. *Br J Audiol* 1998; **22**: 93–104

16 Dillon H, Stroey L. The National Acoustic Laboratories' procedure for selecting the saturation sound pressure level of hearing aids: theoretical derivation. *Ear Hear* 1998; **19**: 255–66

17 Storey L, Dillon H, Yeend I. The National Acoustics Laboratories' procedure for selecting the saturation sound pressure level of hearing aids: experimental validation. *Ear Hear* 1998; **19**: 267–79

18 Barker C, Dillon H. Client preferences for compression threshold in single-channel wide dynamic range compression hearing aids. *Ear Hear* 1999; **20**: 127–39

19 Byrne D. Implications of the National Acoustic Laboratories' (NAL) research for hearing gain and frequency response selection strategies. In: Studebaker GA, I Hochberg I. (eds) *Acoustic Factors Affecting Hearing Aid Performance*, 2nd edn. Boston, MA: Allyn-Bacon, 1980; 119–31

20 Byrne D, Dillon H. The National Acoustic Laboratories' (NAL) new procedure for selecting the gain and frequency response of a hearing aid. *Ear Hear* 1986; **7**: 257–65

21 Byrne D, Dillon H. Future directions in hearing aid selection and evaluation. In: Valentre M, Hosford-Dunn H, Roeser RJ. (eds) *Audiology: Treatment*. New York: Thieme, 2000; 164–91

22 Byrne D. Effects of frequency response characteristics on speech discrimination and perceived intelligibility and pleasantness of speech for hearing-impaired listeners. *J Acoust Soc Am* 1986; **80**: 494–504

23 Keidser G, Dillon H, Byren D. Guidelines for fitting multiple memory hearing aids. *J Am Acad Audiol* 1996; **7**: 406–18

24 Moore BC, Alcantara JI, Glasberg BR. Development and evaluation of a procedure for fitting multi-channel compression hearing aids. *Br J Audiol* 1998; **32**: 177–95

25 Noble W. *Self-assessment of Hearing and Related Functions*. London: Whurr, 1998

26 Brooks DN. Counselling and its effect on hearing aid use. *Scand Audiol* 1979; **8**: 101–7

27 Appollonio I, Carabellese C, Frattola L *et al*. Effects of sensory aids on the quality of life and mortality of elderly people: a multivariate analysis. *Age Ageing* 1996; **25**: 89–96

28 Byrne D, Noble W. Optimising sound localisation with hearing aids. *Trends Amplif* 1998; **3**: 51–73

29 Byrne D, Noble W, LePage B. Effect of long-term bilateral and unilateral fitting of different hearing aid types on the ability to locate sounds. *J Am Acad Audiol* 1992; **3**: 369–82

30 Zurek PM. Binaural advantages and directional effects in speech intelligibility. In: Studebaker GA, I Hochberg I. (eds) *Acoustic Factors Affecting Hearing Aid Performance*, 2nd edn. Boston, MA: Allyn-Bacon, 1980; 255–76

31 Chung S, Stephens S. Factors influencing binaural hearing aid use. *Br J Audiol* 1986; **20**: 129–40

32 Byrne D. Binaural hearing aid fitting: research findings and clinical application. In: Libby ER. (ed) *Binaural Hearing and Amplification*. Chicago, IL: Zenerton, 1980; vol.2: 1–21

33 Chimel R, Jerger J, Murphy E *et al*. Unsuccessful use of binaural amplification by an elderly person. *J Am Acad Audiol* 1997; **8**: 1–10

34 Hakansson B, Carlsson P, Tjellstrom A *et al*. The bone-anchored hearing aid: principal design and audiometric results. *Ear Nose Throat J* 1994; **73**: 670–5

35 Snik AF, Beynon AJ, Mylanus EA *et al*. Binaural application of the bone-anchored hearing aid. *Ann Otol Rhinol Laryngol* 1998; **107**: 187–93

36 Tjellstrom A, Hakansson B. The bone-anchored hearing aid. Design principles, indications, and long-term clinical results. *Otolaryngol Clin North Am* 1995; **28**: 53–72

37 Chasin M. Current trends in implantable hearing aids. *Trends Amplif* 1997; **2**: 84–107

38 Chazan D, Medan Y, Shvadron U. Evaluation of adaptive multi-microphone algorithms for hearing aids. *J Rehabil Res Dev* 1987; **24**: 111–8

39 Snik AF, Dreschler WA, Tange RA *et al*. Short and long term results with implantable transcutaneous and precutaneous bone-conduction devices. *Arch Otolaryngol Head Neck Surg* 1998; **124**: 265–8

40 Yanagihara N, Aritomo H *et al*. Implantable hearing aids. *Arch Otolaryngol Head Neck Surg* 1987; **113**: 869–72

41 Tyler RS, Schum DJ. *Assistive Devices for Persons with Hearing Impairment*. Boston, MA: Allyn-Bacon, 1994

Application of new biological approaches to stimulate sensory repair and protection

Matthew C Holley

Institute of Molecular Physiology, Department of Biomedical Sciences, University of Sheffield, Sheffield, UK

The inner ear governs hearing and balance via six sense organs, each composed of a few thousand mechanosensory hair cells. Most inner ear disorders involve irreversible loss of hair cells and their associated nerves. They are a function of age, genetic abnormalities and environmental factors such as noise and the use of ototoxic drugs. The genetics and cell biology of the inner ear have revealed some key molecular mechanisms of development and sensory degeneration that raise hopes for new therapeutic approaches to the regeneration of sensory function. This review highlights these advances and the approaches that might be taken to effect protection and repair. It concludes with the suggestion that we can expect tangible, practical progress towards the clinic over the next 5–10 years and that, to provide the training and skills required to take full advantage of emerging technologies, we should forge much closer links between specialist clinicians and basic scientists.

The challenge of sensory recovery

Hearing loss affects some 9 million people in the UK (<www.defeatingdeafness.org>). One in every 850 babies are born profoundly deaf and progressive or age-related hearing loss affects more than half of all people over 60 years old. In over 80% of cases, the cause is directly or indirectly related to degeneration and death of sensory hair cells and their associated spiral ganglion neurons (SGNs)[1]. The vestibular sensory epithelia are also located within the inner ear and suffer progressive sensory losses that compromise mobility on a similar scale amongst elderly people.

Loss of auditory hair cells in adult mammals is currently irreversible (see Raphael, this volume) and the development of therapeutic techniques designed to replace them is a challenge. Optimism has been fuelled by discoveries that hair cells can be replaced in non-mammalian vertebrates, especially birds, which have provided some of the most promising mechanistic insights[2]. This has been enhanced by evidence for growth of new hair cells in mammalian vestibular epithelia and lies in

Correspondence to:
Prof. Matthew C Holley,
Institute of Molecular
Physiology, Alfred Denny
Building, Western Bank,
Sheffield S10 2TN, UK

the context of the discovery that many tissues, long considered to be irreparable, contain stem cells that can be coaxed towards the task of functional repair[3].

The causes of sensory loss within the inner ear are diverse, but by far the largest number of cases relate to age or to damage caused by noise or ototoxic drugs[4]. The genetic component is highly variable (see Bitner-Glindzicz, this volume). Sadly, numerous drugs used to treat life-threatening illnesses damage hair cells and their innervation directly. These include aminoglycoside antibiotics and drugs such as cisplatin, which is used for cancer treatment. Thus there is a need not only to seek methods of regenerating lost sensory cells but also to develop protective treatments against ototoxic drugs. Noise damage can obviously be avoided using much simpler protective measures such as ear muffs. However, many young people subject themselves to damaging noise levels, which may lead to significant hearing losses later in life.

There are no clinical treatments for the loss of vestibular hair cells. Loss of auditory hair cells, or cochlear function, can be addressed to some extent by insertion of a cochlear implant, which by-passes the sensory cells and delivers electrical stimuli direct to the SGNs within the auditory nerve[5]. Biotechnologies that enhance the interface between the implant electrode and the auditory nerve may widen the candidature for implants and improve the quality of perception[6].

This article addresses the progress in the development of new biotechnologies for treating sensory loss in the inner ear. It does not offer a comprehensive review of the extensive literature, but should highlight research that best represents progress in the selected areas.

Cellular and molecular therapeutic targets

The selection of cellular targets depends upon the nature of the cell loss and whether the aim is to protect or to regenerate tissue. Protection of hair cells or spiral ganglion neurons (SGNs) requires knowledge of the mechanisms of damage and the factors that govern cell survival or death. To replace lost cells, it is necessary to identify potential precursors and to find the means of inducing either appropriate cell division or differentiation. Much of this kind of work is based upon the assumption that an understanding of basic developmental mechanisms will illuminate potential mechanisms for regeneration. Although this applies to a large degree, there are key differences between the two processes, not least because so many developmentally regulated genes are expressed only transiently during development. Added to this, there are significant differences between species and between sensory epithelia *in vitro* and *in vivo*[7]. Whilst identification of molecular targets depends upon a wide spectrum of experimental preparations, *in vivo* studies with mammals are especially important for progress towards effective clinical application.

Approaches to the protection of hair cells and neurons

Growth factors

The clinical application of growth factors is complicated by wide-spread, potential side-effects and the need to deliver them locally and for long periods[8]. Many neurotrophic factors in man have a serum half-life of minutes or hours, and systemic application requires high dose levels to ensure that effective concentrations reach the desired target. This increases the chances of generating non-specific and undesirable side-effects. However, with respect to protective treatments in the inner ear there are two key advantages. The first is that drugs and other agents, including viral vectors, can be delivered directly into the enclosed environment of the inner ear fluids. The second is that application is required only transiently, during the administration of the ototoxic drug.

A considerable amount of groundwork is required to test applications in animals before proceeding to clinical trials, but current evidence is encouraging. Growth factors can influence cell proliferation, differentiation and survival and numerous studies have been carried out on inner ear epithelia from a variety of different animal species.[9] Much of the work has focused on neurotrophin-3 (NT3) and brain-derived neurotrophic factor (BDNF), which are expressed by hair cells and act on tyrosine kinase receptors (trkB and trkC, respectively) on the sensory neurons[10]. Excitation of these receptors is important for neuronal survival[10,11]. Interestingly, electrical activity in the neurons can induce secretion of BDNF and NT3[12] and it transpires that neuronal survival is dependent upon the presence of hair cells and on electrical stimulation[12–14]. Consequently, the loss of hair cells is associated with a loss of SGNs[15,16].

The progressive loss of SGNs has serious implications for the application of cochlear implants. Although there is little direct evidence from patients for a correlation between implant performance and the degree of innervation[17,18], the timing of implantation appears to be crucial in order to maximize the benefit from the remaining auditory nerve fibres[19]. Thus appropriate drugs that can protect the SGNs may be of potential therapeutic value.

The protective action of growth factors has been assessed in terms of hair cells[20] and nerves[11], but one study showed that a combination of agents directed against both cell types can provide significant functional protection against noise or drug-induced damage[21]. Inner hair cells release glutamate, which excites N-methyl-D-aspartate (NMDA) receptors on the dendrites of the SGNs. NMDA receptors have been implicated in excitotoxic cell death and may be key mediators of damage induced both by noise or by aminoglycosides. NT3 protects SGNs during aminoglycoside treatment in guinea pigs[22] and an NMDA antagonist helps to preserve hair cell morphology, the Preyer reflex and distortion product oto-acoustic emissions (DPOAEs) following similar treatment in the same animal[23]. Applied together, shortly before noise damage or infusion of amikacin into the perilymph, the NMDA antagonist MK801 and NT3 prevent dendritic swelling, preserve the morphology of hair cells and SGNs and significantly decrease threshold shifts in the auditory brain stem responses (ABR)[21]. This kind of study is particularly important, being conducted *in vivo* with measurements of physiological function.

Shinohara *et al*[6] refined the functional analysis by exploring the protective effects of neurotrophic factors in a guinea pig cochlear prosthesis model. Ears were perfused with 10% neomycin for 48 h to induce hearing loss followed by BDNF and ciliary neurotrophic factor (CNTF) for up to 29 days. A platinum electrode placed about 1.5 mm into the cochlea was used to stimulated the SGNs at weekly intervals before the experiment was terminated to allow the histology of the spiral ganglion to be assessed. There was a significant reduction in the electrically evoked ABR thresholds, which correlated with the density of surviving SGNs. The results are clearly very promising although potential side-effects and the longer term efficacy of the treatment will have to be analysed before clinical trials can be undertaken.

Apoptosis

Hair cells assaulted by aminoglycosides or excessive noise suffer a certain degree of damage and then die by apoptosis[24-27]. Apoptosis is a physiological response that controls cell death and may allow epithelial repair without excessive functional disruption, such as decay of the endocochlear potential. Hair cells can be rescued by blocking apoptotic pathways[28] and the associated intracellular signalling cascade involved also provides suitable molecular drug targets. Hair cells damaged either by the aminoglycoside neomycin or by excessive noise activate the c-Jun N-terminal kinase (JNK) pathway leading to apoptosis[26]. Systemic application of CEP-1347, and agent which inhibits the JNK pathway, to guinea pigs *in vivo*, prior to the ototoxic stimuli, reduces hair cell loss in both auditory and vestibular epithelia and decreases temporary threshold shifts in the ABRs[27]. Studies *in vitro* reveal that CEP-1347 is as effective as NT3 as a survival factor for SGNs[26]. This small molecule can be applied systemically and may reach the target cells more effectively, although concerns about side-effects and long-term efficacy remain. Activation of caspases is an early event in apoptosis and caspase inhibitors can protect both mammalian[29] and chick[30] hair cells from ototoxic damage.

Other protective agents

Aminoglycoside toxicity involves the formation of free radicals via the formation of iron complexes, a process that can be countered by treatment with antioxidants or iron chelators[31]. Recent clinical trials in China have shown that aspirin can act as an extremely effective therapeutic antioxidant, providing protection from ototoxic doses of aminoglycosides without the need to reduce the serum levels required for disease treatment[32]. The results of this trial are not yet published, but they promise a realistic, inexpensive treatment for one of the world's most common causes of hearing loss.

Approaches to the regeneration of hair cells and neurons

Replacement of lost cells is a more challenging task than protection. In practice, the latter applies where justified clinical intervention leads to predictable damage. In seeking mechanisms and likely drug targets for cell replacement, it is important to identify competent cells and then to find ways of stimulating their division and/or differentiation. Studies in development and regeneration suggest that supporting cells and hair cells share a common precursor and that mature supporting cells can form hair cells either via division or phenotypic conversion. A number of specific transcription factors involved in cell determination and differentiation in the inner ear have been identified. These molecules do not present attractive drug targets. However, components of associated intracellular signalling pathways that can regulate their function may do so, and it is worth exploiting *in vitro* preparations, including cell lines and epithelial or organotypic cultures to this end.

Growth factors and other agents in vivo

There is some potential for stimulating sensory regeneration in vestibular epithelia. Cell proliferation and the appearance of new hair cells in vestibular epithelia from adult rats was induced *in vivo* by infusion of insulin and TGFβ into the cochlear scala vestibuli[7]. The mean numbers of supporting cells and hair cells labelled with tritiated thymidine within a whole utricular macula after 10 days of treatment was small, only 15 and 3, respectively. The response was enhanced by simultaneous application of gentamicin. Interestingly, similar treatment of vestibular epithelia *in vitro* did not induce proliferation. This may be due to the fact that growth factor responses are integrated with signalling events via the extracellular matrix[9], and it highlights the problems of correlating data from experiments *in vitro* and *in vivo*. It has also been found that insulin and TGFβ induced or enhanced proliferation in most of the surrounding, non-sensory epithelia, including the transition zone, roof of the membranous labyrinth, underlying stroma and squamous mesothelium[33].

The potential side-effects of growth factor therapy may be subtle, but if detrimental effects occur within the inner ear then they may compromise functional recovery. This issue has been addressed by measuring horizontal vestibular-ocular reflexes (HVORs) in adult guinea pigs following treatment with gentamicin[34]. It is significant that in this study the growth factor treatment, consisting of TGFα, IGF-1, retinoic acid and BDNF, was delivered 7 days after the gentamicin and *via* an infusion pump directly into the vestibule. A recovery in HVORs was associated with hair cell recovery, including type 1 cells in the cristae. This is a step forward, but problems relating to the complexity of the growth factor infusion and the longer term stability of recovery still need to be addressed.

The machinery of cell proliferation

Low levels of cell division and hair cell replacement occur in mammalian vestibular epithelia following hair cell loss[35]. Experiments *in vitro* show that small numbers of cells in utricular sensory epithelia from guinea pigs and humans enter S-phase following treatment with aminoglycosides[36]. The effects can be enhanced with various combinations of growth factors[37]. Regeneration of hair cells in the auditory epithelia of birds very obviously involves a proliferative response, which is mediated by cAMP[38]. The intracellular signalling pathways activated by the human recombinant glial growth factor 2 (rhGGF2) have been studied in supporting cell preparations derived from rat utricles[39,40]. Brief exposure to forskolin, which activates adenylyl cyclase and increases cAMP, stimulates some cells to enter the cell cycle. The response is clearly increased in the presence of rhGGF2 and is blocked by inhibitors of membrane receptor recycling[40]. The effects of rhGGF2 involve the activation of phosphoinositol-3-kinase, protein kinase C and mitogen-activated protein kinase and an increase in intracellular calcium, all of which trigger a mitogenic response. It is important to elucidate these intracellular events because the components may offer suitable drug targets. In mammalian epithelia, the cyclin-dependent kinase inhibitor p27[kip1] is expressed in supporting cells and in null mouse mutants the number of hair cells and supporting cells is greater than normal[41,42]. It may be possible to induce proliferative replacement of hair cells by suppressing p27 or associated proteins in supporting cells.

Conversion of supporting cells to hair cells

There is strong evidence that new hair cells can be derived by phenotypic conversion or transdifferentiation of supporting cells both in birds and mammals. Understanding the molecular mechanisms that underlie this process may reveal potential therapeutic targets. One way of addressing the issue is to screen cultures for molecular events in supporting cells following damage to sensory epithelia[43]. FGF receptors are up-regulated in chick epithelial supporting cells[44,45], and a receptor-like protein tyrosine phosphatase (RPTP) is down-regulated[46]. Down-regulation of RPTP is an early event following ototoxic damage and may be linked to release of an inhibitory influence on cell proliferation[46].

Non-sensory epithelial cells within the greater epithelial ridge (GER) can be converted into *bona fide* hair cells when transfected with the basic helix loop helix (bHLH) transcription factor Math1[47]. Supporting cells and non-sensory epithelial cells are less versatile in adult ears. There is no evidence that Math1 can induce the same response in adult supporting cells or in cells that form the epithelial scar following hair cell loss. This is important because cells induced in this way must be located with some precision within the organ of Corti to detect vibration of the basilar membrane.

Gene therapy

Gene transfer provides a potentially powerful method of addressing a variety of problems. It is conceptually seductive, presenting the opportunity to achieve the ultimate in microsurgery. In principle, cells within the ear can be modified to secrete therapeutic gene products, such as growth factors, and they can be re-programmed to develop different functional properties or to correct an inherent genetic defect[48]. In practice, there are many problems to solve on the roads to clinical application, not least the design and delivery of safe, effective vectors that reliably infect suitable target cells and confer appropriate levels of gene expression over a sufficient period of time.

Adenoviral vectors (AdV) are currently the most efficient and specific means of gene transfer to the inner ear. Non-viral vehicles such as plasmids, liposomes and synthetic polymers are much less efficient and certainly less specific. Amongst the different viral vectors applied either *in vitro* or *in vivo*, herpes simplex virus (HSV), vaccinia, lentivirus and adeno-associated virus (AAV) appear to be less effective[49–51]. HSV may be better for infecting neurons[52], but it is not effective for hair cells[49]. However, the literature should be read with care. Different results may not be due to cell targeting but to delivery and access, especially when comparing *in vitro* and *in vivo* data, or to viral titres, which vary between different studies. Cell targeting can be controlled by careful selection of the virus and the promoter used to express the transgene[53]. Nevertheless, glial-derived neurotrophic factor (GDNF) delivered *via* AdV vectors can protect both auditory and vestibular hair cells[54,55] as well as SGNs[56] from aminoglycosides.

Viral vectors are potentially toxic and both viral and transgene proteins may generate immune responses *in vivo*. Thus it is important to make functional assessments of hearing and balance when considering clinical application. Such measurements include distortion product oto-acoustic emissions (DPOAEs)[50], hair cell transducer currents[49], Preyer reflexes or balance tasks[57]. Despite the difficulties, current progress suggests that gene therapy mediated by viral vectors is a significant, evolving field with real therapeutic potential. The transfer of genes that encode growth factors is attractive in the sense that, for secreted products, the target cells are less critical. However, cell targeting is essential if genes that regulate cell fate, such as Math1, are to be used directly.

Cell transplantation

Cell transplantation is a rapidly growing research field, particularly in terms of brain repair. It is hard to predict the outcome of transplantation experiments because interactions between cells and tissues *in vivo* are highly complex. Nevertheless, in some cases the behaviour of transplanted cells has been remarkably successful, revealing a plasticity demanding that this area of research be fully explored.

A great deal of progress has been achieved in the visual system where the first clinical trials for cell transplantation are now being considered[58]. In animals, retinal transplantation of conditionally immortal pigment epithelial cells[59] or neural progenitor cells[60] can lead to sensory recovery that is measurable not only in the retina but also in the superior colliculus[59]. The first animal experiments have recently been attempted in the auditory system, involving repair to the central auditory pathway[61]. Embryonic brain tissue was placed into a lesion in the ventral cochlear tract, resulting in some tissue regeneration and associated recovery of the ABR. Controls lacking the embryonic tissue displayed no recovery at all. Neural stem cells derived from the hippocampus have been implanted into the cochlea[62]. It is suggested that some cells adopted hair cell characteristics although the experimental evidence is at a very preliminary stage.

The choice of cells for transplantation is a key issue. Embryonic stem cells (ESCs) could potentially be used if they can be coaxed into a cochlear lineage. For example, they can be induced to differentiate into neuronal phenotypes in the presence of retinoic acid[3]. The task of inducing auditory sensory or neural phenotypes may be possible with suitable manipulation. An alternative is to isolate cells from the otic placode, otocyst or even at later stages of inner ear development. Several reasonably successful attempts have been made to establish inner ear cell lines[63]. Most lines have been derived from a transgenic animal that carries a conditionally expressed immortalising gene from the SV40 virus. The results show that it is possible to establish conditionally immortal, characterised cell lines that retain an inner ear phenotype. Surprisingly, the cells present realistic candidates for transplantation. Conditionally immortal, embryonic brain cells from the Immortomouse can migrate to sites of damage in the hippocampus and effect both structural and functional repair[64]. This work has led to the development of methods to establish similar conditionally immortalised cells from human tissue. Attempts have been made to identify stem cells from adult, mammalian sensory epithelia[65,66], but this has not yet led to establishment of clonal, characterised cells with predictable phenotypes. The concept of cell transplantation in the ear is thus tangible even if the clinical application remains some way into the future.

Although transplantation of sensory cells into the auditory system seems highly unlikely given the extremely specialised mechanics of the organ of Corti, the task of replacing lost SGNs is more tractable. However, cell replacement is not the only potential application for cell transplantation. Cell lines can be engineered for *ex vivo* gene transfer, that is to deliver secreted products such as growth factors and thus replace neurotrophic functions compromised by the loss of hair cells or supporting cells.

Drug delivery

The method of administering drugs, growth factors or viral vectors to the inner ear depends upon the problem and the desired target cells. It may be systemic[26] or by direct perfusion, often via a mini-pump[67], into cochlear or vestibular chambers[11]. It can also be achieved by diffusion across the round window[68]. The movement of solutes within the inner ear is not uniform and must be modelled carefully to ensure that the appropriate drug doses are applied[69,70]. For example, intratympanic administration of aminoglycosides is used to treat intractable vertigo in patients with Menière's disease[71,72]. At appropriate doses, the drug can target the vestibular epithelia with limited effects on the auditory system. However, functional communication between the cerebrospinal and inner ear fluids can facilitate spread of adenovirus from one innoculated ear to the contralateral ear[73]. These issues are extremely important for any future therapeutic intervention.

Key points for clinical practice

- At present, very few clinicians venture through the oval window. However, the research described in this chapter should hopefully stimulate awareness that many different types of therapeutic intervention are being explored.

- Some interventions may move to clinical trials in the next 5–10 years, others may sink without trace. Regardless of the specific outcome, we should be training more clinicians to understand the structure and function of the inner ear and to take an active part in current research during their training.

- There are numerous potential projects to pursue within a variety of research centres around the world so the trainees of today have every opportunity to equip themselves for future developments.

Acknowledgements

This work was supported by grants from The Wellcome Trust and Defeating Deafness. I thank Andrew Forge, Yehoash Raphael and Marcalo Rivolta for their comments on this manuscript.

References

1 Davis AC. *Hearing in Adults*. London: Whurr, 1995
2 Stone JS, Rubel EW. Cellular studies of auditory hair cell regeneration in birds. *Proc Natl Acad Sci USA* 2000; **97**: 11714–21
3 Guan K, Chang H, Rolletschek A, Wobus AM. Embryonic stem cell-derived neurogenesis. Retinoic acid induction and lineage selection of neuronal cells. *Cell Tissue Res* 2001; **305**: 171–6
4 Forge A, Schacht J. Aminoglycoside antibiotics. *Audiol Neuro-Otol* 2000; **5**: 3–22
5 Rubinstein JT, Miller CA. How do cochlear prostheses work? *Curr Opin Neurobiol* 1999; **9**: 399–404
6 Shinohara T, Bredberg G, Ulfendahl M *et al*. Neurotrophic factor intervention restores auditory function in deafened animals. *Proc Natl Acad Sci USA* 2002; **99**: 1657–60
7 Kuntz AL, Oesterle EC. Transforming growth factor alpha with insulin stimulates cell proliferation *in vivo* in adult rat vestibular sensory epithelium. *J Comp Neurol* 1998; **399**: 413–23
8 Apfel SC. Is the therapeutic application of neurotrophic factors dead? *Ann Neurol* 2002; **51**: 8–11
9 Oesterle EC, Hume CR. Growth factor regulation of the cell cycle in developing and mature inner ear sensory epithelia. *J Neurocytol* 1999; **28**: 877–87
10 Fritzsch B, Pirvola U, Ylikoski J. Making and breaking the innervation of the ear: neurotrophic support during ear development and its clinical implications. *Cell Tissue Res* 1999; **296**: 369–82
11 Miller JM, Chi DH, O'Keeffe LJ, Kruszka P, Raphael Y, Altschuler RA. Neurotrophins can enhance spiral ganglion cell survival after inner hair cell loss. *Int J Dev Neurosci* 1997; **15**: 631–43

12 Hansen, MR, Zha X-M, Bok J, Green SH. Multiple distinct signal pathways, including an autocrine neurotrophic mechanism, contribute to the survival-promoting effect of depolarization on spiral ganglion neurons *in vitro. J Neurosci* 2001; **21**: 2256–67

13 Mitchell A, Miller JM, Finger PA, Heller J, Raphael Y, Altschuler RA. Effects of chronic high rate electrical stimulation on the cochlea and eighth nerve in the deafened guinea pig. *Hear Res* 1997; **105**: 30–43

14 Miller AL. Effects of chronic stimulation on auditory nerve survival in ototoxically deafened animals. *Hear Res* 2001; **151**: 1–4

15 Leake PA, Hradek GT, Rebscher SJ, Snyder RL. Chronic intracochlear electrical stimulation induces selective survival of spiral ganglion neurons in neonatally deafened cats. *Hear Res* 1991; **54**: 251–71

16 Dodson HC, Mohuiddin A. Response of spiral ganglion neurones to cochlear hair cell destruction in the guinea pig. *J Neurocytol* 2000; **29**: 525–37

17 Nadol Jr JB. Patterns of neural degeneration in the human cochlea and auditory nerve: implications for cochlear implantation. *Otolaryngol Head Neck Surg* 1997; **117**: 220–8

18 Nadol Jr JB, Shiao JY, Burgess BJ *et al*. Histopathology of cochlear implants in humans. *Ann Otol Rhinol Laryngol* 2001; **110**: 883–91

19 Blamey P, Arndt P, Bergeron F *et al*. Factors affecting auditory performance of postlinguistically deaf adults using cochlear implants. *Audiol Neuro-Otol* 1996; **1**: 293–306

20 Shoji F, Miller AL, Mitchell A, Yamasoba T, Altschuler RA, Miller JM. Differential protective effects of neurotrophins in the attenuation of noise-induced hair cell loss. *Hear Res* 2000; **146**: 134–42

21 Duan M, Agerman K, Ernfors P, Canlon B. Complementary roles of neurotrophin 3 and a N-methyl-D-aspartate antagonist in the protection of noise and aminoglycoside-induced ototoxicity. *Proc Natl Acad Sci USA* 2000; **97**: 7597–602

22 Ernfors P, Duan ML, El-Shamy WM, Canlon B. Protection of auditory neurons from aminoglycoside toxicity by neurotrophin-3. *Nat Med* 1996; **2**: 463–467

23 Basile AS, Huang JM, Xie C, Webster D, Berlin C, Skolnick P. N-methyl-D-aspartate antagonists limit aminoglycoside antibiotic-induced hearing loss. *Nat Med* 1996; **2**: 1338–43

24 Forge A. Outer hair cell loss and supporting cell expansion following chronic gentamicin treatment. *Hear Res* 1985; **19**: 171–82

25 Huang T, Cheng AG, Stupak H *et al*. Oxidative stress-induced apoptosis of cochlear sensory cells: otoprotective strategies. *Int J Dev Neurosci* 2000; **18**: 259–70

26 Pirvola U, Xing-Qun L, Virkkala J *et al*. Rescue of hearing, auditory hair cells, and neurons by CEP-1347/KT7515, an inhibitor of c-Jun N-terminal kinase activation. *J Neurosci* 2000; **20**: 43–50

27 Ylikoski J, Xing-Qun L, Virkkala J, Pirvola U. Blockade of c-Jun N-terminal kinase pathway attenuates gentamicin-induced cochlear and vestibular hair cell death. *Hear Res* 2002; **163**: 71–81

28 Forge A, Li L. Apoptotic death of hair cells in mammalian vestibular sensory epithelia. *Hear Res* 2000; **139**: 97–115

29 Liu W, Staecker H, Stupak H, Malgrange B, Lefebvre P, Van De Water TR. Caspase inhibitors prevent cisplatin-induced apoptosis of auditory sensory cells. *Neuroreport* 1998; **9**: 2609–14

30 Matsui JI, Ogilvie JM, Warchol ME. Inhibition of caspases prevents ototoxic and ongoing hair cell death. *J Neurosci* 2002 **22**: 1218–27

31 Sha SH, Schacht J. Antioxidants attenuate gentamicin-induced free radical formation *in vitro* and ototoxicity *in vivo*: D-methionine is a potential protectant. *Hear Res* 2000; **142**: 34–40

32 Huang W, Chen Y, Zha D *et al*. Prevention of aminoglycoside-induced hearing loss by aspirin: preliminary data from a clinical study. *Assoc Res Otolaryngol Midwinter Meeting* 2002; Abst 262, p 69

33 Kuntz AL, Oesterle EC, Transforming growth factor-alpha with insulin induces proliferation in rat utricular extrasensory epithelia. *Otolaryngol Head Neck Surg* 1998; **118**: 816–24

34 Kopke RD, Jackson RL, Li G *et al*. Growth factor treatment enhances vestibular hair cell renewal and results in improved vestibular function. *Proc Natl Acad Sci USA* 2001; **98**: 5886–91

35 Forge A, Li L, Corwin JT, Nevill G. Ultrastructural evidence for hair cell regeneration in the mammalian inner ear. *Science* 1993; **259**: 1616–9

36   Warchol ME, Lambert PR, Goldstein BJ, Forge A, Corwin JT. Regenerative proliferation in inner ear sensory epithelia from adult guinea pigs and humans. *Science* 1993 **259**: 1619–22

37   Zheng JL, Helbig C, Gao WQ. Induction of cell proliferation by fibroblast and insulin-like growth factors in pure rat inner ear epithelial cell cultures. *J Neurosci* 1997; **17**: 216–26

38   Navaratnam DS, Su HS, Scott SP, Oberholtzer JC. Proliferation in the auditory receptor epithelium mediated by a cyclic AMP-dependent signalling pathway. *Nat Med* 1996; **2**: 1136–9

39   Montcouquiol M, Corwin JT. Brief treatments with forskolin enhance s-phase entry in balance epithelia from the ears of rats. *J Neurosci* 2001; **21**: 974–82

40   Montcouquiol M, Corwin JT. Intracellular signals that control cell proliferation in mammalian balance epithelia: key roles for phosphatidylinositol-3 kinase, mammalian target of rapamycin, and S6 kinases in preference to calcium, protein kinase C, and mitogen-activated protein kinase. *J Neurosci* 2001; **21**: 570–80

41   Lowenheim H, Furness DN, Kil J *et al*. Gene disruption of p27(Kip1) allows cell proliferation in the postnatal and adult organ of Corti. *Proc Natl Acad Sci USA* 1999; **96**: 4084–8

42   Chen P, Segil N. p27(Kip1) links cell proliferation to morphogenesis in the developing organ of Corti. *Development* 1999; **126**: 1581–90

43   Lomax MI, Huang L, Cho Y, Gong TL, Altschuler RA. Differential display and gene arrays to examine auditory plasticity. *Hear Res* 2000; **147**: 293–302

44   Lee KH, Cotanche DA. Localization of the hair-cell-specific protein fimbrin during regeneration in the chicken cochlea. *Audiol Neuro-Otol* 1996; **1**: 41–53

45   Bermingham-McDonogh O, Stone JS, Reh TA, Rubel EW. FGFR3 expression during development and regeneration of the chick inner ear sensory epithelia. *Dev Biol* 2001; **238**: 247–59

46   Kruger RP, Goodyear RJ, Legan PK *et al*. The supporting-cell antigen: a receptor-like protein tyrosine phosphatase expressed in the sensory epithelia of the avian inner ear. *J Neurosci* 1999; **19**: 4815–27

47   Zheng JL, Gao WQ. Overexpression of Math1 induces robust production of extra hair cells in postnatal rat inner ears. *Nat Neurosci* 2000; **3**: 580–6

48   Dazert S, Battaglia A, Ryan AF. Transfection of neonatal rat cochlear cells *in vitro* with an adenovirus vector. *Int J Dev Neurosci* 1997; **15**: 595–600

49   Holt JR, Johns DC, Wang S *et al*. Functional expression of exogenous proteins in mammalian sensory hair cells infected with adenoviral vectors. *J Neurophysiol* 1999; **81**: 1881–8

50   Luebke AE, Steiger JD, Hodges BL, Amalfitano A. A modified adenovirus can transfect cochlear hair cells *in vivo* without compromising cochlear function. *Gene Ther* 2001; **8**: 789–94

51   Staecker H, Gabaizadeh R, Federoff H, Van De Water TR. Brain-derived neurotrophic factor gene therapy prevents spiral ganglion degeneration after hair cell loss. *Otolaryngol Head Neck Surg* 1998; **119**: 7–13

52   Staecker H, Li D, O'Malley Jr BW, Van De Water TR. Gene expression in the mammalian cochlea: a study of multiple vector systems. *Acta Otolaryngol* 2001; **121**: 157–63

53   Luebke AE, Foster PK, Muller CD, Peel AL. Cochlear function and transgene expression in the guinea pig cochlea, using adenovirus- and adeno-associated virus-directed gene transfer. *Hum Gene Ther* 2001; **12**: 773–81

54   Yagi M, Magal E, Sheng Z, Ang KA, Raphael Y. Hair cell protection from aminoglycoside ototoxicity by adenovirus-mediated overexpression of glial cell line-derived neurotrophic factor. *Hum Gene Ther* 1999; **10**: 813–23

55   Suzuki M, Yagi M, Brown JN, Miller AL, Miller JM, Raphael Y. Effect of transgenic GDNF expression on gentamicin-induced cochlear and vestibular toxicity. *Gene Ther* 2000; **7**: 1046–54

56   Yagi M, Kanzaki S, Kawamoto K *et al*. Spiral ganglion neurons are protected from degeneration by GDNF gene therapy. *J Assoc Res Otolaryngol* 2000; **1**: 315–25

57   Dazert S, Aletsee C, Brors D, Gravel C, Sendtner M, Ryan A. *In vivo* adenoviral transduction of the neonatal rat cochlea and middle ear. *Hear Res* 2001; **151**: 30–40

58   Lund RD, Kwan AS, Keegan DJ, Sauve Y, Coffey PJ, Lawrence JM. Cell transplantation as a treatment for retinal disease. *Prog Retin Eye Res* 2001; **20**: 415–49

59   Lund RD, Adamson P, Sauve Y *et al*. Subretinal transplantation of genetically modified human cell lines attenuates loss of visual function in dystrophic rats. *Proc Natl Acad Sci USA* 2001; **98**: 9942–7

60   Young MJ, Ray J, Whiteley SJ, Klassen H, Gage FH. Neuronal differentiation and morphological integration of hippocampal progenitor cells transplanted to the retina of immature and mature dystrophic rats. *Mol Cell Neurosci* 2000; **16**: 197–205

61   Ito J, Murata M, Kawaguchi S. Regeneration and recovery of the hearing function of the central auditory pathway by transplants of embryonic brain tissue in rats. *Exp Neurol* 2001; **169**: 30–5

62   Ito J, Kojima K, Kawaguchi S. Survival of neural stem cells in the cochlea. *Acta Otolaryngol* 2001; **121**: 140–2

63   Rivolta MN, Holley MC. Cell lines from the inner ear. *J Neurobiol* 2002; In press

64   Virley D, Ridley RM, Sinden JD *et al*. Primary CA1 and conditionally immortal MHP36 cell grafts restore conditional discrimination learning and recall in marmosets after excitotoxic lesions of the hippocampal CA1 field. *Brain* 1999; **122**: 2321–35

65   Zhao H-B. Long-term natural culture of cochlear sensory epithelia of guinea pigs. *Neurosci Lett* 2001; **315**: 73–6

66   Malgrange B, Belachew S, Thiry M *et al*. Proliferative generation of mammalian auditory hair cells in culture. *Mech Dev* 2002; 112: 79–88

67   Praetorius M, Limberger A, Muller M *et al*. A novel microperfusion system for the long-term local supply of drugs to the inner ear: implantation and function in the rat model. *Audiol Neuro-Otol* 2001; **6**: 250–8

68   Goycoolea MV. Clinical aspects of round window membrane permeability under normal and pathological conditions. *Acta Otolaryngol* 2001; **121**: 437–47

69   Ghiz AF, Salt AN, DeMott JE, Henson MM, Henson Jr OW, Gewalt SL. Quantitative anatomy of the round window and cochlear aqueduct in guinea pigs. *Hear Res* 2001; **162**: 105–12

70   Salt AN, Ma Y. Quantification of solute entry into cochlear perilymph through the round window membrane. *Hear Res* 2001; **154**: 88–97

71   Hibi T, Suzuki T, Nakashima T. Perilymphatic concentration of gentamicin administered intratympanically in guinea pigs. *Acta Otolaryngol* 2001; **121**: 336–41

72   Hoffer ME, Kopke RD, Weisskopf P, Gottshall K, Allen K, Wester D. Microdose gentamicin administration via the round window microcatheter: results in patients with Menière's disease. *Ann NY Acad Sci* 2001; **942**: 46–51

73   Stover T, Yagi M, Raphael Y. Transduction of the contralateral ear after adenovirus-mediated cochlear gene transfer. *Gene Ther* 2000; **7**: 377–83

Auditory development and the role of experience

David R Moore

University Laboratory of Physiology, Oxford, UK

The human ear is functionally mature shortly after birth, but the central auditory system continues to develop for at least the first decade of life. Current interest focuses on the relation between the very late developing aspects of hearing and other aspects of cognition and behaviour. While active neural input to the brain is essential during the very early stages of development, auditory experience is now thought to be a powerful influence on central function throughout an individual's lifespan. Studies of sound localization and hearing with two ears have shown the capacity of the auditory system to adapt to altered environmental cues, even into adulthood. This environmental influence may either be harmful, as during conductive deafness, or beneficial, as evidenced by the positive outcomes of auditory training.

Hearing in humans begins around the 22nd week of gestation (*see* Moore and Jeffery[1]). At this stage, behavioural responses to sounds are produced only by intense airborne stimulation, since the fetus is in a highly sound-attenuated environment, the outer and middle ears are fluid-filled[2], and the cochlea and central auditory pathway are structurally and functionally immature. Following birth, sensitivity to sound is rapidly acquired, and many simple aspects of hearing achieve maturity during the first year. However, some aspects, such as sound localization and temporal processing, that seem to require more extensive processing in the central auditory system, do not achieve mature performance for many years, even into adolescence.

Many factors contribute to the relatively slow development of hearing: the environment, poor sound conduction, and incomplete neural development. Of these, it is neural development that has received the most attention, that has seen the most significant advancement in understanding, over the last 10 years, and that will form the focus of this review. I will present a synthesis of recent findings and thinking on the role that experience plays in shaping auditory function. The two volumes of the *Springer Handbook of Auditory Research* dealing with development[3] and plasticity[4] of hearing are more general accounts. Here, I will define 'experience' broadly to include the effects of both sensorineural and conductive hearing loss, as well as exposure to

Correspondence to:
Prof. David R Moore,
University Laboratory of
Physiology, Parks Road,
Oxford OX1 3PT, UK

'passive' auditory environments and 'active' auditory training and learning. While early auditory experience is still considered especially critical for normal development, a major change of thought in the last 10 years has been the recognition of a life-time dependency on auditory input, and the ability of the mature system to respond to clinical or experimental manipulation of that input.

Development of the auditory nervous system

The neural basis of hearing begins in the cochlear hair cells, where transduction channels in the tips of stereocilia pass K^+ and other cations in response to mechanical displacement of the organ of Corti (*see* reviews by Richardson and by Ashmore, this volume). The electrical driving force behind the transduction current, the endocochlear potential of the scala media, begins to function only a short period before the onset of functional hearing[5]. At the same time, the cochlear partition is maturing structurally, in a basal-to-apical direction. Paradoxically, the earliest neural responses recorded from the central auditory system are evoked by low frequency sounds (*e.g.* Aitkin and Moore[6]). This appears to result from an immaturity of cochlear mechanics, such that the peak of the travelling wave along the cochlear partition produced by a given frequency occurs more basally than is the case in adults[7]. Other significant neural developments in the cochlea include changes in the size and shape of the hair cells, and the acquisition of mature synaptic function. These latter developments impair initial auditory function by limiting, respectively, the highest stimulus frequency at which auditory neurones can phase lock, and the maximum rate of firing of single auditory nerve fibres[8]. In short, there are known structural and functional restrictions on the ability of the cochlea to function at all before a certain age, and to function in an adult-like way for some further period. It is not completely clear how long these developmental processes take in humans, but peripheral auditory function appears to mature by the end of the first few post-natal months (Fig. 1A)[9,10].

Developmental changes of function in the central auditory system, by contrast, appear to continue for several years. Neurones throughout the system show mature responses to single tones relatively soon after cochlear function begins[12] and, indeed, the capacity for neural function may precede that of cochlear function (*see* Romand[13]). However, hearing of some more complex sounds, such as temporally separated pairs[14,15], and performance on higher demand listening tasks (*e.g.* sound localization[16]) may remain immature well into the second decade of life (*see* Ponton *et al*[11]). One important, and increasingly recognised, issue in the interpretation of

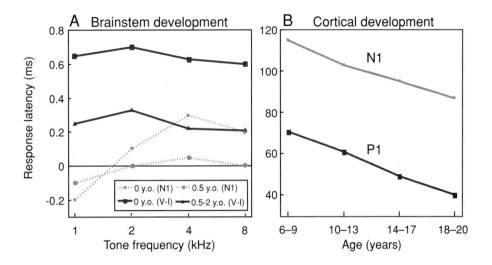

Fig. 1 Development of human central auditory physiology. Auditory evoked potentials recorded from (A) the auditory nerve (wave N_1 of the compound action potential) were, in terms of response latency (shown here, relative to adult values) and amplitude to tone stimuli, mature by the sixth postnatal month (0.5-year-old [y.o.]). The difference in latency between waves V and I of the auditory brainstem response (V–I) is a measure of conduction time from the cochlea to the midbrain. A substantial reduction in this conduction time occurred between a group tested at birth (0 y.o.) and a group tested at 6–24 months. Extrapolation of the V–I data yielded a final maturation age of 15–24 months, with responses to lower frequency tones developing more rapidly. In the auditory cortex (B), the N_1 and P_1 responses (see text) to click stimuli underwent substantial development into the second decade of life. Again, the measure is response latency, referenced to values for adult listeners. Adapted from Ponton et al[9,11].

behavioural studies of hearing is the extent to which performance reflects sensory and non-sensory factors. Cognitive influences (*e.g.* attention) may be developing in parallel with sensation and, without appropriate experimental control, give a misleading impression of immature function in the auditory system. On the other hand, a strict distinction between sensory and non-sensory influences on perception, even at relatively low levels of the brain, has recently been called into question by neuro-imaging studies of the human visual cortex[17]. Nevertheless, physiological studies in anaesthetised animals[18] and in awake humans[11] of neural responses to dichotic (*i.e.* binaurally discordant) or rapidly presented sounds suggest that much of the immaturity of hearing seen after birth does have a sensory basis, in the conventional sense.

The protracted immaturity of the human central auditory system (Fig. 1B) could be caused by several known factors. Both morphological[19] and physiological studies[9,11] indicate that development beyond the second to third year is a property of the higher, thalamocortical auditory system.

While cortical cyto-architecture develops early, myelination of the thalamic fibres innervating the auditory cortex begins around one year of age and progresses until the fourth year. Expression of cortical neuro-filament protein, forming the basis of the axonal cytoskeleton, continues to change through to the age of 5–10 years[19]. Conduction pathways are, therefore, immature for a protracted period of postnatal life and this will, of course, affect neural functions, such as auditory temporal processes. However, recent auditory evoked potential studies suggest that human thalamocortical function, as measured by the long-latency (40–200 ms) $P_1 - N_1 - P_2$ response sequence, continues to develop 'well into adolescence' according to Ponton *et al*[11]. Although the later components of these compound responses are notoriously difficult to localize, the P_1 response is thought to originate predominantly from the lateral portion of Heschl's gyrus and, therefore, represents a relatively

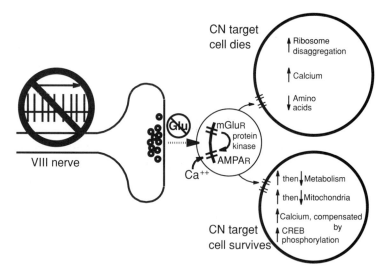

Fig. 2 Auditory experience may be thought of as neural activity generated in the cochlea and transmitted to the brain. Removal of auditory (VIIIth) nerve activity early in life abolishes glutamate (Glu) neurotransmission and causes some auditory brain stem neurones to die and some to survive. In the chicken cochlear nucleus (CN), the cellular processes underlying this experience-dependent regulation have been worked out in some detail. In the synapse, de-activation of metabotropic glutamate receptors (mGluRs) signals an increase in intracellular calcium levels via the AMPAR type of glutamate receptors. Neurones destined to die undergo other rapid responses to the de-activation, including ribosomal disaggregation and a decrease in amino acid incorporation. If input is restored within 1–2 days, the neurones can return to normal. Neurones that do not die nevertheless undergo a number of responses including soma shrinkage and an increase, followed by a decrease, of oxidative metabolism and mitochondrial density. Recently, an increased phosphorylation of a transcription factor (CREB) has been demonstrated. This may lead to compensation for the activity deprivation and thence to neurone survival. Again, if input is restored, the neurones can return to normal. Adapted from Garden *et al*[48] and Zirpel *et al*[49].

'low' level of auditory processing. Nevertheless, the P_1 and N_1 responses do not reach maturity until 14–15 years of age. The very late development of these responses, which involve a decrease in both amplitude and latency, may be related to decreasing synaptic density and dendritic elaboration in the auditory cortex[20]. However, insufficient anatomical data are available in the 5–15-year-old age range to form more definite conclusions.

The nature of auditory experience

We generally think of auditory experience as the sounds we hear. But neuroscientists think in terms of neural activity generated in the cochlea and transmitted to the brain (Fig. 2). Environmental sound (*e.g.* speech) will modulate and increase auditory nerve activity, conductive hearing loss (*e.g.* otosclerosis, otitis media) will decrease and desynchronize nerve activity, and sensorineural loss will reduce and broaden, or abolish nerve activity from damaged parts of the cochlea. The brain is affected by these input fluctuations in two ways. The first is, of course, that it will pass the information to, and through, the various centres of the auditory system for processing, and on into the cortex for understanding, integration and action (*see* Palmer and Summerfield, this volume). The second is that it will change the way in which the brain processes future input. These latter changes may be either beneficial, as occurs during developmental shaping of speech processing circuits, or detrimental, as when lack of stimulation produced by (untreated) deafness leads to neurodegeneration. In the following sections, I discuss in more detail recent thinking about these two contrasting roles of auditory experience in shaping the function of the auditory brain.

Bad auditory experience

The notion of 'critical' or 'sensitive' periods of development is well over 100 years old, but it is one that has undergone substantial recent revision. In hearing, there has been much progress in defining and characterizing a very early period during which clinical, surgical or chemical de-afferentation, resulting in total abolition of nerve activity, leads to wide-spread neurodegeneration in brain centres normally receiving direct input from the deaf ear (Fig. 2). In the cochlear nucleus of rodents, 50–70% of neurones have been found to die following cochlear removal before postnatal day (P) 10, where hearing begins at about P12[21,22]. This apoptotic neurone death is but the end stage of a complex cascade of intracellular events that is triggered within minutes

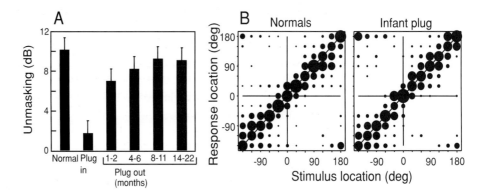

Fig. 3 Unilateral or asymmetric conductive hearing loss, as seen in middle ear disease in children and otosclerosis in adults, can lead to poor binaural hearing. In the laboratory, these diseases are modelled using ear plugs in experimental animals to control for variability and to investigate mechanisms. Ferrets receiving several months of unilateral ear plugging had reduced binaural unmasking for several more months after the plug was removed (A; adapted from Moore *et al*[27]). Sound localization abilities (B; from King *et al*[24]) show adaptation to the plug during plugging (as shown in the figure) but, surprisingly, there is no lasting impairment after plug removal. The latter result suggests that, in this case, altered experience leads to the formation of a parallel neural representation ('map') of space, rather than to re-ordering of an existing map.

of activity withdrawal. However, just before the time at which hearing normally begins, the short-term dependence of auditory neurones on afferent activity abruptly stops. Thereafter, total deafening leads to shrinkage of neurones, probably due to membrane responses to axon retraction, but little or no death of target neurones, at least over a time course of months to years. One rationale for early cochlear implantation has been the need to provide trophic support for central auditory neurones in the absence of afferent activity. The early cessation of extreme sensitivity to de-afferentation suggests the importance of providing that support very early in development, and a reduced urgency for support thereafter.

Sensitive periods for some other aspects of auditory system plasticity have been more difficult to establish, especially where the change in auditory experience has consisted of a conductive hearing loss or a modification of the auditory environment. In addition, there has been a general realisation in neuroscience over the last decade that some aspects of the brain's susceptibility to experience-dependent plasticity are maintained throughout life. This will come as no surprise to those familiar with the well-known capacity in the elderly for recovery from stroke. However, there has been a great increase recently in the power of methods available for observing and measuring the plasticity. The new technology includes functional magnetic resonance imaging (fMRI) in humans (see Griffiths, this volume), and direct, optical imaging of the living brains of animals[23].

The plasticity of binaural and spatial hearing has been studied behaviourally, using psycho-acoustic methods, and physiologically[24]. Although binaural hearing may be adversely affected by unilateral or asymmetric hearing loss, there is no clear evidence, in mammals, for an elevated susceptibility of the developing binaural system to abnormal experience. Clinically, both otosclerosis in adults and otitis media with effusion (OME) in children perturb binaural hearing. More surprisingly, poor auditory function at any age may persist beyond the time of the peripheral pathology[25,26]. These effects have also been demonstrated in the laboratory. For example, prolonged ear plugging can lead to poor sound localization and binaural unmasking, a measure of the detection of sounds in noisy environments (Fig. 3)[24,27]. When the plug is inserted, some adaptation (recovery of function) may occur but, following removal of the plug, performance may remain impaired. These results suggest that impoverished auditory experience produces a protracted difficulty in detecting sounds in noisy environments. This difficulty may contribute to the early language processing problems that have been reported[28] in some children with severe, recurrent OME.

Good auditory experience

The adaptive plasticity of the brain appears capable both of mediating recovery of auditory function after hearing loss and of improving function following auditory training. Children who have had recurrent OME, and who have persistent, impaired binaural hearing, gradually recover normal binaural function[29,30]. Adult human listeners who have the normal cues for sound localization distorted gradually 'adapt' to the new cues and regain normally accurate localization[31,32]. Most interestingly, ferrets that have had their auditory spatial localization disrupted by unilateral ear plugging gradually improve their localization if left in the home cage[33]. If, however, they are given additional training in sound localization, the improvement occurs more rapidly.

Each of these cases provides compelling evidence for an experience-dependent improvement in spatial hearing following earlier maladjust-ment. That the improvement is at least partly mediated by auditory system neural plasticity is suggested by animal experiments showing that a neural 'map' of auditory space in the midbrain is shifted by manipulating the input from the ears in a way that is predictable from the localization behaviour. In the barn owl, for example, recent experiments[34] have shown frequency-specific changes in the tuning of midbrain neurones to the binaural cues underlying sound localization following several months of wearing an acoustic device that alters the time and level cues independently. Other experiments on the plasticity of spatial hearing mechanisms in mammals suggest that neurones in both the midbrain[35] and the auditory cortex[36] are influenced by prior auditory experience.

Enhanced auditory experience has recently been shown to be a useful therapeutic tool. For many years, it has been known that subjects in psycho-acoustic and other sensory tasks improve their performance with practice. When those practice effects have been applied to training listening skills in children with language impairments, dramatic results have been reported[37,38]; (but see review by Bailey and Snowling, this volume). While the therapeutic effectiveness of this approach appears to be impressive, it is unclear whether the technique works through auditory perceptual learning or, more indirectly, through building up attention and other more general sensorimotor skills. Perceptual learning is thought to be highly specific to the trained stimulus, at least for some types of task[39]. A recent study that trained adults in the time and level cues for sound localization[40] has shown that the long-term, intensive training that is often considered necessary to obtain robust improvements is specific both for the stimulus frequency used during training and the type of cue trained. These findings suggest that sensory training will only be practically effective if the trained stimuli closely resemble the skill that the training is designed for. In the case of language training, this seems to indicate the use of appropriate linguistic stimuli rather than simpler signals of the type usually used in auditory research.

Deprivation followed by enhancement of 'auditory' experience in profoundly deaf people fitted with cochlear implants is thought to lead to the same cycle, and mechanisms, of neurodegeneration and recovery found in other examples of adaptive plasticity[41]. Traditionally, the focus of interest in implantation has centred on the design of the speech processor and how that interfaces with remaining neural elements in the cochlea. It is now more widely recognised that both the problem (deafness) and the solution (implantation) are also dependent on the central auditory system. For example, recent studies have shown that activation of the auditory cortex in congenitally deaf cats is substantially enhanced by long-term electrical stimulation of the cochlea. Animals deafened and stimulated at later ages seem not to respond as well to implantation, but it is unclear to what extent that limitation is due to more peripheral effects of the deafening[42].

Neuro-imaging techniques are beginning to capture the changes in brain activation in humans that accompany impaired or enhanced auditory experience. Unilateral, congenital deafness leads to changes in the symmetry of auditory cortex fMRI activation produced by stimulation of the functional ear[43]. Experience of cochlear implantation in adults following post-lingual deafness modifies activation of the auditory and temporal cortices[44]. Individuals with impaired auditory and/or linguistic function have correlated perturbations of sound processing in the auditory cortex[45,46]. Audiovisual training, matching simple non-linguistic sound sequences to patterns of rectangles on a computer screen, has been found to improve both reading skills and an electrophysiological indicator of cortical function (the 'mismatch negativity') in dyslexic children[47]. While these efforts to study the 'mechanisms' of auditory system plasticity are exciting, the results need to be interpreted with considerable caution. As noted above, it is not always clear just what aspect of the life experience of the affected individuals has led to the impaired, or enhanced, function. It is also uncertain how the changes in observed activation relate specifically to auditory function. From the viewpoint of auditory experience, it is also sometimes unclear what the direction of causation is when relating patterns of activation to hearing. Nevertheless, careful improvements in experimental design, and continually evolving technology, including data from two or three techniques (*e.g.* fMRI **and** auditory evoked potentials) for a single listener, hold the promise of significant advances in understanding the neural basis of auditory system plasticity over the coming few years.

Acknowledgements

I thank the Medical Research Council, the Wellcome Trust, Defeating Deafness, the John Ellerman Foundation, and the National Health Service for supporting our research. Doug Hartley, Sarah Hogan, Andy King, Carl Parsons, Jan Schnupp, Travis Tierney and Huib Versnel collaborated on work from our laboratory described in this paper.

References

1 Moore DR, Jeffery G. Development of auditory and visual systems in the fetus. In: Thorburn GD, Harding R. (eds) *Textbook of Fetal Physiology*. Oxford: Oxford University Press, 1994; 278–86

2 Sohmer H, Perez R, Sichel JY, Priner R, Freeman S. The pathway enabling external sounds to reach and excite the fetal inner ear. *Audiol Neurootol* 2001; **6**: 109–16

3 Rubel EW, Popper AN, Fay. RR (eds) *Development of the Auditory System. Springer Handbook of Auditory Research*, vol. 9, New York: Springer, 1998

4 Parks TN, Rubel EW, Popper AN, Fay RR. (eds) *Plasticity of the Auditory System. Springer Handbook of Auditory Research*, vol. 10. New York: Springer, 2002

5 Rübsamen R, Lippe WR. The development of cochlear function. In: Rubel EW, Popper AN, Fay RR. (eds) Development of the Auditory System. Springer Handbook of Auditory Research, vol. 9, New York: Springer, 1998; 193–270

6 Aitkin LM, Moore DR. Inferior colliculus. II. Development of tuning characteristics and tonotopic organization in central nucleus of the neonatal cat. *J Neurophysiol* 1975; **38**: 1208–16

7 Mills DM, Rubel EW. Development of the base of the cochlea: place code shift in the gerbil. *Hear Res* 1998; **122**: 82–96

8 Kettner RE, Feng JZ, Brugge JF. Postnatal development of the phase-locked response to low frequency tones of auditory nerve fibers in the cat. *J Neurosci* 1985; **5**: 275–83

9 Ponton CW, Eggermont JJ, Coupland SG, Winkelaar R. Frequency-specific maturation of the eighth nerve and brain-stem auditory pathway: evidence from derived auditory brain-stem responses (ABRs). *J Acoust Soc Am* 1992; **91**: 1576–86

10 Eggermont JJ, Brown DK, Ponton CW, Kimberley BP. Comparison of distortion product otoacoustic emission (DPOAE) and auditory brain stem response (ABR) traveling wave delay measurements suggests frequency-specific synapse maturation. *Ear Hear* 1996; **17**: 386–94

11 Ponton CW, Eggermont JJ, Kwong B, Don M. Maturation of human central auditory system activity: evidence from multi-channel evoked potentials. *Clin Neurophysiol* 2000; **111**: 220–36

12 Sanes DH, Walsh EJ. The development of central auditory processing. In: Rubel EW, Popper AN, Fay RR. (eds) *Development of the Auditory System. Springer Handbook of Auditory Research*, vol. 9, New York: Springer, 1998; 271–314

13 Romand R. *Development of Auditory and Vestibular Systems*. New York: Academic Press, 1983

14 Trehub SE, Schneider BA, Henderson JL. Gap detection in infants, children, and adults. *J Acoust Soc Am* 1995; **98**: 2532–41

15 Hartley DE, Wright BA, Hogan SC, Moore DR. Age-related improvements in auditory backward and simultaneous masking in 6- to 10-year-old children. *J Speech Lang Hear Res* 2000; **43**: 1402–15

16 Litovsky RY. Developmental changes in the precedence effect: estimates of minimum audible angle. *J Acoust Soc Am* 1997; **102**: 1739–45

17 Ress D, Backus BT, Heeger DJ. Activity in primary visual cortex predicts performance in a visual detection task. *Nat Neurosci* 2000; **3**: 940–5

18 Eggermont JJ. Differential maturation rates for response parameters in cat primary auditory cortex. *Aud Neurosci* 1996; **2**: 309–27

19 Moore JK, Guan YL. Cytoarchitectural and axonal maturation in human auditory cortex. *J Assoc Res Otolaryngol* 2001; **2**: 297–311

20 Huttenlocher PR, Dabholkar AS. Regional differences in synaptogenesis in human cerebral cortex. *J Comp Neurol* 1997; **387**: 167–78

21 Tierney TS, Russell FA, Moore DR. Susceptibility of developing cochlear nucleus neurones to deafferentation-induced death abruptly ends just before the onset of hearing. *J Comp Neurol* 1997; **378**: 295–306

22 Mostafapour SP, Del Puerto NM, Rubel EW. *bcl-2* Overexpression eliminates deprivation-induced cell death of brainstem auditory neurons. *J Neurosci* 2002; **22**: 4670–4

23 Versnel H, Mossop JE, Mrsic-Flögel T, Ahmed B, Moore DR. Optical imaging of intrinsic signals in ferret auditory cortex: responses to narrow-band sound stimuli. *J Neurophysiol* 2002; In press

24 King AJ, Parsons CH, Moore DR. Plasticity in the neural coding of auditory space in the mammalian brain. *Proc Natl Acad Sci USA* 2000; **97**: 11821–8

25 Hall JW, Grose JH. Short-term and long-term effects on the masking level difference following middle ear surgery. *J Am Acad Audiol* 1993; **4**: 307–12

26 Hogan SC, Moore DR. Impaired binaural hearing in children produced by a threshold level of middle ear disease. *J Assoc Res Otolaryngol* 2002; In press

27 Moore DR, Hine JE, Jiang ZD, Matsuda H, Parsons CH, King AJ. Conductive hearing loss produces a reversible binaural hearing impairment. *J Neurosci* 1999; **19**: 8704–11

28 Bluestone CD, Klein JO. *Otitis Media in Infants and Children*, 2nd edn. Philadelphia, PA: WB Saunders, 1995

29 Hall JW, Grose JH, Pillsbury HC. Long-term effects of chronic otitis media on binaural hearing in children. *Arch Otolaryngol Head Neck Surg* 1995; **121**: 847–52

30 Hogan SC, Meyer SE, Moore DR. Binaural unmasking returns to normal in teenagers who had otitis media in infancy. *Audiol Neurootol* 1996; **1**: 104–11

31 Hofman PM, Van Riswick JG, Van Opstal AJ. Relearning sound localization with new ears. *Nat Neurosci* 1998; **1**: 417–21

32 Shinn-Cunningham BG, Durlach NI, Held RM. Adapting to supernormal auditory localization cues. I. Bias and resolution. *J Acoust Soc Am* 1998; **103**: 3656–66

33 King AJ, Kacelnik O, Mrsic-Flögel TD, Schnupp JW, Parsons CH, Moore DR. How plastic is spatial hearing? *Audiol Neurootol* 2001; **6**: 182–6

34 Knudsen EI, Zheng W, DeBello WM. Traces of learning in the auditory localization pathway. *Proc Natl Acad Sci USA* 2000; **97**: 11815–20

35 Schnupp JW, King AJ, Carlile S. Altered spectral localization cues disrupt the development of the auditory space map in the superior colliculus of the ferret. *J Neurophysiol* 1998; **79**: 1053–69

36 Mrsic-Flögel TD, King AJ, Jenison RL, Schnupp JW. Listening through different ears alters spatial response fields in ferret primary auditory cortex. *J Neurophysiol* 2001; **86**: 1043–6

37 Merzenich MM, Jenkins WM, Johnston P, Schreiner C, Miller SL, Tallal P. Temporal processing deficits in language-learning impaired children ameliorated by training. *Science* 1996; **271**: 77–81

38 Tallal P, Miller SL, Bedi G *et al.* Language comprehension in language-learning impaired children improved with acoustically modified speech. *Science* 1996; **271**: 81–4

39 Wright BA, Buonomano DV, Mahncke HW, Merzenich MM. Learning and generalization of auditory temporal-interval discrimination in humans. *J Neurosci* 1997; **17**: 3956–63

40 Wright BA, Fitzgerald MB. Different patterns of human discrimination learning for two interaural cues to sound-source location. *Proc Natl Acad Sci USA* 2001; **98**: 12307–12

41 Shepherd RK, Illing RB. Cochlear implants and brain plasticity. *Audiol Neurootol* 2001; **6**: 299–396

42 Kral A, Hartmann R, Tillein J, Heid S, Klinke R. Delayed maturation and sensitive periods in the auditory cortex. *Audiol Neurootol* 2001; **6**: 346–62

43 Scheffler K, Bilecen D, Schmid N, Tschopp K, Seelig J. Auditory cortical responses in hearing subjects and unilateral deaf patients as detected by functional magnetic resonance imaging. *Cereb Cortex* 1998; **8**: 156–63

44 Giraud AL, Truy E, Frackowiak R. Imaging plasticity in cochlear implant patients. *Audiol Neurootol* 2001; **6**: 381–93

45 Temple E, Poldrack RA, Protopapas A *et al.* Disruption of the neural response to rapid acoustic stimuli in dyslexia: evidence from functional MRI. *Proc Natl Acad Sci USA* 2000; **97**: 13907–12

46 Ahissar E, Nagarajan S, Ahissar M, Protopapas A, Mahncke H, Merzenich MM. Speech comprehension is correlated with temporal response patterns recorded from auditory cortex. *Proc Natl Acad Sci USA* 2001; **98**: 13367–72

47 Kujala T, Karma K, Ceponiene R *et al.* Plastic neural changes and reading improvement caused by audiovisual training in reading-impaired children. *Proc Natl Acad Sci USA* 2001; **98**: 10509–14

48 Garden GA, Canady KS, Lurie DI, Bothwell M, Rubel EW. A biphasic change in ribosomal conformation during transneuronal degeneration is altered by inhibition of mitochondrial, but not cytoplasmic protein synthesis. *J Neurosci* 1994; **14**: 1994-2008.

49 Zirpel L, Janowiak MA, Veltri CA, Parks TN. AMPA receptor-mediated, calcium-dependent CREB phosphorylation in a subpopulation of auditory neurons surviving activity deprivation. *J Neurosci* 2000; **20**: 6267-75.

Cochlear implants and brain stem implants

Richard T Ramsden

Department of Otolaryngology, Head and Neck Surgery, Manchester Royal Infirmary, Manchester, UK

This chapter describes the development of two implantable prosthetic neuro-stimulators which, in the last 20 years, have revolutionised the management of severe-to-profound sensorineural deafness. We have witnessed their rapid evolution from the realms of esoteric laboratory abstraction, with many critics and little perceived clinical use, to a routine treatment which is safe, effective and, indeed, cost effective. It is one of the great triumphs of biomedical and surgical collaboration, and is without any doubt the greatest ever advance in the treatment of deafness.

The anatomy and physiology of the auditory pathways have been described in a previous special issue[1]. To summarise, a sound wave entering the ear causes the tympanic membrane and ossicular chain to vibrate. The stapes, the smallest and innermost of the three ossicles moves in-and-out in the oval window and is the interface between the middle and inner ears. The mechanical movements of the middle-ear sound-conducting apparatus are transmitted to the inner-ear fluids and a wave, the travelling wave of von Bekesy, passes up the cochlea to reach a maximum at a point determined by its frequency. For the process to continue, the physical energy of the travelling wave has to be converted into electrical energy that can be propagated through the auditory nerve to the brain stem and from there to the higher auditory centres. This process of transduction occurs in the organ of Corti. Depolarisation in the inner hair cells initiates transmission through the first order neurones, the cell bodies of which are in the spiral ganglion. The synapse with the second order neurone occurs in the cochlear nucleus which is situated in the lower pons cranial to the foramen of Luschka. The more cranial nuclear projections in the brain stem and auditory cortex are complex and a detailed understanding of their anatomy is not necessary for the understanding of this essay.

Many disease processes may lead to loss of hair cells in the organ of Corti. The commonest is the natural process of ageing in which there is a progressive loss of cells typically starting in the basal turn of the cochlea and advancing apically, accompanied by a hearing loss that initially affects the high frequencies and, with time, the middle and lower frequencies. These cells are incapable of spontaneous regeneration

Correspondence to:
Prof. Richard T Ramsden,
Professor of
Otolaryngology,
Department of
Otolaryngology, Head and
Neck Surgery, Manchester
Royal Infirmary,
Oxford Road,
Manchester M13 9WL, UK

(although there are hopes that some time in the next few decades neurotropic factors may be identified that might make this dream a possibility). Chronic noise exposure is another good example of progressive hair cell loss. In neither of these conditions does the hair cell loss become complete, so total hearing loss is unlikely and treatment with hearing aids may be effective. There are, however, a number of conditions in which total or near total loss of the organ of Corti may occur and the most common are listed in Table 1. It will be seen that these are all acquired conditions and may affect both adults and children. To these must be added a number of causes of total deafness that are present at birth or soon after birth, and, of these, recessively inherited non-syndromic deafness is the commonest. Whatever the cause, the absence of the organ of Corti prevents transduction and, although all other components of the auditory system may be intact, profound deafness results.

The cochlear implant is a device that takes over the role of mechano-electric transduction and delivers to the auditory nerve a processed signal that can be transmitted to the auditory cortex and interpreted as sound. There are two recognizable components of a typical cochlear implant system: (i) the implanted electrode array with associated microcircuitry; and (ii) the external component that refines the raw signal before delivering it to the implanted electrode. In the early days, the cochlea was regarded as inviolable, and fairly simple single channel analogue systems were inserted on to the surface of the cochlea. The modern electrode system is multichannel with up to 22 electrodes and is inserted into the scala tympani of the cochlea. It takes advantage of the highly developed tonotopicity of the cochlea with an orderly progression from high frequencies at the basal end of the cochlea to low frequencies at the apical, like a piano keyboard. Digitised processing is now almost universal. The external component comprises a microphone that sends an electrical signal to the 'brains' of the system – the speech processor.

Table 1 Causes of acquired severe/profound cochlear deafness

- Idiopathic (cause cannot be identified)
- Meningitis
- Viral infection of the inner ear (*e.g.* measles, mumps, rubella, CMV)
- Bacterial labyrinthitis complicating middle ear sepsis
- Menière's disease
- Ototoxic drugs (*e.g.* aminoglycoside antibiotics)
- Skull base fracture
- Cochlear otosclerosis
- Auto-immunity
- Iatrogenic (*e.g.* following stapedectomy)

There are many different strategies employed by the various manufacturers, but the aim of speech processing is to manipulate the raw signal so that the most important features necessary for speech recognition are preserved and delivered to the ear. Underlying early speech processing strategies was the recognition that there are various bands (or formants) of spectral energy in speech. Low frequency information corresponds to the vowel sounds and contributes to the prosodic patterns of speech. The higher frequencies convey consonant information which is essential for speech recognition. Modern strategies try to convey the time-varying spectral patterns that are characteristic of speech by analyzing the signal in short time frames and signalling the most prominent spectral peaks in each frame. The other factor that influences the fidelity of the signal delivered to the ear is the rate at which speech is sampled and digitized by the speech processor. Of the current generation of cochlear implant systems, the maximum stimulus rate, summed across all electrodes and using pulsatile stimulation is approximately 96,000 s^{-1}. The processed signal is transmitted through the intact skin by a process of inductive coupling. An external coil is held magnetically over an internal coil that is part of the implanted component of the system. A microchip decodes the incoming wave form and directs it to the appropriate intracochlear electrode or electrodes depending on the frequency of the sound, and at a rate determined by the specification of the individual processing programme.

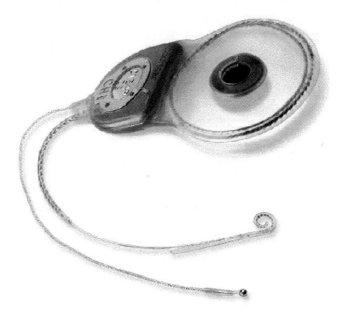

Fig. 1 Implanted component of the Nucleus CI24 system.

Devices implanted in the body should be reliable, safe and last for many years – in the case of a child, that means life (Fig. 1). Experience gained from pacemaker technology has proved invaluable, particularly in providing water-tight ceramic or silastic sealing systems for the electronics and cumulative failure rates of as little as 3% at 10 years are quoted by most manufacturers. Many implant programmes round the world have been operating for 15 years and most devices have continued to function without trouble. Implants that do fail can be replaced usually without difficulty and without loss in performance. Most of the important recent advances in implant design relate to speech processing strategies rather than the design of the implantable component. This means that performance with an early implant system can be improved by replacing or modifying the external component, rather than removing and replacing the intracochlear electrode. Advances in electrode design have been somewhat less spectacular. At present, the major manufacturers are pre-occupied with developing so-called 'modiolus-hugging' electrodes. As their name suggests, these are designed to lie close to the spiral ganglion and to the residual neural elements within the cochlea that the implant aims to stimulate. Their alleged advantages are more precise stimulus delivery and reduced power consumption. Neither of these claims can, as yet, stand up to close scrutiny, and many surgeons have fears that the new electrodes may traumatize the cochlea.

Who is suitable for a cochlear implant?

There are two main groups of candidates for implantation: (i) postlingually deafened adults; and (ii) prelingually or congenitally deaf children. To understand the issues relating to these two groups, it helps to understand the process of speech and language development in the normally hearing child. At birth, the child is not capable of speech, but by the age of a year babbling commences and by 18 months recognizable words begin to appear. From then on lexical, grammatical and semantic skills are acquired at a staggering rate, and this capacity remains immense during childhood. During this time, the auditory pathways are in a state of maximum plasticity. This facility wanes as the teens approach and is almost lost by mid-teenage. A normally hearing child, deprived of the sound of human speech during this critical period, and restored to it in adult life would be unable to acquire normal speech despite having normal peripheral auditory function. This phenomenon is similar to that observed in strabismic children who develop amblyopia[2]. Adults who lose their hearing after the critical period already have a programmed auditory cortex. A cochlear implant rapidly re-activates dormant neural

Table 2 Factors to be considered in cochlear implant assessment

- Severity of hearing loss
- Benefit from hearing aids
- Age and duration of deafness
- Linguistic status
- Imaging of cochlea and auditory pathways (CT, MRI)
- General health
- Cognitive impairment
- Expectations and motivation

networks. This is clearly observable in the many adults who can converse almost effortlessly within hours of 'switch-on'. Additional improvement occurs in many as a result of subsequent cortical re-organization. For an implant to be effective in a congenitally or prelingually deafened child, it has to be inserted while the auditory system is still plastic or programmable. There is convincing evidence that the earlier a child is implanted the better the improvement in auditory performance[3]. The extent of neuronal survival is clearly an important determinant of outcome, and it must also be recognized that electrical stimulation (from the implant) prevents further neural degeneration. Most cochlear implant programmes like to implant children as early as possible usually around the age of 2 years.

Implant candidates are assessed in some detail by the implant team (Table 2). Cochlear implant technology is expensive and the process of rehabilitation involves the skills of many professionals. As a result, the cost to the National Health Service of an implant with assessment, surgery and 2 years of rehabilitation is in the region of £30,000. An appropriate and rigorous selection process is, therefore, desirable. A number of criteria are considered.

Degree of deafness

This is always the first and most important consideration – is the hearing loss bad enough to warrant an implant or could as good a result be obtained with conventional hearing aids? Criteria are changing as implant technology improves. Fifteen years ago, the typical implantee was a postlingually deafened adult with a pure tone threshold of 100–110 dB and no speech discrimination (profound deafness). Now, teams are implanting patients who are still deriving some limited benefit from their hearing aids. Their maximum speech discrimination score in the best-aided condition might well be in the region of 20–40% (using material such as Bench, Kowal, Bamford sentences). In the paediatric population, there are problems in assessing hearing thresholds and thus candidacy. Behavioural audiometry may be difficult or impossible. Objective audiometry, notably the Auditory Brain Stem Response (ABR), is widely used in assessment, but cannot as yet give accurate information about the low frequency thresholds. Speech audiometry is clearly out of the question in a prelingually deaf child with no lexical base. For these reasons, assessment of the rate of development of auditory performance over time is often necessary, particularly acquisition of language using hearing aids during a trial period which may last several months.

Age of the patient and duration of deafness

In postlingually deafened adults, age is relatively unimportant. Duration of deafness is, however, and the longer the period of auditory isolation the less good the outcome is likely to be[4]. It is impossible to set firm rules but a 55-year old, deaf for 40 years is a less favourable prospect than a 70-year-old, deaf for 5 years. The age of a congenitally deaf child is important for the reasons explained above. It is unlikely that a congenitally totally deaf child over the age of 7 years would do well with an implant, and congenitally deaf adolescents are bad candidates.

Imaging

High quality CT and MR imaging is essential to provide details of the anatomy of the cochlea and its connections, and may reveal a number of absolute or relative contra-indications to implantation. Congenital malformations (dysplasias) or acquired conditions such as cochlear obliteration, temporal bone fracture or otosclerosis should be reliably identifiable using the current generation of scanners.

General health

Common-sense rules about suitability for general anaesthesia and reasonable life expectancy apply. Of particular importance is an evaluation of central or cognitive function which may reveal potential difficulties with information processing with the implant. This is an issue after meningitis and with deaf and multiply handicapped children, more and more of whom are being referred for assessment. Each child has to be looked at on his or her merits.

Motivation, expectations and cultural issues

It is important that individuals contemplating implantation for themselves or for their children should have a realistic view of what the outcomes are likely to be. Exalted expectations are often perpetuated by the tabloid press. It is the job of the team to temper enthusiasm with realism, based on what can be predicted from knowledge of the individual subject. It is particularly important for parents to have some idea of the on-going nature of rehabilitation and that hard work is needed by them as well as the rehabilitation team and the child's teachers over a period of many years.

Many of these factors are only relative contra-indications, but taken together they allow the team to give an informed opinion to the patient or to parents of a child about likely outcome, and enlighten the discussions that precede a final decision about whether to proceed with surgery.

Surgery

The operation to insert the internal component of the cochlear implant system, the actual implant, has to be meticulously performed, but is well within the capability of most otologists. Through a small postauricular incision, a cortical mastoidectomy is performed and the middle ear is entered through the facial recess – the so-called posterior tympanotomy. The stapes can then usually be easily identified and 2 mm below it is the round window niche. The scala tympani of the basal turn of the cochlea is entered by drilling in front of the round window niche with a 1–1.5 mm microdrill. Usually a perilymph-filled cavity is encountered into which the electrode array can be gently introduced. As discussed previously, the latest generation of electrode arrays has a mechanism to carry it close to the modiolus and the spiral ganglion. The package comprising the receiver coil and the microchip is recessed into a bony well in the outer table of the skull, and the overlying pericranium usually provides sufficient stability without the need for anchoring ties. The operation takes about 1.5 h and, at the end of the procedure, the electrical integrity of the device can be tested by a number of measures including neural response telemetry. Using this technique, whole nerve action potentials are recorded from the auditory nerve in response to stimulation of individual electrodes within the cochlea. The information thus obtained may help the rehabilitation team in the initial estimation of threshold values of stimulation at the time of switch-on of the device, as well as confirming the integrity of each channel in the array. The incidence of postoperative complications is very low. Although the facial nerve is in the surgical field, as indeed it is with most tympanomastoid surgery, damage to it is very rare with an incidence of under 0.5%.

Special surgical problems

Surgical difficulties may be encountered in a number of well recognized conditions.

Inner ear dysplasia

The most extreme form of dysplasia, aplasia, is a contra-indication to implantation and would be picked up on pre-operative imaging. At the other end of the scale, the Mondini deformity and the large vestibular aqueduct syndrome are usually not difficult to implant. Between these extremes, the common cavity deformity in which there is little differentiation of the cochlea beyond the primitive otocyst stage is challenging, with the possibility of inadvertently inserting the implant into the posterior cranial fossa through the inner ear. Associated with this is a high risk of CSF fistula. Furthermore, in such cases of dysplasia, the facial nerve may be abnormally placed and be at increased risk. Aplasia of the auditory nerve is rare, but needs to be recognised (on MR imaging) as it is an absolute contra-indication to cochlear implantation.

Cochlear obliteration (osteoneogenesis)

In a number of conditions, the cochlear lumen may become obliterated, either by fibrous tissue or new bone, making insertion of the implant difficult, if not impossible. Meningitis, otosclerosis and skull-base fracture are associated with the deposition of new bone. Autoimmune ear disease may be associated with intracochlear fibrosis. Modified surgical techniques and electrodes have been developed to deal with these problems.

Chronic middle ear and mastoid disease

Insertion of a foreign object into the body is contra-indicated in the presence of active infection. Tympanomastoid disease, if present, including cholesteatoma must be eliminated at a first stage operation and the implant inserted at a subsequent date.

Switch-on and tuning

About 1 month after the operation, when the skin is well healed, the implant is connected to the external component and tuned up. Each electrode in the cochlea has an electrical threshold at which the stimulus is just perceived as sound. It also has a higher level at which the stimulus just ceases to be comfortable. These are the T and C levels and the difference between them is referred to as the 'dynamic range'.

The process of establishing T and C levels for all 22 electrodes and entering them into the memory of the speech processor is called 'mapping' and requires the skills of the audiological and rehabilitation members of the cochlear implant team. Mapping is usually straight-forward in adults, but can require considerable skill and patience with small prelingual children whose lack of language means that they have to be programmed using conditioning techniques. If one sets the levels too low, nothing will be heard; if too high, a non-auditory response such as pain or facial twitching may occur, which will upset the child and ensure the end of his or her co-operation in the whole mapping process. Mapping has to be repeated on a number of occasions in the first weeks and months since the psychophysical features of the auditory system change as a result of stimulation by the implant.

Outcomes

Nearly all implanted postlingually deafened adults achieve some degree of open set speech understanding using the implant alone (*i.e.* without lip reading); most achieve a high level of performance within a matter of weeks and can use the telephone with a fair degree of proficiency. Cochlear implantation in adults has been shown to be cost effective. Summerfield and Marshall calculated the cost per quality adjusted life year (QALY) for cochlear implantation and a number of other common conditions. As can be seen in Table 3, cochlear implantation compares very favourably[5].

It is becoming increasingly clear that the majority of congenitally or prelingually deaf children implanted by the age of 2 years are able to take their place in main stream schools after 3 years of implant use and training, albeit with some degree of support. Speech perception and

Table 3 The cost per quality adjusted life year (QALY) for cochlear implantation and a number of other common conditions

Treatment	Cost/QALY (US$)	Cost/QALY (UK£)
Cochlear implant	15,593	11,440
Coronary artery bypass graft (3 vessel disease)	11,255	2090
Heart transplantation	38,970	7840
Coronary artery bypass graft (1 vessel)	64,033	18,830
Peritoneal dialysis	83,011	19,870
Haemodialysis	86,198	21,970

production continue to improve with time and most develop the accents and modulations of their geographical regions and peer groups.

The auditory brain stem implant (ABI)

This development from cochlear implant technology is indicated for totally deaf individuals who have no auditory nerves and who are thus not candidates for a cochlear implant. In practice, this patient group comprises almost exclusively sufferers from neurofibromatosis type 2 (NF2) who have been deafened as a result of bilateral vestibular schwannomas (acoustic neuromas) or from the surgery to remove them. Other possible indications may emerge such as cochlear nerve agenesis or the unimplantable cochlea from excessive ossification. The ABI has an electrode carrier with 20 small disc electrodes (Fig. 2) and is inserted on to the surface of the cochlear nucleus in the lateral recess of the fourth ventricle, accessed through the foramen of Luschka. Technically, this is not easy, as surgical landmarks are not always obvious. The correct position of the implant is verified by eliciting the electrically evoked auditory brain stem response (EABR). Adjacent cranial nerves (facial, glossopharyngeal, accessory and trigeminal) are monitored to minimise the risk of non-auditory stimulation. From the point of view of neuro-anatomy, there is a major problem with the frequency maps, or tonotopicity, of the cochlear nucleus compared with the cochlea. A surface electrode will function most effectively if the frequency map is distributed across the surface of the nucleus. In the cochlear nucleus, the map is disposed obliquely through the depths of the nucleus, and to take advantage of this arrangement a penetrating electrode has been developed but as yet it has not been used in clinical trials.

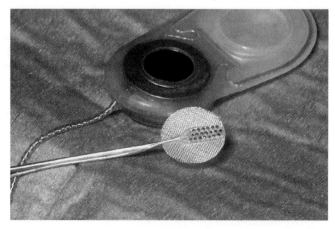

Fig. 2 The auditory brain stem implant with 20 disc electrodes on dacron carrier.

Multicentre trials with the surface electrode array have been carried out in North America and in Europe[6,7]. They indicate that outcomes with the ABI are not as good as typical cochlear implant results. Nevertheless, most patients gained an awareness of environmental sounds and found the ABI enhanced their lip reading scores. A small, but important, number obtained reasonable-to-good open set speech perception using the implant alone and some obtain limited telephone use. Unwanted non-auditory side-effects such as facial twitching, pain in the throat, face or body may occur with some electrodes, but these can be programmed-out at mapping sessions.

Future developments

The near future should see the development of totally implantable devices that use either an intrinsic power source or implanted batteries that can be recharged remotely through intact skin. Similarly, remote re-programming would be possible. Research is also well advanced into mechanisms for delivering drugs or neurotrophic factors to the cochlea and auditory system through the intracochlear electrode[8]. Of course, if hair cells could be encouraged to regenerate, which again is the subject of much research, cochlear implantation would become a curiosity of medical history.

References

1   Haggard MP, Evans EF. Hearing. *Br Med Bull* 1987; **43**
2   Ryugo DK, Limb CJ, Redd EE. Brain plasticity. In: Niparko J. (ed) *Cochlear Implants: Principles and Practices*. Philadelphia, PA: Lippincott Williams and Wilkins, 2000
3   O'Neill CO, O'Donoghue GM, Archbold SM, Nikolopoulos TP, Sach T. Variations in gains in auditory performance from paediatric cochlear implantation. *Otol Neurotol* 2002; **23**: 44–8
4   Summerfield AQ, Marshall DH. *Cochlear Implantation in the UK 1990–1994*. London: HMSO, 1995; 144
5   Summerfield AQ, Marshall DH. *Cochlear Implantation in the UK 1990–1994*. London: HMSO, 1995; 227–8
6   Otto SR, Shannon RV, Brackmann DE *et al*. The multichannel auditory brainstem implant: performance in 20 patients. *Otolaryngol Head Neck Surg* 1998; **118**: 291–303
7   Nevison B, Laszig R, Sollmann W-P *et al*. Results from a European clinical investigation of the Nucleus multichannel auditory brainstem implant. *Ear Hear* 2002; In press
8   Clark GM. Cochlear implants in the third millennium. *Am J Otol* 1999; **20**: 4–8

Mechanisms of tinnitus

David M Baguley

Audiology Department, Addenbrooke's Hospital, and Centre for the Neural Basis of Hearing, Physiological Laboratory, University of Cambridge, Cambridge, UK

The generation of tinnitus is a topic of much scientific enquiry. This chapter reviews possible mechanisms of tinnitus, whilst noting that the heterogeneity observed within the human population with distressing tinnitus means that there may be many different mechanisms by which tinnitus can occur. Indeed, multiple mechanisms may be at work within one individual. The role of the cochlea in tinnitus is considered, and in particular the concept of discordant damage between inner and outer hair cells is described. Biochemical models of tinnitus pertaining to the cochlea and the central auditory pathway are considered. Potential mechanisms for tinnitus within the auditory brain are reviewed, including important work on synchronised spontaneous activity in the cochlear nerve. Whilst the number of possible mechanisms of tinnitus within the auditory system is considerable, the identification of the physiological substrates underlying tinnitus is a crucial element in the design of novel and effective therapies.

Hypotheses regarding mechanisms of tinnitus generation abound. Given the heterogeneity observed in the tinnitus population[1], it may be considered that no single theory, model or hypothesis will explain the presence of tinnitus in all those affected. Thus, the mechanisms described in this chapter are not mutually exclusive, and multiple mechanisms may be present in an individual with tinnitus. The focus of this review is upon physiological mechanisms of tinnitus generation rather than the psychological impact that tinnitus may have, or therapies and treatments.

The word tinnitus derives from the Latin *tinnire* meaning 'to ring', and in English is defined as 'a ringing in the ears'[2]. In an attempt at a scientific definition, McFadden[3] considered that: 'tinnitus is the conscious expression of a sound that originates in an involuntary manner in the head of its owner, or may appear to him to do so'. This definition has been widely adopted.

Tinnitus is a common experience in adults and children. Adult data from the MRC Institute of Hearing Research[4] indicate that, in the UK, 10% of adults have experienced prolonged spontaneous tinnitus, and that in 5% of adults tinnitus is reported to be moderately or severely annoying. In 1% of the adult population, tinnitus has a severe effect on quality of life. The incidence data from the MRC study indicate that 7% of the UK adult population have consulted their doctor about tinnitus, and 2.5% have

Correspondence to:
Mr David M Baguley,
Audiology Department
(Box 94), Addenbrooke's
Hospital, Hills Road,
Cambridge CB2 2QQ, UK

attended a hospital with regard to tinnitus. Up to one-third of children experience occasional tinnitus, and in approximately 10% tinnitus has been bothersome[5].

A complex relationship between epidemiological factors and tinnitus has been identified[4]. The prevalence of tinnitus increases with age and with hearing impairment. Women are more likely to report tinnitus than men, and occupational noise and lower socio-economic class are also associated with increased tinnitus. These factors are not independent of each other, and further work is needed in this area.

A large number of descriptors of tinnitus have been reported, the most common being hissing, sizzling and buzzing, these reflecting the clinical finding that tinnitus is usually high pitched. An individual may localise tinnitus to one ear or other, to both, within the head or occasionally external to the head. In a clinical context, many individuals may hear more than one tinnitus sound.

Tinnitus is an element of the symptom profile of several significant otological pathologies (such as otosclerosis, vestibular schwannoma and Menière's disease) that necessitate medical or surgical treatment. Whilst such conditions are rare within both the general and tinnitus-complaint populations, there is a consensus that an informed clinical opinion should be sought by an individual with troublesome tinnitus (especially when unilateral) in order to exclude such pathologies. This review does not consider pathology-specific mechanisms other than the cochlear dysfunction implicated in sensorineural hearing loss.

Cochlear models

Any model which considered the cochlea in isolation from the rest of the auditory pathway in relation to tinnitus would not now be considered adequate, but there are situations where cochlear dysfunction has been implicated in tinnitus generation.

Spontaneous oto-acoustic emissions

The concept that a normal healthy cochlea may produce low intensity tonal or narrow-band sound in the absence of any acoustic stimulation (spontaneous oto-acoustic emissions, SOAEs) was introduced by Gold in 1948[6] as an element of a model of active processes within the cochlea. The identification of such activity[7] (see Kemp this volume) was greeted with enthusiasm by the scientific community concerned with tinnitus as 'our hope was that they corresponded to their owner's tinnitus and thus, at long last, we could measure tinnitus objectively'[8].

This hope was not well founded, as it became clear that whilst 38–60% of normal-hearing adults have measurable SOAEs, the majority of such individuals are not aware of this activity[9]. Penner and Burns[10] noted that when SOAEs do occur in the ear of a tinnitus patient, they rarely correspond to the judged frequency of the tinnitus. These authors considered that if a SOAE could be suppressed by a suitable low-level external tone without affecting the tinnitus perception, and, conversely, if tinnitus could be masked in an individual without affecting the SOAE, then the inference of physiological independence could be made. This suppression/masking paradigm has been used to determine the incidence of tinnitus complaint caused by SOAEs. Penner[11] found that 4.1% of a series of tinnitus patients ($n = 96$) had tinnitus originating as an SOAE. Baskill and Coles[12] found an incidence of 2%, and Coles (cited in Penner[13]) of 4.5%.

One additional piece of evidence that SOAEs are not largely responsible for tinnitus generation is as follows. SOAEs are largely abolished by aspirin (salicylate)[14], but tinnitus perception is not generally improved by salicylate, there being only one report of such an experience[15], this in a case where SOAE and tinnitus were demonstrably linked. Penner[13] notes that the treatment of SOAE-generated tinnitus with salicylate is done at the risk of ototoxic hearing loss and the possible generation of new tinnitus perceptions.

Discordant damage of IHC and OHC

Jastreboff[16] noted that intense noise and ototoxic agents initially damage the basal turn of the cochlea, and outer hair cells (OHCs), and only later affect inner hair cells (IHCs) if continued or repeated, IHCs being more resistant to such damage[17]. The inference was made that, within a partially affected organ of Corti, there will be an area with both OHCs and IHCs affected, an area with OHCs are affected but IHCs are intact, and an area with both intact. In the second of these three categories, the coupling between the tectorial membrane and the basilar membrane would be affected, to the extent that the tectorial membrane might directly impinge upon the cilia of the IHCs, thus causing them to depolarise. Clinical support for such modification of auditory afferent activity leading to tinnitus perception has been cited, in that some patients with tinnitus and high-frequency hearing loss match their tinnitus frequency to the point at which the loss begins[18,19]. The role that increased neural activity in the auditory periphery may have in tinnitus generation is considered in detail below. Jastreboff[20] went on to consider not only the afferent activity generated by the IHCs, but also the possibility that afferent activity of the IHCs might be interpreted in the light of attempted (but failed) reduction of cochlear gain via OHCs, giving rise to increased perceived intensity. It was further suggested that this model might apply to both permanent and temporary discordant damage, the example of temporary damage being temporary tinnitus associated with temporary threshold shift following noise exposure. Chery-Croze et al[21] noted that, in an area where IHC damage was present, any efferent inhibition of the OHCs in that area will be reduced due to the reduced afferent input. That efferent innervation may be shared with neighbouring OHCs partnering undamaged IHCs, due to the diffuse nature of efferent innervation (one fibre for 20–30 OHCs), and so the undamaged area neighbouring the damaged IHCs may also have reduced efferent inhibition, giving rise to a highly active area of the basilar membrane, resulting in tonal tinnitus.

LePage[22] suggested an alternative mechanism by which an area of the basilar membrane with damaged OHCs but intact IHCs might contribute to tinnitus generation. The role of the normal OHCs in fixing the operating point of IHCs was considered, that is an ability of OHCs to control the sensitivity of IHCs by setting the operating point on the IHCs' transfer characteristic to a value which the brain normally interprets as no sound. This point would not actually correspond to zero sound input, but a sound level regarded as background. A loss of motility in OHCs might reduce the ability to set the operating point of the IHCs appropriately, thus causing a 'virtual' sound input, so that this normally inaudible activity might be perceived as tinnitus. If this were to occur over a short length of the basilar membrane, the perception would be interpreted according to the tonotopic frequency normally transduced at that point, and hence would be tonal. LePage notes that if there were functional OHCs adjacent to the dysfunctional OHCs, then no loss of audiometric sensitivity might be evident. Zenner and Ernst[23] suggested that tinnitus generated by such a mechanism should be classified as 'DC motor tinnitus'.

A further role for OHC in tinnitus has been suggested by Patuzzi[24], who noted that OHC dysfunction may cause excessive release of neurotransmitter from IHCs following an increase in the endocochlear potential. This phenomenon might then lead to a 'rate tinnitus', so called because of the excessive rate of glutamate release from IHCs. Patuzzi predicted that the tinnitus percept would have a 'hiss' quality.

Biochemical models

A biochemical model of peripheral tinnitus has recently been proposed[25] based partly on the clinical observation that adult humans with distressing tinnitus have experiences of agitation, stress and anxiety, and partly on cochlear neurochemistry. Endogenous dynorphins (associated with stress) are postulated to potentiate the excitatory function of glutamate within the cochlea, mimicking the action of sodium salicylate in increasing spontaneous neural activity.

The biochemistry of the central auditory system has also been considered in the tinnitus literature. A role for serotonin (5-HT) in persistent tinnitus was postulated by Simpson and Davies[26], based on the consideration that disrupted or modified 5-HT function might cause a reduction in auditory filtering abilities and in tinnitus habituation (see later). The identification of a role of 5-HT in persistent distressing tinnitus is important as it may facilitate the development of effective pharmacological intervention. The need for investigation of the effect of selective serotonin re-uptake inhibitors upon tinnitus is urgent[27].

Non-cochlear mechanisms of tinnitus generation

Considerable attention has been paid to the possible involvement of cochlear mechanisms in tinnitus generation, but in recent years the interest of the scientific community has shifted towards retro-cochlear and central mechanisms[16,28–31]. In many cases, the models and hypotheses proposed do not preclude a role for the cochlea, but have as their primary concern neural mechanisms of tinnitus generation and persistence.

Jastreboff neurophysiological model

In a review of tinnitus from a neurophysiological perspective, Jastreboff[16] considered a role for 'signal recognition and classification circuits' in persistent tinnitus, that function as neural networks becoming tuned to the tinnitus signal, even when that signal is transitory, fluctuating or intermittent. It was suggested that cochlear processes might be involved in the generation of weak tinnitus-related activity, but since the majority of individuals with normal hearing perceive tinnitus-like sound in quiet surroundings[32], it was not necessary for a lesion of the auditory system to be present for tinnitus to be heard. The Jastreboff 'neurophysiological model', which involves the auditory perceptual, emotional and reactive systems involved in tinnitus, was published in 1996[33] and in slightly more detailed form (Fig. 1) in 1999[34]. In many individuals after a short period of awareness of tinnitus-related activity, a process of habituation occurs, such that the activity is no longer consciously perceived. However, in cases where there is some 'negative emotional re-inforcement', described as fear, anxiety or tension, limbic system and autonomic activation cause the activity to be enhanced and perception

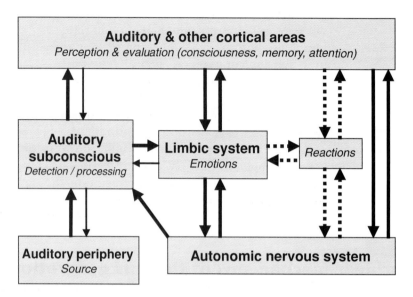

Fig. 1 Diagrammatic representation of the Jastreboff neurophysiological model[34] (with permission).

persists. The distinction between the perception of, and the behavioural and emotional reaction to, tinnitus was explicit, as was the potential for a feed-back loop between these processes. A treatment protocol arising from this perspective, and based upon facilitating habituation to both the tinnitus signal and to the reaction to that perception, has been entitled Tinnitus Retraining Therapy[33]. The Jastreboff model has been widely accepted as a synthesis that has utility for patients, clinicians and researchers alike. Whilst direct empirical evidence to support this model has not been forthcoming, the concepts involved are congruent with a modern understanding of the auditory system. A potential criticism is that the model does not represent the full complexity and dynamism of the human auditory system, but if the primary aim was a model of tinnitus that was easily understood by patients then this may have been intentional.

Increased neural activity

Evans *et al*[35] noted that then contemporary theories of tinnitus generation made the assumption, either implicit or explicit, that it was associated with spontaneous overactivity of the cochlear nerve. This was at odds with the literature which indicated that experimentally induced chronic cochlear pathology resulted in a decrease in such spontaneous activity. Such a decrease had been reported by Kiang *et al*[36] on the basis of a study involving kanamycin-deafened cats. Evans *et al*[35], however, reported that doses of salicylate in the cat equivalent to blood-concentration doses known to induce tinnitus in humans (in excess of 300–400 mg/l) had the effect of increasing spontaneous activity. Tyler[37] noted the different methodology of these studies, and that the recording from single units in the cochlear nerve might miss hyperactivity occurring elsewhere. Eggermont[30] also considered the discrepancy between these findings, and concluded that increased spontaneous activity in the human cochlear nerve was unlikely to be involved in tinnitus generation (assuming that animal data can be applied to humans) since tinnitus-inducing events in humans are as likely to reduce spontaneous activity as increase it.

Increased neural activity at levels above the cochlear nerve may be implicated in tinnitus generation. Increases in spontaneous activity in the dorsal cochlear nucleus (DCN) in the golden hamster after intense sound exposure have been reported[38–40]. Salvi *et al*[41] subjected chinchillas to intense sound exposure (2 kHz tone, 105 dB SPL, 30 min) and reported increases of spontaneous activity in the inferior colliculus and the dorsal cochlear nucleus; in addition, they noted tonotopic re-organisation in these structures. Increased activity in the inferior colliculus has also been reported after salicylate administration in the rat[42] and the guinea pig[43]. Chen *et al*[44] studied the effect of intense sound exposure (125 dB SPL, 10 kHz tone, 4 h) on spontaneous activity in the DCN of the rat. They found an increase in bursting spontaneous activity and a decrease in regular (simple spiking) spontaneous activity. The authors suggested that such activity might represent increased auditory efferent activity.

Increased cortical activity in the gerbil following salicylate administration has been demonstrated using 2-deoxyglucose methods[45] and c-fos immunochemistry[46], one study[43] using impulse noise as well as salicylate to induce cochlear dysfunction. Wallhausser-Franke and Langner[47] also noted evidence of increased activity in the amygdalae of these animals, and considered this a response to induced tinnitus, though they noted that the changes may have been produced by the stress of the animals. Langner and Wallhauser-Franke[48] proposed a model for tinnitus generation based on these findings. The lack of increased activity in the ventral cochlear nucleus (VCN)[49] after salicylate administration was claimed as evidence that the reported effects of salicylate are not due to increased afferent activity in the cochlear nerve. The altered activity reported in the DCN was suggested to result either from increased efferent activity from the cortex or inferior colliculus (IC), or from a lack of inhibition from other cochlear nucleus units. The amplification of spontaneous activity within this feedback loop, influenced also by processes of attention (involving the reticular formation) and the limbic system (specifically the amygdala) was thought to be the cause of tinnitus perception.

A mechanism of disinhibition in the IC and DCN has been proposed[30,50]. In the DCN type II/III, interneurones act in an inhibitory manner upon spontaneously active type IV neurones[30]. If these inhibitory interneurones have reduced afferent input due to peripheral auditory dysfunction, there may be a loss of inhibition of the spontaneous activity of the type IV neurones, thus resulting in abnormally high spontaneous activity which might be audible. Eggermont[30] furthered this proposal, suggesting, after Moller[51], additional disinhibition in the IC.

Synchronisation of spontaneous neural activity

Eggermont[30] has reviewed the evidence for a theory that tinnitus may result from the imposition of a temporal pattern upon stochastic cochlear nerve activity. Hudspeth and Corey[52] reported that, in the saccular hair cells of the bull frog, an increase in the concentration of extracellular calcium could lead to increased firing. Eggermont[29] proposed that if such a calcium-induced increase were present in dysfunctional human cochleae, then it might lead to enhanced neurotransmitter release from IHC, and thence to increased activity in auditory nerve fibres, some of the spikes occurring in bursts. This pattern of activity (burst-firing) may mimic that seen in response to sound stimulation. Burst-firing can occur in the cat auditory nerve after exposure to kanamycin[36], and in the rat inferior colliculus after salicylate administration[42]. Increased burst-firing in the rat DCN following intense sound exposure has also been reported[44]. Kaltenbach[31] argued that a link between such bursting activity and tinnitus perception is problematic, in the light of the finding of Ochi and Eggermont[53,54] that, in the cat, no increase in cortical bursting activity is demonstrated after administration of salicylate or quinine. It is possible, however, that bursting activity in the auditory periphery could be re-coded as a rate change in more central nuclei.

Eggermont[50] proposed that the synchronised activity of a small number of fibres in the auditory periphery may give rise to a sensation of sound, and thus of tinnitus. Moller[55] drew an analogy with hemifacial spasm and trigeminal neuralgia patients, noting that the surgical decompression of vessels impinging upon the Vth cranial nerve relieved trigeminal neuralgia, and upon the VIIth cranial nerve relieved hemifacial spasm. Moller noted that these cranial nerves were sensitive to such compression at the root entry zone, where they were covered by myelin. He hypothesised that compression of the nerve caused cross-talk between nerve fibres, the breakdown of the myelin insulation of the nerve fibres establishing ephaptic coupling between them. This concept was applied to the cochlear-vestibular nerve, which is covered by central myelin for the majority of its length, and hence is vulnerable to compression from blood vessels or tumours impinging upon the nerve, such as vestibular schwannoma. Such compression and consequent ephaptic coupling might lead to tinnitus perception, if synchronisation of the stochastic firing in the human cochlear nerve is perceived as sound. Eggermont[29] modelled the effect of ephaptic interaction between fibres of the auditory nerve, and proposed that the effect of the interaction was to increase the number of interspike intervals around 10 ms. He concluded that the ephaptic interaction model had a 'potential real-life parallel in the demyelinating effects of tumours of the eighth nerve' (e.g. vestibular schwannoma).

Several terms have been used for such measures of synchronised activity – ensemble spontaneous neural activity (ESNA)[56], average spectrum of electrophysiological cochlear activity (ASECA)[57], ensemble spontaneous activity (ESA)[58], and spectrum of background neural noise (SNN)[59]. Evidence for synchronised spontaneous neural activity associated with tinnitus is emergent. Martin et al[60] recorded spontaneous auditory nerve activity from 10 cats pre- and post-salicylate administration using an incoherent spectral averaging technique, which allows the identification of continuous signals that have consistent frequency characteristics. It was noted that the results needed to be interpreted with caution because of the physiological stress salicylate places upon the animal. Marked changes in the spectral analysis of auditory nerve activity pre- and post-salicylate administration were reported, with a new peak of activity centred at or near 200 Hz being identified in all post-administration recordings. A higher-frequency, broader peak was also identified. Two animals in whom saline was administered did not demonstrate the new peaks of activity. Cazals et al[61] reported the effects of long-term salicylate administration in the guinea pig. Changes (specifically an immediate decrease followed by a progressive increase) in spontaneous activity recorded from the round window predated changes in hearing sensitivity, which the authors felt was an indication of high-frequency salicylate-induced tinnitus as this would be expected in humans under such conditions. Martin[56] described spectral average recordings from the cochlear nerve of 14 human adult patients undergoing cerebellopontine angle surgery. In 12 patients with tinnitus, a prominent peak in the spectral average near 200 Hz was reported (see Fig. 2). Further animal studies report that ESNA is influenced by contralateral acoustic stimulation[62].

The origin of peaks within the spectrum of spontaneous neural activity recorded from guinea pigs undergoing salicylate administration was explored by McMahon and Patuzzi[63]. They questioned the assumption of Cazals and Huang[57] that the peaks are indicative of synchronous

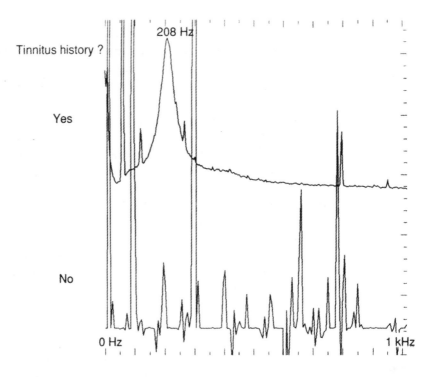

Fig. 2 Comparison of power spectra of spontaneous auditory nerve activity recorded from a patient with pre-operative tinnitus (upper) and a patient with no pre- or postoperative tinnitus (lower). It should be noted that the sharp spikes in both traces are the result of 60 Hz noise and its harmonics. From Martin[56], with permission.

activity. Two spectral peaks were identified. A peak at 170 Hz was thought to be consistent with the 200 Hz peak previously reported by Martin[56] in humans (see Fig. 2). A spectral peak at 900 Hz was thought to arise from resonance of the primary afferent nerve membrane, with a potential contribution from neurones with similar membrane properties in the ventral cochlear nucleus. Evidence favouring the existence of these two peaks has also been reported by Searchfield *et al*[64]. McMahon and Patuzzi suggested that the peaks of spontaneous activity recorded at 200 Hz and 900 Hz may in future be used to determine the location of physiological generators of tinnitus.

Medial efferent system involvement

Eggermont[50] suggested that the efferent system might influence the perceived intensity of tinnitus, and associated annoyance, based on the observation that stressful situations may exacerbate tinnitus, and that techniques such as biofeedback may reduce tinnitus. In addition, the connection of the auditory efferent system with the reticular formation within the brain stem had been linked with the persistence of tinnitus as an alerting stimulus by Hazell and Jastreboff[19]. Jastreboff and Hazell[61] additionally suggested a role for the efferent system in modulating a cochlear mechanism of tinnitus generation.

Veuillet *et al*[66] investigated the possibility that dysfunction of the medial efferent system was involved in tinnitus perception by measuring the suppressive effect of contralateral noise upon transient evoked oto-acoustic emissions (TEOAE) in subjects with tinnitus localised to one ear only. The hypothesis that efferent dysfunction in the tinnitus ear would result in a smaller suppressive effect of noise upon TEOAE amplitude than in the non-tinnitus ear was only marginally supported. Large intersubject variability in the suppressive effect was noted.

Lind[67] also measured the suppressive effect of contralateral broad-band noise on TEOAE in 20 patients with unilateral tinnitus and symmetrical hearing, finding no significant difference between the suppression effect in tinnitus and non-tinnitus ears.

An alternative mechanism of efferent system involvement in tinnitus perception has been suggested by Robertson *et al*[68], following experimental evidence that, in the guinea pig, olivocochlear inputs to the cochlear nucleus can be excitatory, thus directly affecting ascending activity in the auditory pathway, separately from influence upon the cochlea. Efferent dysfunction might, therefore, be implicated in tinnitus perception generated at a brain stem level. However, a review[69] of tinnitus experience following vestibular nerve section in humans, which involves ablation of the medial efferent pathway in the inferior vestibular nerve, indicated that total medial efferent dysfunction was not associated with troublesome or exacerbated tinnitus.

Somatic modulation

The modulation of tinnitus by somatosensory input was considered by Levine[70]. Patients were first interviewed about their experiences of somatic modulation of their tinnitus, such as changes in pitch or intensity associated with face stroking or head movements. They were then asked to perform manoeuvres of a few seconds' duration to test for somatic effects, including teeth clenching, pressure on the occiput, forehead, vertex and temples, head turning and shoulder abductions. In the interview, 16 of 70 patients reported that they could somatically modulate their tinnitus (23%). On testing, however, 48 patients (68%) reported modulation of their tinnitus with at least one of the manoeuvres. The pattern of modulation reported was highly variable

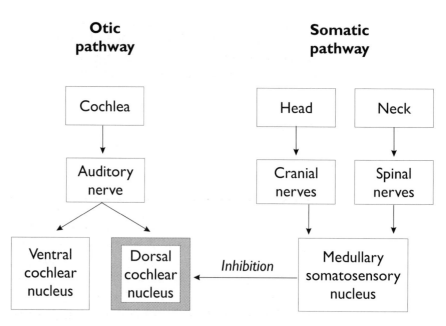

Fig. 3 Schematic diagram of suggested interaction between somatic and otic pathways (following Levine[72] with permission).

involving changes in intensity (both increase and decrease) and pitch. In all cases, these changes were transient. The results led Levine to conclude that 'somatic modulation appears to be a fundamental attribute of tinnitus', and to propose interactions between auditory perception and somatosensory input at the dorsal cochlear nucleus. Higher centres where such interaction also occurs (such as the SOC and IC) were not considered as somatically modifiable tinnitus is largely localised to one or other ear, and it was thought that binaural interactions in the SOC and higher centres would not have given rise to tinnitus heard to just one side. Levine[71,72] also noted that cranial nerves V, VII, IX and X converge in the medullary somatosensory nuclei (MSN; Fig. 3) and that anatomical links between the MSN and the DCN had previously been described[73]. The ability of some mammals to incorporate information about pinna position in sound localisation is indicative of such a pathway[74]. Levine hypothesised that decreases in inhibitory MSN input to the DCN (specifically inhibition) might result in disinhibition of DCN activity leading to increased activity and the perception of tinnitus. Levine[71] noted potential criticisms of this model. The DCN may not be the site of somatic and auditory interaction involved in tinnitus. The argument that the lateralisation of the tinnitus perception being evidence for the role of DCN somatic modulation of tinnitus is strong, but a role of the extralemniscal pathway in interactions between somatic and auditory pathways, as proposed by Moller et al[75], is also worthy of consideration and would allow unilateral tinnitus perception. Another potential criticism is that, whilst the anatomical links between the MSN and DCN have been identified in the cat, the situation is humans is less clear, and in particular no pathway from the cunate/spiral tract of cranial nerve V to the DCN has been identified.

Analogies with pain

Analogy with chronic pain

Analogies between pain and tinnitus have been made many times in the literature (see House & Brackmann[76] and Evans[77] for early examples). It has been noted that: (i) pain, like tinnitus, can arise from a great variety of lesions; (ii) there is no one specific mechanism for pain perception; (iii) pain is a subjective phenomenon that is difficult to quantify; and (iv) treatment of pain symptoms is difficult and often ineffective[79,80]. More specifically, Moller[1,80,81] considered the analogy between tinnitus and chronic pain in terms of peripheral generation and of central persistence once the acute injury has resolved. Whilst chronic pain is often a consequence of peripheral injury, that injury may not in itself account for the sustained nature of chronic pain. Moller[81] considered that the involvement of the CNS in such sustained perception was indicated by the relevant literature (see Basbaum & Jessell[82] for a comprehensive review). Such involvement implies plasticity within the CNS. Similarly, while tinnitus is often associated with peripheral auditory dysfunction, that dysfunction may not account for the sustained and distressing tinnitus perception. Emotional and environmental influences upon pain perception have been noted[82]. The consequent large variation between individual experience of pain, makes the development of effective therapy very difficult.

Cortical re-organisation, tinnitus, and analogies with phantom pain

The possible analogy between tinnitus and phantom limb pain was first drawn by Goodhill in 1950[83]. The concept that cortical re-organisation similar to that involved in phantom limb pain[84] might occur in auditory cortical areas following change in the auditory periphery was first reviewed in detail by Meikle[85] and more recently by Salvi et al[86]. The precise tonotopicity that has been demonstrated in the central auditory pathways means that de-afferentation of a specific portion of the cochlea will, in the short-term, lead to reduced activity in the cortical area with corresponding characteristic frequency (CF). If similar measurements are made some months later, that area is again responsive to sound, but many neurones now have CFs adjacent to that of the lesioned region[86]. This phenomenon has been demonstrated in animals[87,88] (one study in particular reported that even a modest noise induced hearing loss resulted in significant cortical re-organisation[89]) and in humans[90,91]. One consequence of this re-organisation is that a disproportionately large number of neurones will be sensitive to frequencies at the upper and lower borders of the hearing loss. Salvi et al[86] proposed that spontaneous activity in these areas might be perceived as tinnitus. Meikle[85] suggested that the mechanism of such re-organisation might be the disinhibition of previously weak synaptic connections, and that the area of re-organisation might be limited to 1–2 mm, leading her to suggest that cortical re-organisation effects larger than this might represent re-organisation at a lower level in the auditory pathway where the tonotopic maps are smaller (the inferior colliculus for example). Re-organisation of the tonotopic map in the IC of the chinchilla following a high-frequency cochlear lesion has been demonstrated[92].

Evidence for re-organisation of the auditory cortex being a mechanism of tinnitus generation in humans was reported by Mulnickel et al[93] and Dietrich et al[91]. Whilst these studies involve small numbers of subjects, there are early indications that the identification of tinnitus mechanisms involving re-organisation and plasticity within the central auditory system may facilitate the development of novel pharmacological therapies for tinnitus[60,94].

The future

This review indicates that there are many potential mechanisms for tinnitus, and so the population of people with troublesome tinnitus will be heterogeneous in aetiology and experience, as is observed in clinical practice. It is envisaged that the objective of tinnitus mechanism research in coming years will be to determine the validity and relevance of the hypotheses regarding tinnitus generation to the clinical population, and to use that evidence to design effective clinical treatments.

Key points for clinical practice

- There are multiple potential mechanisms of tinnitus, and this accounts for the heterogeneity evident in the clinical population.

- The development of new and effective treatments will be greatly facilitated by identification of mechanisms in humans.

- The analogy between tinnitus and phantom limb pain, and the possibility of a role for 5-HT dysfunction in tinnitus, indicate the possibility of effective clinical intervention in tinnitus where these mechanisms are evident.

Acknowledgements

Discussions with Ian Winter and his detailed critical review of the manuscript were extremely helpful in writing this chapter. Brian Moore was a kind and diligent editor. Thanks also are due to David Moffat, Ross Coles and Jonathan Hazell for nurturing my interest in tinnitus.

References

1 Moller AR. Similarities between chronic pain and tinnitus. *Am J Otol* 1997; **18**: 577–85
2 Allen RE. *Concise Oxford Dictionary of Current English*. Oxford: Clarendon Press, 1990
3 McFadden D. *Tinnitus: Facts, Theories and Treatments*. Report of working group 89. Committee on Hearing, Bioacoustics and Biomechanics. National Research Council. Washington DC: National Academy Press, 1982
4 Davis AC, Rafaie EA. Epidemiology of tinnitus. In: Tyler RS. (ed) *Tinnitus Handbook*. San Diego, CA: Singular, 2000; 1–24
5 Baguley DM, McFerran DJ. Current perspectives on tinnitus. *Arch Dis Child* 2002; **86**: 141–3
6 Gold T. Hearing. II. The physical basis of the action of the cochlea. *Proc R Soc Edinb* 1948; 135: 492–8
7 Kemp DT. Stimulated acoustic emissions from within the human auditory system, *J Acoust Soc Am* 1978; **64**: 1386–91
8 Coles RRA. Classification of causes, mechanisms of patient disturbance, and associated counselling. In: Vernon JA, Moller AR. (eds) Mechanisms of tinnitus. Boston, MA: Allyn and Bacon, 1995; 11–20
9 Wilson JP, Sutton GJ. Acoustic correlates of tonal tinnitus. *Ciba Found Symp* 1981; **85**: 82–100
10 Penner MJ, Burns EM. The dissociation of SOAEs and tinnitus. *J Speech Hearing Res* 1987; **30**: 396–403
11 Penner MJ. An estimate of the prevalence of tinnitus caused by spontaneous otoacoustic emissions. *Arch Otolaryngol Head Neck Surg* 1990; **115**: 871–5
12 Baskill JB, Coles RRA. Current studies of tinnitus caused by spontaneous otoacoustic emissions. In: Aran J-M, Dauman R. (eds) *Proceedings of the Fourth International Tinnitus Seminar*. Amsterdam: Kugler, 1992
13 Penner MJ. Spontaneous otoacoustic emissions and tinnitus. In: Tyler RS. (ed) *Tinnitus Handbook*. San Diego, CA: Singular, 2000; 203–20
14 Long GR, Tubis A. Modification of spontaneous and evoked emissions and associated psychoacoustic microstructure by aspirin consumption. *J Acoust Soc Am* 1988; **84**: 1343–53
15 Penner MJ, Coles RRA. Indications for aspirin as a palliative for tinnitus caused by SOAEs : a case study. *Br J Audiol* 1992; **26**: 91–6
16 Jastreboff PJ. Phantom auditory perception (tinnitus): mechanism of generation and perception. *Neurosci Res* 1990; **8**: 221–54
17 Stypulkowski PH. Mechanisms of salicylate ototoxicity. *Hear Res* 1990; **46**: 113–46
18 Hazell JWP. A cochlear model for tinnitus. In: Feldmann H. (ed) *Proceedings Third International Tinnitus Seminar, Münster 1987*. Karlsruhe: Harsch, 1987; 121–8
19 Hazell JWP, Jastreboff PJ. Tinnitus. I. Auditory mechanisms: a model for tinnitus and hearing impairment. *J Otolaryngol* 1990; **19**: 1–5
20 Jastreboff PJ. Tinnitus as a phantom perception: theories and clinical implications. In: Vernon JA, Moller AR. (eds) *Mechanisms of Tinnitus*. London: Allyn and Bacon, 1995; 73–94
21 Chery-Croze S, Truy E, Morgon A. Contralateral suppression of transiently evoked otoacoustic emissions and tinnitus. *Br J Audiol* 1994; **28**: 255–66
22 LePage EL. A model for cochlear origin of subjective tinnitus: excitatory drift in the operating point of inner hair cells. In: Vernon JA, Moller AR. (eds) *Mechanisms of Tinnitus*. London: Allyn and Bacon, 1995; 115–48

23 Zenner HP, Ernst A. Cochlear motor tinnitus, transduction tinnitus and signal transfer tinnitus: three models of cochlear tinnitus. In: Vernon JA, Moller AR. (eds) *Mechanisms of Tinnitus*. London: Allyn and Bacon, 1995; 237–54

24 Patuzzi R. Outer hair cells, EP regulation and tinnitus. In: Patuzzi R. (ed) *Proceedings VIIth International Tinnitus Seminar*. Perth: University of Western Australia, 2002; 16–24

25 Sahey TL, Nodar RH. A biochemical model of peripheral tinnitus. *Hear Res* 2001; **152**: 43–54

26 Simpson JJ, Davies WE. A review of evidence in support of a role for 5-HT in the perception of tinnitus. *Hear Res* 2000; **145**: 1–7

27 Dobie R. Randomized clinical trials for tinnitus: not the last word? In: Patuzzi R. (ed) *Proceedings VIIth International Tinnitus Seminar*. Perth: University of Western Australia, 2002; 3–6

28 Moller AR. Pathophysiology of tinnitus. *Ann Otol* 1984; **93**: 39–44

29 Eggermont JJ. On the pathophysiology of tinnitus: a review and peripheral model. *Hear Res* 1990; **48**: 111–24

30 Eggermont JJ. Psychological mechanisms and neural models. In: Tyler RS. (ed) *Tinnitus Handbook*. San Diego, CA: Singular, 2000; 85–122

31 Kaltenbach JA. Neurophysiologic mechanisms of tinnitus. *J Am Acad Audiol* 2000; **11**: 3, 125–37

32 Heller MF, Bergman M. Tinnitus aurium in normally hearing persons. *Ann Otol Rhinol Laryngol* 1953; **62**: 73–83

33 Jastreboff PJ, Gray WC, Gold SL. Neurophysiological approach to tinnitus patients. *Am J Otol* 1996; **17**: 236–40

34 Jastreboff PJ. The neurophysiological model of tinnitus and hyperacusis. In: Hazell JWP. (ed) *Proceedings of the Sixth International Tinnitus Seminar*. London: Tinnitus and Hyperacusis Centre, 1999; 32–8

35 Evans EF, Wilson JP, Borerwe TA. Animal models of tinnitus. *Ciba Found Symp* 1981; **85**: 108–38

36 Kiang NYS, Moxon EC Levine RA. Auditory-nerve activity in cats with normal and abnormal cochleas. In: Wolstenholme GEW, Knight J. (eds) *Sensorineural Hearing Loss*. London: Churchill Livingstone, 1970; 241–76

37 Tyler RS. Does tinnitus originate from hyperactive nerve fibers in the cochlea? *J Laryngol Otol* 1984; **Suppl 9**: 38–44

38 Kaltenbach JA, Godfrey DA, McCaslin DL, Squire AB. Changes in spontaneous activity and chemistry of the cochlear nucleus following intense sound exposure. In: Reich GE, Vernon JE. (eds) *Proceedings of the Fifth International Tinnitus Seminar*. Portland, OR: American Tinnitus Association, 1996; 429–40

39 Kaltenbach JA, McAslin DL. Increases in spontaneous activity in the dorsal cochlear nucleus following exposure to high intensity sound: a possible neural correlate of tinnitus. *Auditory Neurosci* 1996; **3**: 57–78

40 Kaltenbach JA, Heffner HE, Afman CE. Effects of intense sound on spontaneous activity in the dorsal cochlear nucleus and its relation to tinnitus. In: Hazell JWP. (ed) *Proceedings of the Sixth International Tinnitus Seminar*. London: Tinnitus and Hyperacusis Centre, 1999; 133–8

41 Salvi RJ, Wang J, Powers NL. Plasticity and reorganisation in the auditory brainstem: implications for tinnitus. In: Reich GE, Vernon JE. (eds) *Proceedings of the Fifth International Tinnitus Seminar*. Portland, OR: American Tinnitus Association, 1996; 457–66

42 Chen G, Jastreboff PJ. Salicylate induced abnormal activity in the inferior colliculus of rats. *Hear Res* 1995; **82**: 158–78

43 Jastreboff PJ, Sasaki CT. Salicylate induced changes in spontaneous activity of single units in the inferior colliculus of the guinea pig. *J Acoust Soc Am* 1986; **80**: 1384–91

44 Chen K, Chang H, Zhang J, Kaltenbach JA, Godfrey DA. Altered spontaneous activity in rat dorsal cochlea nucleus following loud tone exposure. In: Hazell JWP. (ed) *Proceedings of the Sixth International Tinnitus Seminar*. London: Tinnitus and Hyperacusis Centre, 1999; 212–7

45 Wallhausser-Franke E, Braun S, Langner G. Salicylate alters 2-DG uptake in the auditory system : a model for tinnitus? *Neuroreport* 1996; **7**: 1585–8

46 Wallhausser-Franke E. Salicylate evokes *c-fos* expression in the brainstem, implications for tinnitus. *Neuroreport* 1997; **8**: 725–8

47 Wallhausser-Franke E, Langner G. Central activation patterns after experimental tinnitus induction in an animal model. In: Hazell JWP. (ed) *Proceedings of the Sixth International Tinnitus Seminar*. London: Tinnitus and Hyperacusis Centre, 1999; 155–62

48 Langner G, Wallhausser-Franke E. Computer simulation of a tinnitus model based on labelling of tinnitus activity in the auditory cortex. In: Hazell JWP. (ed) *Proceedings of the Sixth International Tinnitus Seminar*. London: Tinnitus and Hyperacusis Centre, 1999; 20–5

49 Zhang JS, Kaltenbach JA. Increases in spontaneous activity in the dorsal cochlear nucleus of the rat following exposure to high intensity sound. *Neurosci Lett* 1998; **250**: 197–200

50 Eggermont JJ. Tinnitus: some thoughts about its origin. *J Laryngol Otol* 1984; **Suppl 9**: 31–7

51 Moller AR. Pathophysiology of tinnitus. In: Vernon JA, Moller AR. (eds) *Mechanisms of Tinnitus*. Boston, MA: Allyn and Bacon, 1995; 207–17

52 Hudspeth AJ, Corey DP. Sensitivity, polarity and conductance change in the response of vertebrate haircells to controlled mechanical stimuli. *Proc Natl Acad Sci USA* 1977; **74**: 2407–11

53 Ochi K, Eggermont JJ. Effects of salicylate on neural activity in cat auditory cortex. *Hear Res* 1996; **95**: 63–76

54 Ochi K, Eggermont JJ. Effects of quinine on neural activity in cat primary auditory cortex. *Hear Res* 1997; **105**: 105–18

55 Moller AR. Pathophysiology of tinnitus. *Ann Otol* 1984; **93**: 39–44

56 Martin WH. Spectral analysis of brain activity in the study of tinnitus. In: Vernon JA, Moller AR. (eds) *Mechanisms of Tinnitus*. London: Allyn and Bacon, 1995; 163–80

57 Cazals Y, Huang ZW. Average spectrum of cochlear activity: a possible synchronized firing, its olivo-cochlear feedback and alterations under anesthesia. *Hear Res* 1996; **101**: 81–92

58 Lenarz T, Schreiner C, Snyder C, Ernst RL. Neural mechanisms of tinnitus: the pathological ensemble of spontaneous activity of the auditory system. In: Vernon JA, Moller AR. (eds) *Mechanisms of Tinnitus*. London: Allyn and Bacon, 1995; 101–33

59 McMahon CM, Patuzzi RB. The origin of the 900 Hz spectral peak in spontaneous and sound-evoked round window electrical activity. Hear Res 2002; In press

60 Martin WH, Schwegler JW, Scheibelhoffer J, Ronis ML. Salicylate-induced changes in cat auditory nerve activity. *Laryngoscope* 1993; **103**: 600–4

61 Cazals Y, Horner KC, Huang ZW. Alterations in average spectrum of cochleoneural activity by long-term salicylate treatment in the guinea pig : a plausible index of tinnitus. *J Neurophysiol* 1998; **80**: 2113–20

62 Popelar J, Erre JP, Syka J, Aran JM. Effects of contralateral acoustical stimulation on three measures of cochlear function in the guinea pig. *Hear Res* 2001; **152**: 128–38

63 McMahon CM, Patuzzi RB. Spectral peaks in spontaneous and sound evoked cochlear electrical activity and tinnitus. In: Patuzzi R. (ed) *Proceedings VIIth International Tinnitus Seminar*. Perth: University of Western Australia, 2002; 34–8

64 Searchfield G, Munoz DJB, Towns EC, Thorne PR. Ensemble spontaneous activity of the cochlear nerve: cochlear pathology and tinnitus. In: Patuzzi R. (ed) *Proceedings VIIth International Tinnitus Seminar*. Perth: University of Western Australia, 2002; 53–5

65 Jastreboff PJ, Hazell JWP. A neurophysiological approach to tinnitus: clinical implications. *Br J Audiol* 1993; **27**: 7–17

66 Veuillet E, Collet L, Disnat F, Morgon A. Tinnitus and medial cochlear efferent system. In: Aran J-M, Dauman R. (eds) *Tinnitus 91*. Amsterdam: Kugler, 1992; 205–9

67 Lind O. Transient evoked otoacoustic emissions and contralateral suppression in patients with unilateral tinnitus. *Scand Audiol* 1996; **25**: 167–72

68 Robertson D, Winter IM, Mulders WHAM. Influence of descending neural pathways on responses in the mammalian cochlear nucleus. In: Patuzzi R. (ed) *Proceedings VIIth International Tinnitus Seminar*. Perth: University of Western Australia, 2002; 31–3

69 Baguley DM, Axon P, Winter IM, Moffat DA. The effect of vestibular nerve section upon tinnitus: a review. Clin Otolaryngol 2002; In press

70 Levine RA. Somatic modulation appears to be a fundamental attribute of tinnitus. In: Hazell JWP. (ed) *Proceedings of the Sixth International Tinnitus Seminar*. London: Tinnitus and Hyperacusis Centre, 1999; 193–7

71 Levine RA. Somatic (craniocervical) tinnitus and the dorsal cochlear nucleus hypothesis. *Am J Otolaryngol* 1999; **20**: 351–62

72 Levine RA. Diagnostic issues in tinnitus: a neuro-otological perspective. *Semin Hear* 2001; **22**: 23–36

73 Young ED, Nelken I, Conley RA. Somatosensory effects on neurons in dorsal cochlear nucleus. *J Neurophysiol* 1995; **73**: 743–65

74 Nelken I, Young ED. Why do cats need a dorsal cochlear nucleus? *J Basic Clin Physiol Pharmacol* 1996; **7**: 199–220

75 Moller AR, Moller MB, Yokota M. Some forms of tinnitus may involve the extralemniscal auditory pathway. *Laryngoscope* 1992; **102**: 1165–71

76 House JW, Brackmann DE. Tinnitus: surgical treatment. *Ciba Found Symp* 1981; **85**: 204–16

77 Evans EF. Chairman's closing remarks. In: *Ciba Found Symp* 1981; **85**: 295–9

78 Tonndorf J. The analogy between tinnitus and pain: a suggestion for a physiological basis of chronic tinnitus. *Hear Res* 1987; **28**: 71–95

79 Tonndorf J. The analogy between tinnitus and pain: a suggestion for a physiological basis of chronic tinnitus. In: Vernon JA, Moller AR. (eds) *Mechanisms of Tinnitus*. London: Allyn and Bacon, 1995; 231–6

80 Moller AR. Pathophysiology of severe tinnitus and chronic pain. In: Hazell JWP. (ed) *Proceedings of the Sixth International Tinnitus Seminar*. London: Tinnitus and Hyperacusis Centre, 1999; 26–31

81 Moller AR. Similarities between severe tinnitus and chronic pain. *J Am Acad Audiol* 2000; **11**: 115–24

82 Basbaum AI, Jessell TM. The perception of pain. In: Kandel ER, Schwartz JH, Jessell TM. (eds) *Principles of Neural Science*, 4th edn. New York: McGraw Hill, 2000; 472–91

83 Goodhill V. The management of tinnitus. *Laryngoscope* 1950; **60**: 442–50

84 Kandel ER. From nerve cells to cognition: the internal cellular representation required for perception and action. In: Kandel ER, Schwartz JH, Jessell TM. (eds) *Principles of Neural Science*, 4th edn. New York: McGraw Hill, 2000; 381–410

85 Meikle MB. The interaction of central and peripheral mechanisms in tinnitus. In: Vernon JA, Moller AR. (eds) *Mechanisms of Tinnitus*. London: Allyn and Bacon, 1995; 181–206

86 Salvi RJ, Lockwood AH, Burkard R. Neural plasticity and tinnitus. In: Tyler RS. (ed) *Tinnitus Handbook*. San Diego, CA: Singular, 2000; 123–48

87 Rajan R, Irvine DRF, Wise LZ, Heil P. Effect of unilateral partial cochlear lesions in adult cats on the representation of lesioned and unlesioned cochleas in primary auditory cortex. *J Comp Neurol* 1993; **338**: 17–49

88 Robertson D, Irvine DRF. Plasticity of frequency organization in auditory cortex of guinea pigs with partial unilateral deafness. *J Comp Neurol* 1989; **282**: 456–71

89 Komiya H. Eggermont JJ. Spontaneous firing activity of cortical neurons in adult cats with reorganised tonotopic map following pure-tone trauma. *Acta Otolaryngol* 2000; **120**: 750–6

90 Harrison RV, Nagasawa A, Smith DW, Stanton S, Mount RJ. Re-organisation of auditory cortex after neonatal high frequency cochlear hearing loss. *Hear Res* 1991; **54**: 11–9

91 Dietrich V, Nieschalk M, Stoll W, Rajan R, Pantev C. Cortical re-organisation in patients with high frequency cochlear hearing loss. *Hear Res* 2001; **158**: 95–101

92 Salvi RJ, Wang J, Powers NL. Plasticity and re-organisation in the auditory brainstem: implications for tinnitus. In: Reich GE, Vernon JE. (eds) *Proceedings of the Fifth International Tinnitus Seminar*. Portland, OR: American Tinnitus Association, 1996; 457–66

93 Mulnickel W, Elbert T, Taub E, Flor H. Re-organisation of auditory cortex in tinnitus. *Proc Natl Acad Sci USA* 1998; **95**: 10340–3

94 Davies WE. Future prospects for the pharmacological treatment of tinnitus. *Semin Hear* 2001; **22**: 89–99

Under-rated neuro-otological symptoms: Hoffman and Brookler 1978 revisited

Adolfo M Bronstein

Department of Neuro-otology, Division of Neuroscience and Psychological Medicine, Imperial College Faculty of Medicine, Charing Cross Hospital, London, UK

In 1978, Hoffman and Brookler published an article in *The Laryngoscope* to challenge prevailing views on the lack of diagnostic power of certain symptoms often reported by patients to neuro-otologists. Some of these 'under-rated neuro-otological symptoms' include complaints of non-rotational dizziness, blurred and double vision, and the development of visual motion hypersensitivity in patients with balance disorders. In this review, I revisit these visual symptoms in the light of new findings from our laboratory. Double vision due to skew eye deviation can indeed occur in peripheral vestibular disease when there is a large, acute peripheral imbalance of vestibular function. It is more frequent and severe in brain stem disease. In both cases, it is explained by disruption of the torsional vestibular ocular reflex. It is usually assumed that damage to the otolith underlies the emergence of skew diplopia, but recent evidence shows that the vertical canal system is likely to be partly responsible as well. The other 'under-rated symptom' revisited here is what patients describe as dizziness when watching moving objects or whilst walking in visually busy surroundings such as supermarkets. Recent work has shown that this 'visual vertigo' emerges in patients who, in addition to suffering from a vestibular disorder, have increased visual dependence. Visual dependence denotes subjects who preferentially use vision, as opposed to vestibular or proprioceptive input, for spatial orientation and postural control. We do not know as yet what makes some vestibular patients become extremely visually dependent. However, we have provided evidence for Hoffman and Brookler's impression that visually triggered complaints should not be summarily dismissed, as they often point to an underlying vestibular disorder.

Correspondence to:
Prof. Adolfo M Bronstein,
Academic Department of
Neuro-otology, Division
of Neuroscience and
Psychological Medicine,
Imperial College
Faculty of Medicine,
Charing Cross Hospital,
Fulham Palace Road,
London W6 8RF, UK

Excellent monographs on the subject of vertigo and vestibular disorders have appeared recently[1,2]. For this reason, I will not review the whole subject of balance disorders, but rather concentrate on a few poorly understood vestibular symptoms which have been the subject of recent research. Indeed, this article was inspired by Hoffman and Brookler's paper in 1978, called *Underrated Neuro-otological Symptoms*[3]. This publication, which exudes clinical finesse, was structured around case reports and set out to dispel the erroneous belief that certain symptoms reported by patients are not useful in the diagnosis of labyrinthine disorders. It shows that in the practice of medicine nothing replaces the combination of a good capacity for observation with the paying of careful attention to the patients' own description of their symptoms.

Some of these under-rated symptoms are complaints of dizziness, light-headedness or a floating sensation. Although presented in different ways, one of the myths in neuro-otology is that these are 'lesser' symptoms than 'proper' rotational vertigo. Whilst it is true that spinning vertigo usually implies disorder of the labyrinth or its immediate central connections, the reverse implication, that these underrated symptoms do not support the diagnosis of vestibular disease, is certainly not true. As Hoffman and Brookler indicate, anyone who has done a sufficient number of caloric tests knows that people use all sorts of terms to describe the vestibular sensation induced by caloric stimulation: faintness, rocking, staggering, light headedness, waviness as well as rotational vertigo, of course. One of my patients, clearly not bothered at all by the procedure, said 'it's like going to the pub but much cheaper'. The obvious conclusion in their paper was that: 'the complaint of dizziness, be it nondescript of rotatory vertigo, must be taken seriously and thoroughly investigated'.

In this paper, I will revisit the two underrated neuro-otological symptoms which, in Hoffman and Brookler's opinion, relate to the visual system.

Double vision and skew eye deviation in vestibular disease

The first neuro-otological visual symptom Hoffman and Brookler discussed is the vestibular patient who complains of blurred vision and, in extreme cases, of double vision. Whilst diplopia should always raise the possibility of brain stem involvement, Hoffman and Brookler quote Lord Brain's article of 1938[4]: 'it is important to remember that double vision may occur as a result of vestibular disorder, lest this symptom should be attributed to ophthalmoplegia and ascribed to a lesion of the nervous system. The two images are seen one above the other and the diplopia is doubtless due to skew deviation of the eyes, a disorder of ocular posture emanating from the labyrinth and sometimes occurring transitorily, as Cairns and I have shown after resection of the auditory nerve.' I suspect that this statement was basically ignored for some 40 years, between 1938 and 1978 to be precise.

The issue has been re-examined by Riordan-Eva et al[5] in a robust study including 18 patients who underwent vestibular nerve section for intractable vertigo or acoustic neuroma. Patients were assessed pre- and postoperatively ophthalmologically and with measurements of the subjective visual vertical (i.e. the task of aligning a luminous straight line in the dark to the perceived gravitational vertical). It was found that 5 patients developed an ocular skew deviation (that is, a vertical squint due to a supranuclear, vertical, disconjugate misalignment of the eyes). Only three reported frank diplopia, lasting 1 day to 6 months. There was an association between large changes in ocular torsional position (ocular tilt) and tilts of the visual vertical. In turn, this was associated with lesser degrees of canal paresis on pre-operative caloric assessment. The results indicate that, as expected, the larger the vestibular imbalance produced by the surgery, the larger the tilts in ocular position and, consequently, in subjective visual vertical. They also suggest that the presence of vertical skew deviation is dependent on the presence of a large torsional change. Although prevalent wisdom dictates that such ocular skew and torsional changes are due to the acute asymmetry induced in the otolith control of eye position, alternative sources such as asymmetry in vertical canal function were mentioned.

It may be helpful to examine why the vestibular system needs to be involved in the control of vertical ocular conjugacy in the first place. Figure 1 is taken from the work of Lopez et al[6]. Imagine that you tilt your head slowly towards your right shoulder. As you do so, you begin to loose good visual contact with the vertically oriented visual world (e.g. try to read this article with your head tilted maximally towards the right or left shoulder). *Prima facie*, a good compensatory vestibulo-ocular mechanism would be to counter-rotate the eyes conjugately in the opposite direction to the head tilt and to produce a disconjugate skew deviation so that both eyes lie parallel to the horizon as we tilt (see Fig. 1). Although such mechanism is present

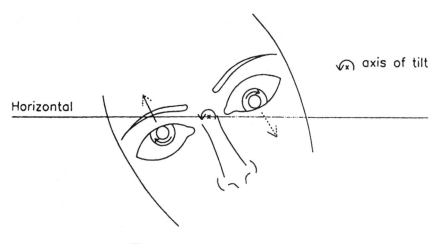

Tilt about naso—occipital axis

Fig. 1 Diagram showing the compensatory eye movements which could be expected during a right ear down head tilt. The vertical ocular disconjugacy induced is usually called a skew deviation. From Lopez et al[6] with permission.

in animals with laterally placed eyes, like the rabbit, its existence and underlying mechanisms in man are not entirely clear.

Lopez *et al*[6] examined patients with spontaneous torsional nystagmus and identified the site of lesion in the contralateral vestibular nuclei, in the pontomedullary junction. In addition to this topographic finding, the

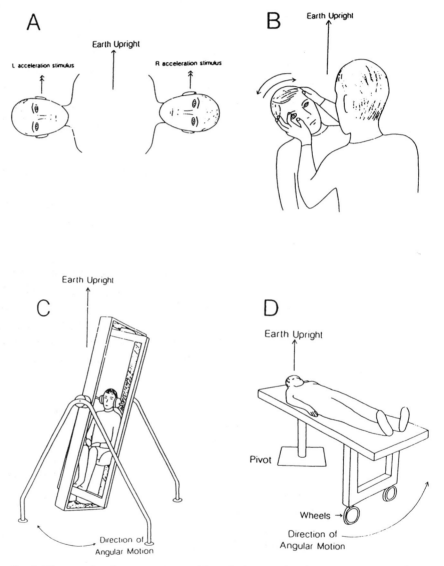

Fig. 2 Diagram showing manoeuvres able to induce torsional eye movements and, therefore, capable of modulating a pathological torsional nystagmus. In (A), a simple head tilt to right or left produces a change in the direction of action of the gravitational vector on the otoliths. In (B), the clinical manoeuvre used to induce ocular counter-rolling activates both otolith and vertical semicircular canals; the gymbals system shown in (C) is similar. In (D), only the vertical canals are activated during rotation since the head is not re-oriented with respect to gravity. From Lopez *et al*[6] with permission from *Brain*.

authors examined the physiological modulation of the nystagmus during predominantly otolith manoeuvres (static tilt) or predominantly vertical semicircular canal manoeuvres (head rolling movements; Fig. 2). Since the nystagmus was mainly modulated by the latter manoeuvres, the authors concluded that the pathophysiological basis of torsional nystagmus is a functional asymmetry in the central projections of the semicircular canal system. But it was also noted that many of the patients had ocular skew deviations as well. The presence of skew deviations in patients with a disorder of the central semicircular canal system (rather than of the otolithic gravitational system) was puzzling. For this reason, it was decided to investigate the normal physiological basis for this phenomenon, namely whether the normal vertical canal system participates in the control of ocular vertical alignment.

In a series of experiments by Jauregui-Renaud *et al*[7,8], normal subjects were whole-body rotated in roll (*i.e.* about the visual axis) with the rotational axis placed either earth-horizontal (subjects upright; Fig. 2C) or earth-vertical (subjects supine; Fig. 2D). In the first condition, the compensatory vestibulo-ocular response is mediated by the otoliths, as they continuously change orientation with respect to the gravitational field, and by the semicircular canals. In the second condition, since the otolith do not undergo re-orientation with respect to gravity, the response is only mediated by the vertical canals. For these experiments, eye movements have to be recorded not with electro-oculography (EOG, ENG) but with techniques able to measure vertical, horizontal and torsional movements, such as the scleral coil technique or video-oculography (3-D VOG). The results showed clearly that a dynamic skew deviation occurs during the roll oscillation and that there was no difference in the magnitude of the skew when subjects were oscillated supine or upright. The conclusion is that the vertical semicircular canal system exerts a dominant influence on vertical, divergent ocular movements. Therefore, lesions to this system, central or peripheral, have the potential to produce pathological skew deviations in man and, consequently, diplopia. In further studies, it was shown that, during whole body velocity steps in the roll plane, the magnitude of the physiological skew deviation decays with a time constant of approximately 5 s[9]. This time constant is identical to the time constant of the vertical semicircular canal system, measured by eye movement[9] or psychophysical[10] techniques, further indication of the prominent role of the vertical canal system in the origin of the dynamic skew eye deviation.

Returning to 'under-rated neuro-otological symptoms', it is clear that double vision can occur in peripheral vestibular disease, as a result of acute disruption to otolith and vertical canal mechanisms controlling vertico-torsional ocular alignment. Good clinical practice still dictates, however, that care should be exercised before attributing diplopia to labyrinthine disease. Furthermore, clinically obvious skew ocular deviations must be considered as secondary to CNS lesions disrupting central otolith and/or vertical canal pathways. In this regard, lesions in the vicinity of the vestibular nuclei in the pontomedullary junction usually produce hypodeviation of the ipsilateral eye (*e.g.* a left medullary lesion produces a skew eye deviation in which the left eye is lower than the right) and mid-brain lesions induce skew deviations with the ipsilateral eye uppermost[11]. When this rule of thumb does not explain the clinical findings, other mechanisms may be at work. For instance, patients may have paroxysmal skew deviations due to 'irritative' lesions of the brain stem which produce an abnormal increase of activity in saccadic-related areas[12]. Since the brain stem saccadic centres are also responsible for the generation of the fast phases of nystagmus, such skew deviations can be considered to arise from abnormally overactive quick components of vertico-torsional nystagmus. Also, cerebellar lesions (*e.g.* in the uvula) can produce disinhibition and instability in the vestibular vertico-torsional system[13], leading to paroxysmal nystagmus with skew deviation and disabling oscillopsia (moving images) and diplopia (double vision).

Visual influences on vestibular symptoms

The other under-rated visual neuro-otological symptom discussed by Hoffman and Brookler is exemplified by their 'case 6', a woman with a cerebello-pontine angle lesion who presented with intolerance to visual motion.

Indeed, many patients state that their dizziness or unsteadiness is triggered or increased in surroundings with profuse visual motion or repetitive visual patterns. Patients may dislike traffic, moving crowds, supermarket aisles, watching car chases in movies, ironing striped shirts, or driving on motorways, with many patients displaying several of these triggers. Undoubtedly, in some of these patients the diagnosis is one of anxiety, phobia or panic. But this is not true for all of them, particularly when, as in patient 6 of Hoffman and Brookler, such symptoms develop after a vestibular insult. The origin of these symptoms, termed 'space and motion discomfort'[14], 'visuo-vestibular mismatch'[15], 'visual vertigo syndrome'[16] or 'motorist disorientation syndrome'[17] by different authors, has been recently investigated by Guerraz *et al*[18].

To begin with, it should be remembered that, as soon as the vestibular system is damaged, a neural process of recovery called vestibular compensation gets under way. Guerraz *et al*[18] speculated that, if the process of compensation from vestibular lesions is dependent on alternative sources of sensory information (visual, proprioceptive), individual differences in the functional status of these systems should have a critical influence on the clinical outcome of a vestibular disorder. Since most of these patients do

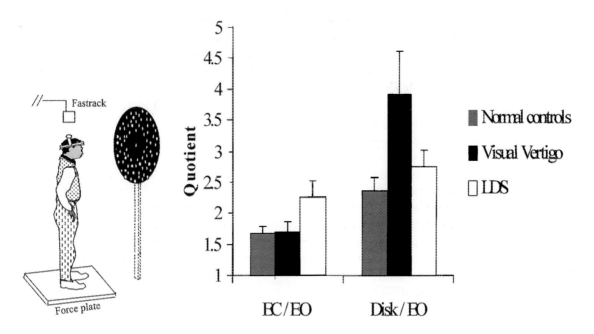

Fig. 3 Diagram illustrating the large rotating disk used to destabilise posture, whilst recording head sway with an electro-magnetic device (fastrak) and force platform posturography (Left). The body sway results show sway path expressed as ratios between two conditions in normal control subjects, bilateral labyrinthine defective subjects (LDS) and patients with visually induced dizziness (visual vertigo). The eyes closed/eyes open ratio (EC/EO), or Romberg quotient, represents the stabilising power of vision, *i.e.* how unstable subjects become with eyes closed relative to eyes in a stationary environment. The Disk/EO ratio indicates how unstable subjects become when viewing the rotating disk in comparison with eyes open in the stationary environment (the destabilising power of vision). Note that the visual vertigo patients are selectively unstable during disk rotation. Reproduced with permission from *Current Opinion in Neurology*[20].

not have clinically obvious visual or somatosensory disorders, Guerraz *et al*[18] explored the possibility that minor idiosyncratic differences present in normal people could be the underlying cause. Specifically, it was decided to investigate if patients with visual vertigo were 'visually dependent'.

In essence, a visually dependent person is someone who relies more on vision than on gravito-inertial (vestibulo-proprioceptive) cues for spatial orientation. Visually independent people do just the opposite and can quite happily disregard misleading visual information. Visually dependent and independent people represent the two ends of a continuum in the normal population. However, a patient with a vestibular disorder **and** visual dependency is more likely to be made dizzy by excessive or disorienting visual stimuli than a visually independent subject.

In order to examine the role of visual dependence, a group of patients with dizziness triggered by visual stimuli (visual vertigo) were probed with psychophysical and postural tasks of the type shown in Figure 3. Essentially, the tests measured how much a large field rotating disk (Fig. 3) and a statically tilted luminous frame (not shown) can alter the perception of verticality whilst seated, and postural balance whilst standing up. Questionnaires were used to measure spontaneous dizziness and autonomic symptoms as well as handicap and trait anxiety levels. In addition to visual vertigo patients, two control groups were tested – a normal control group, and a group of bilateral labyrinthine defective subjects with absence of vestibular function. The latter were included as a positive control group since labyrinthine defective subjects are by definition visually dependent.

The main results of this study were: (i) the majority of the visual vertigo patients were thought to have a peripheral vestibular disorder; (ii) levels of anxiety were similar in the two patient groups (visual vertigo and labyrinthine defective); and (iii) visual vertigo patients had abnormally large perceptual and postural responses to the tilted frame and the rotating disk, *i.e.* they were visually dependent. Furthermore, when the postural sway induced by the rotating disk was expressed relative to the static baseline sway, the visual vertigo patients had significantly larger responses than those in the labyrinthine defective group (Fig. 3).

Conclusions and key points for clinical practice

- The findings support the view that patients whose dizzy symptoms are precipitated by disorienting visual surroundings are likely to have suffered a vestibular episode **and** be visually dependent.

- This combination should be highly debilitating for visual vertigo patients in disorienting visual environments when both visual and vestibular signals are unreliable.

- Clinical experience indicates that vestibular rehabilitation including repetitive optokinetic stimulation can be extremely beneficial in these patients. A formal trial has just been completed by Pavlou et al[19] with very encouraging results.

- The fact that a patient may have additional anxiety or phobic symptoms should not prompt the clinician to think that **all** symptoms in that patient are psychological. Not surprisingly, I also agree with Hoffman and Brookler in this matter.

References

1   Brandt T. *Vertigo: Its Multisensory Syndromes*, 2nd edn. London: Springer, 1991
2   Baloh RW, Honrubia V. *Clinical Neurophysiology of the Vestibular System*, 3rd edn. London: Oxford University Press 2001
3   Hoffman RA, Brookler KH. Underrated neurotological symptoms. *Laryngoscope* 1978; **88**: 1127–38
4   Brain RW. Vertigo: its neurological, otological, circulatory, and surgical aspects. *BMJ* 1938; **2**: 605

5   Riordan-Eva P, Harcourt JP, Faldon M, Brookes GB, Gresty MA. Skew deviation following
    vestibular nerve surgery. *Ann Neurol* 1997; **41**: 94–9

6   Lopez L, Bronstein AM, Gresty MA, Rudge P, du Boulay EP. A neuro-otological and MRI study of
    thirty five cases. *Brain* 1992; **115**: 1107–24

7   Jauregui-Renaud K, Faldon M, Clarke A, Bronstein AM, Gresty MA. Skew deviation of the eyes in
    normal human subjects induced by semicircular canal stimulation. *Neurosci Lett* 1996; **205**: 135–7

8   Jauregui-Renaud K, Faldon M, Clarke AH, Bronstein AM, Gresty MA. Otolith and semicircular
    canal contributions to the human binocular response to roll oscillation. *Acta Otolaryngol* 1998;
    118: 170–6

9   Jauregui-Renaud K, Faldon M, Gresty AM. Horizontal ocular vergence and the three-dimensional
    response to whole-body roll motion. *Exp Brain Res* 2001; **136**: 79–92

10 Grunfeld EA, Okada T, Jauregui-Renaud K, Bronstein AM. The effect of habituation and plane or
    rotation on vestibular perceptual responses. *J Vestib Res* 2002; **10**: 193–200

11 Brandt T, Dieterich M. Perceived vertical and lateropulsion: clinical syndromes, localization, and
    prognosis. *Neurorehabil Neural Repair* 2000; **14**: 1–12

12 Bentley CR, Bronstein AM, Faldon M *et al*. Fast eye movement initiation of ocular torsion in
    mesodiencephalic lesions. *Ann Neurol* 1998; **43**: 729–37

13 Radtke A, Bronstein AM, Gresty MA *et al*. Paroxysmal alternating skew deviation and nystagmus
    after partial destruction of the uvula. *J Neurol Neurosurg Psychiatry* 2001; **70**: 790–3

14 Furman JM, Jacob RG. A clinical taxonomy of dizziness and anxiety in the otoneurological setting.
    J Anxiety Disord 2001; **15**: 9–26

15 Longridge NS, Mallinson AI, Denton A. Visual vestibular mismatch in patients treated with
    intratympanic gentamicin for Menière's disease. *J Otol* 2002; **31**: 5–8

16 Bronstein AM. Visual vertigo syndrome: clinical and posturography findings. *J Neurol Neurosurg
    Psychiatry* 1995; **59**: 472–6

17 Page NG, Gresty MA. Motorist's vestibular disorientation syndrome. *J Neurol Neurosurg
    Psychiatry* 1985; **48**: 729–35

18 Guerraz M, Yardley L, Bertholon P *et al*. Visual vertigo: symptom assessment, spatial orientation
    and postural control. *Brain* 2001; **124**: 1646–56

19 Pavlou M, Lingeswaran A, Davies RA, Gresty MA, Bronstein AM. Machine-based vs. customised
    rehabilitation for the treatment of chronic vestibular patients. (Abstract Book) Monduzzi Editore.
    1st World Congress of the International Society of Physical and Rehabilitation Medicine. 2001; 139

20 Bronstein AM. Visual and psychological aspects of vestibular disease. *Curr Opin Neurol* 2002; **15**:
    1–3

Otoacoustic emissions, their origin in cochlear function, and use

David T Kemp

UCL Centre for Auditory Research, Institute of Laryngology and Otology, London, UK

Otoacoustic emissions (OAEs) are sounds of cochlear origin, which can be recorded by a microphone fitted into the ear canal. They are caused by the motion of the cochlea's sensory hair cells as they energetically respond to auditory stimulation. OAEs provide a simple, efficient and non-invasive objective indicator of healthy cochlear function and OAE screening is widely used in universal new-born hearing screening programmes. As part of the audiological diagnostic test battery, OAEs can contribute to differential audiological diagnosis, they can be used to monitor the effects of treatment and they can be helpful in the selection of hearing aids and of surgical options. As a research tool, OAEs provide a non-invasive window on intracochlear processes and this has led to new insights into the mechanisms and function of the cochlea and also to a new understanding of the nature of sensory hearing impairment. This chapter provides a broad introduction to OAEs and their applications together with a detailed description of the relationship between OAEs and cochlear mechanisms.

Otoacoustic emissions (OAEs) are sounds which arise in the ear canal when (paradoxically) the tympanum receives vibrations transmitted **backwards** through the middle ear **from** the cochlea. These vibrations occur as a by-product of a unique and vulnerable cochlear mechanism which has become known as the 'cochlear amplifier' and which contributes greatly to the sensitivity and discrimination of hearing. Figure 1A shows an example of a strong, but otherwise typical, transient evoked otoacoustic emission (TEOAE) produced by a healthy new-born ear in response to a click stimulus.

OAE recordings are made *via* an ear canal probe which is deeply inserted into the ear canal as shown in Figure 2. Click stimuli of around 84 dB SPL peak equivalent (p.e) level normally evoke a robust TEOAE response only if hearing threshold is 20 dB HL or better[1-3]. Unlike other audiometric tests, it is not necessary for the stimulus to be near to threshold levels to detect departures from normal function using OAEs. Middle ear status affects OAEs and can prevent their detection[4].

The oscillatory sound pressure waveform seen in TEOAE responses (as in Fig. 1A) actually corresponds to the motion of the eardrum being

*Correspondence to:
Prof. David T Kemp, UCL
Centre for Auditory
Research, Institute of
Laryngology and
Otology,
330 Gray's Inn Road,
London WC1X 8EE, UK*

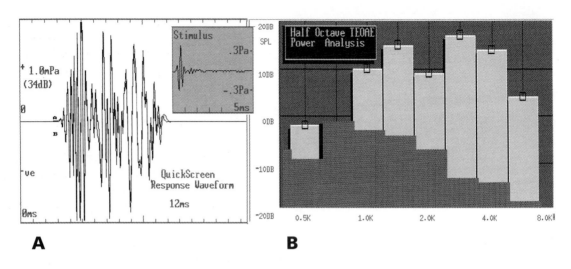

A   **B**

Fig. 1 A strong TEOAE response from a new-born infant. (A) The TEOAE wave form in response at an acoustic click stimulus (shown inset) peaking at 84 dB SPL. The oto-acoustic response level exceeds 30 dB SPL. (B) A frequency analysis of the same TEOAE response showing the energy present per half-octave band. The lower shaded area indicates noise contamination. The wave form is blanked from 0–3.5 ms to remove stimulus artefacts, and again after 12 ms when the next stimulus was applied. A 'non-linear' pattern of different stimulus intensity is usually employed to minimise stimulus artefacts[46]. Multiple stimulus presentations and response averaging are usually required to extract TEOAE responses from background noise. Stimulus repetition rates of 50–100 s^{-1} are usual and recording times vary from a few seconds to a few minutes.

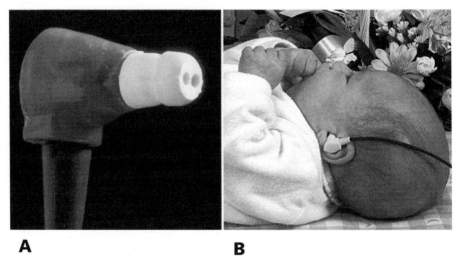

A   **B**

Fig. 2 (A) A TEOAE probe containing miniature sound source and microphone transducers. The soft disposable tip carries sound ports for the stimulus and for the microphone. DPOAE probes have an additional stimulus port. In some probes, all ports feed a single sound tube. (B) The probe needs to be deeply inserted in the ear canal for maximum OAE capture and noise exclusion, with the cable positioned so as to avoid noise production on movement.

pushed backwards and forwards by fluid pressure fluctuations generated inside the cochlea. The sealing of the ear canal by the probe increases the recorded OAEs' sound pressure below 3 kHz, as otherwise drum vibrations would simply move air in and out of the ear canal. The response is long and complex because responses from different parts of the cochlea arrive at the ear canal at different times and at different frequencies. Although clicks are 'wide-band' stimuli, exciting the whole of the cochlea, TEOAE responses can give a frequency specific indication of cochlear status. By splitting the response into frequency bands after recording (Fig. 1B) separate responses from different parts of the cochlea are obtained. TEOAE responses are strongest and easiest to detect in the primary speech frequency band, 1–4 kHz. In young ears, TEOAEs extend up to 6–7 kHz[5], but many clinically normal adult ears give weak TEOAEs (less than 3 dB SPL), with no substantial response above 4 kHz.

TEOAEs are highly sensitive to cochlear pathology and in a frequency-specific way. Frequencies at which hearing thresholds exceed 20–30 dB HL are typically absent in the TEOAE response[1,6,7]. Because of their sensitivity to cochlear dysfunction, TEOAEs have found wide-spread application in new-born hearing screening programmes[8]. Healthy infant ears typically produce strong OAE levels of 15 dB SPL to more than 30 dB SPL. Little signal processing is required to extract these responses from noise and fully validated frequency-specific measurements can often be made in a few seconds. This contrasts with recordings of the auditory brain-stem response (ABR), which require electrodes and which must be extracted from the relatively much stronger EEG background signal over a longer period of signal averaging. However, OAE signals are very sensitive to minor conductive losses caused by middle ear fluid and ear canal debris in neonates, so that sometimes, in the first few hours after birth, an ABR can be recorded when an OAE cannot. Also, since the ABR is sensitive to both cochlear and retro-cochlear pathology, ABR testing would appear to be preferable to OAE for infant screening. However, in practice, sensory hearing impairment in the low-risk new-born population appears to be overwhelmingly of the sensory transmissive type (see below), which is readily detectable by measurement of OAEs. This, together with favourable ergonomic and economics factors, means that OAEs are a reliable and highly cost-effective tool for universal new-born hearing programmes. Nevertheless, where there is a known risk of neurological damage, ABR testing is also essential.

The healthy ear produces OAEs not only to in response to clicks, but to any applied sound including tones. A second method of OAE recording, using tonal stimulation and called 'distortion product otoacoustic emissions' (DPOAEs) is in wide-spread clinical use[9]. Non-linear intermodulation between the two stimulus tones inside the cochlea generates several new acoustic frequency components, which can travel

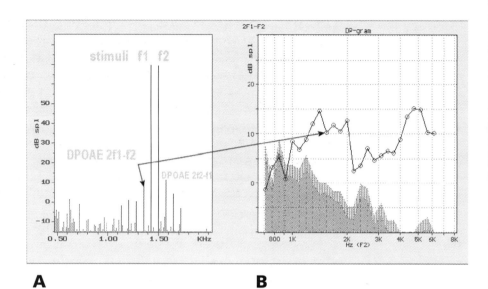

A   **B**

Fig. 3 Distortion product OAE recording requires the application of two pure tone stimuli. The lower frequency tone is commonly applied at a level of 60–70 dB SPL while the higher frequency tone is applied at a lower level of 50–70 dB SPL. (A) The sound spectrum in a healthy human ear canal during stimulation by two closely spaced pure tones, f1 = 1425 Hz and f2 = 1500 Hz, both at 70 dB SPL. The spectral lines between 1100–1800 Hz on either side of the stimulus lines are intermodulation tones created by the cochlea. Each is separated from its neighbour by an interval of [f2–f1]. Clinical DPOAE analysis typically tracks the level of just one of these distortion products (f_{dp} = f1–[f2–f1] = 2f1–f2) as f1 and f2 are stepped across the frequency range of interest. (B) This allows a 'DP-gram' to be constructed. A stimulus frequency separation f2/f1 ~ 1.2 results in the strongest DPOAEs. The lower shaded portion (right) indicates the noise contamination.

to the ear canal. Healthy ear canal distortion levels can be above 20 dB SPL. Figure 3 provides an example of a clinical DPOAE analysis and illustrates its derivation.

Non-linear intermodulation between two tones is a purely mechanical process and distortion products satisfy the frequency relationship $f_{dp} = f_1 + N(f_2 - f_1)$ where N is any positive or negative whole number[10]. Each distortion component can be separated from the stimuli by preset signal frequency analysis. The intensity of one particular component at $f_{dp} = f_1 + (-1)[f_2 - f_1]$, (simplifying to $2f_1 - f_2$) is used as an indicator of cochlear status, plotted as a function of frequency in the 'DP-gram' (see Fig. 3B). DPOAE generation is much reduced and usually absent if there is significant sensory hearing loss[11].

The TEOAE and DPOAE techniques compliment each other. DPOAEs offer a wider frequency range of observation (above 10 kHz) with less sensitivity to minor and sub-clinical conditions in adults. More powerful excitation is practical with continuous tones (up to 75 dB SPL), allowing

DPOAEs to be recorded with moderate losses when no TEOAE can be detected. However, DPOAE recordings provide no greater frequency specificity than TEOAEs despite the use of pure tones. At best, both responses reflect the intrinsic frequency resolution of the cochlea, which is around one-quarter octave (see also Fig. 5).

Although OAEs are a good indicator of hearing loss, it is important to remember that an OAE examination is not a hearing test. It is a test of an essential and vulnerable cochlear function as described below. It is tempting to believe that OAE intensity relates directly to cochlear 'strength', but this is not so. Like electrophysiological measurements of auditory function, the observed OAE response intensity can be strongly affected by the quality of the coupling between sensor and patient (*i.e.* the OAE probe fit or electrode placement) and by spurious non-auditory factors which determine the external field produced by internal physiological activity. Intensity is a primary factor in OAE detectability but, like the ABR, it is the **presence** of a detectable OAE response to a particular stimulus that is clinically important and not its strength.

Measurement of DPOAEs at multiple stimulus levels can establish the OAE 'growth rate'. Healthy ears tend to exhibit a DPOAE growth rate of 1 dB of OAE per 1 dB of stimulus or less. Ears with some impairment show steeper growth while instrumental artefacts tend to have the greatest rates of growth. Single DPOAE observations can be misleading and results needs to be averaged across a frequency range. Estimates of the degree of threshold elevation have been attempted using DPOAE intensity and growth functions[12,13], but obtaining the 'threshold of detectability' of DPOAE against background noise adds little further information. While DPOAEs relate to threshold across a population, they are at best a very unreliable and imprecise indicator of an individual's hearing threshold. This is because, unlike the ABR, OAEs are presynaptic responses. Their origin precedes the 'threshold' imposed by the inner hair cell's transduction process. Use of higher stimulus intensities increases OAE detectability and can provide useful evidence of residual hair cell activity, but does not probe any deeper into the auditory pathway.

The field of OAE research has grown enormously since their discovery 25 years ago[3,10]. Comprehensive overviews of OAEs, measurement technology and applications can be found elsewhere[9,14]. The purpose of this chapter is to present and explain OAEs to potential users in the context of cochlear function and from this to derive a logical basis for their clinical application.

How do otoacoustic emissions arise?

Detectable OAE sound pressure is produced by motions of the eardrum which are extremely small. For example, an eardrum oscillation of only

10^{-10} m (the diameter of an atom of hydrogen) will create a 'large' OAE of intensity 34 dB SPL (1 mPa) in a 1-ml ear canal volume. A common misconception is that OAEs are 'radiated' by the cochlea and transmitted through the middle ear cavity. This is not the case. Motions of the oval and round window membranes during OAE generate negligible sound pressure, because their areas are too small and their motions oppose each other.

To understand how OAEs arise, why vibrations emerge from the cochlea, and why OAEs are indicative of good hearing, it is necessary to consider what normally happens as stimulation enters the cochlea.

The cochlea as a stimulus delivery system

The importance of the outer and middle ear mechanisms in collecting sound energy and conveying it to the cochlea is well understood. Pathology in these areas affects hearing through stimulus attenuation, which can be severe but never profound. Unlike sensory loss, conductive loss introduces no distortion, so it can be very effectively corrected by amplification.

Even healthy ears have a slight 'conductive loss' because not all of the available sound energy enters the cochlea. The proportion which does enter the cochlea depends on how efficiently the middle ear mechanism couples the low acoustic impedance of air to the high mechanical impedance of the fluid-filled cochlea. The round window plays an important role in releasing cochlear fluid pressure caused by stapes displacement thereby greatly reducing the cochlear input impedance. This increases cochlear fluid motion which eventually excites the inner hair cells (Fig. 4). In contrast, acoustic pressure in the cochlear perilymph is almost instantly transmitted to every cell, but causes no sound sensation.

Fluid motion in the basal regions of scala vestibuli and tympani, synchronously with stapes vibration, necessarily displaces the basilar membrane (BM). Only the basal part of the BM moves initially because, although quite stiff, it has little inertia. Being narrow in relation to the cochlear duct, it moves relatively little fluid mass.

Induced transverse oscillations of the basal BM begins to propagate apically. Oscillatory exchanges occur between fluid motion energy and the energy held in elastic BM displacement. Adjacent BM sections are excited as fluid displaced from, for example, the upward motion of the BM at one place forces the next more apical and less stiff place downwards and so on, resulting in a travelling wave (Fig. 5A). The travelling wave (TW) conveys stimulus energy towards the apex at less than 1/100th of the speed of sound in air. For example, the 2 cm journey of a 500-Hz stimulus to its cochlear place takes around 10 ms, accounting for the substantial latency of OAEs[15].

The BM becomes progressively less elastically stiff and wider away from the base. Less elastic stiffness means less force opposing displacement, so

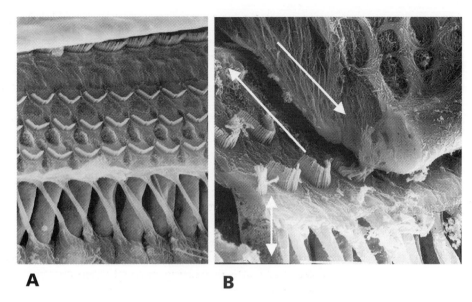

Fig. 4 Two scanning electron micrograph views of the organ of Corti and its sensory hair cells (courtesy of Prof. A. Forge) showing the extremely orderly arrangement of sensory cells and the reason for heavy viscous damping. (**A**) Stereocilia of the inner (back row) and outer (front three rows) hair cells which protrude from the reticula lamina. Sectioning (front) shows the separated cylindrical OHC bodies within the rigid box-like structure. (**B**) A freeze-etched specimen showing the tectorial membrane (TM) in its functional position (with some damage in preparation). The tectorial membrane is anchored to a non-vibrating point near the modiolus and also rests on the stereocilia of the outer hair cells. The organ of Corti moves as a whole with BM motion, causing linear and shear motion relative to the TM. This results in oscillatory radial fluid flow within the narrow sub-tectorial space between scala media and the inner sulcus. The flow impinges on IHC stereocilia, which do not touch the TM but form an almost continuous 'fence' to arrest any fluid flow (see rear of A). Their deflection excites the IHCs causing transduction of stimulus information into neural code. This fluid motion takes place in the very narrow space (less than 10 μm) and it is here that viscosity readily absorbs energy from the travelling wave. OHC stereocilia are deflected against the TM into which they are embedded, the buttressed 'W' configuration ensuring that considerable force can be exchanged. Excitation of the OHCs generates synchronous mechanical forces which are then transmitted to the BM replacing lost energy and sustaining the TW.

TW amplitude can increase. Increased width and fluid contact area means more inertia, which acts to sustain motion and so opposes the elastic forces restraining displacement. Consequently, wave amplitude increases with distance along the BM. It is potentially maximum at the place where (for the particular stimulus frequency) the force of inertia equals and cancels the elastic restoring force, *i.e.* at 'resonance'.

Because inertial forces increase with frequency, the place along the BM at which this peak in TW amplitude occurs is progressively nearer to the base for higher frequency stimuli. The forward speed of the TW also reduces as inertial forces increase and stiffness decreases, and it eventually comes to a

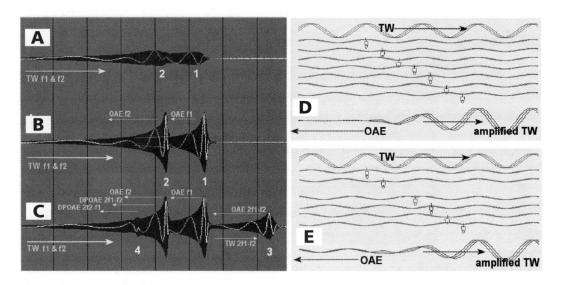

Fig. 5 (A–C) A schematic illustration of the development of the TW along the BM and the sources of OAE. Panels show computed TW envelopes and instantaneous wave patterns in response to two prolonged pure tones with frequencies f1 and f2 (f2/f1 = 1.5). The TW progresses from the base (left) towards the apex (right). In (**A**), natural damping absorbs most of the stimulus energy before any clear separate excitation peaks for f1 and f2 can develop. This corresponds to the 'dead' cochlea as studied by von Békésy. Sharp 'images' of stimuli f1 and f2 can be seen in (**B**), where damping has been largely removed by linear OHC amplification. In reality, OHC motility is non-linear and this results in intermodulation distortion products being created under the entire f2 envelope (including 2f1–f2 and 2f2–f1) as in (**C**), which then travel to their frequency places at points 3 and 4.(**D,E**) Show how OHC energy is fed into the TW to replace that lost by damping, and how OAEs can arise. In (D), seven uniformly spaced electromotile hair cells each 'radiate' a new bi-directional travelling wave exactly in synchrony with the stimulus TW (top), which has unrealistically constant amplitude for the purposes of this schematic. In the forward (apical) direction, these wavelets are automatically in synchrony resulting in an 'amplified' TW (bottom of (D)). OHC wavelets in the reverse (basal) direction cancel each other so that no OAE is generated. In (E) the array is unbalanced, *e.g.* by a missing or less active hair cell. Amplification still occurs, but the imbalance results in a basal-ward TW (bottom trace). A 'place fixed' or 'stimulus frequency' OAE (SFOAE) is created. More complete cochlear models have shown that, in order to recreate experimentally observed TW envelopes, amplification needs to occur over only a limited region of the BM, somewhat basally to the actual TW peak. SFOAEs probably emanate from this same region, as indicated in (B), but there is no guarantee of this. In the non-linear case (C), DP energy can escape in a similar way to SFOAEs, *i.e.* from places 3 and 4 in (C), to form DPOAEs. But with f2/f1 between ~1.15–1.3, a substantial amount of the DP 2f1–f2 escapes directly from inside the f2 envelope, as indicated in (C). These are termed 'wave fixed' emissions[23,25,47]. This figure emphasises the complex origins of OAEs and reasons why frequency-specific OAEs are not strictly 'place' specific.

virtual stop at 'resonance'. A good way to understand the characteristic TW shape (Fig. 5B) is to realise that, as its longitudinal (*i.e.* apical) velocity reduces, its energy must become compressed into a smaller length of BM. Consequently, its transverse oscillations must increase in amplitude.

Increased transverse motion in the wave causes increased viscous drag in the organ of Corti (see Fig. 4), which removes energy at an increasingly rapid rate. At some place, 'energy loss' begins to dominate 'energy concentration' and the wave intensity falls precipitously as its energy is absorbed by the organ of Corti. The overall result is an asymmetric peak of excitation for each frequency component (Fig. 5B).

The cochlea as an imaging system

The TW envelope represents the excitation intensity applied to the organ of Corti as a function of distance along the length of the cochlea. The organ of Corti mechanism then converts BM motion to fluid motion across the IHC stereocilia, leading to neural excitation (see Fig. 4). The tonotopic re-distribution of stimulus energy achieved by the TW is essential in the mammalian cochlea because it facilitates the neural representation of stimulus frequencies well above the maximum nerve fibre firing rate of around 2 kHz. Although the TW is usually credited with frequency separation, the TW envelope is also an 'image' or 'map' of acoustic intensity against acoustic 'source size'. This follows because acoustic radiation efficiency is strongly related to the size of the radiating object, with sound from large objects tending to be dominated by low frequencies and peaking near the apex and with sounds from small objects tending to be dominated by high frequencies, peaking at the base. The functional significance of this is obvious.

Thought of as an 'imaging system', it becomes clearer why the 'quality' or 'sharpness' of the TW envelope is paramount. The resolution of the cochlear imaging mechanism can be characterised by the 'height' and 'width' of the TW excitation peak for each pure-tone component (see Fig. 5A,B).

The need for a 'cochlear amplifier'

In discovering the travelling wave, von Békésy observed the cadaver cochlea to have very poor 'imaging' qualities[16]. He found the travelling wave peak in response to a pure tone stimulus to extend over a third or more of the entire cochlear length (see Fig. 5A). In the healthy living cochlea, the TW peak for low-level pure tone stimulation is much sharper[17,18]. The TW peak covers less than 1 mm and a shift in frequency of just one-third of an octave moves the TW peak to stimulate an entirely different set of sensory cells (see Ashmore, this volume).

The reason for the poor imaging quality of a dead (or deaf) cochlea (Fig. 5A) is high levels of viscous damping. If viscous damping is low, then the TW peak will be sharp and its amplitude will be large. Hearing will be more sensitive and cochlear frequency resolution (and selectivity) will be more acute in a cochlea with less damping.

It is not that cochlear fluids become any 'thicker' or more viscous than water in the deaf or dead cochlea. These viscous losses are physically inevitable because: (i) sensory cells must absorb stimulus energy to operate; and (ii) in order to reach the inner hair cells, cochlear fluid motion must take place in the extremely constricted sub-tectorial space (Fig. 4B). The energy lost from the TW due to viscous fluid drag in the subtectorial space plus energy absorbed by the hair cell themselves is very substantial. In fact the majority of the incident stimulus energy is actually lost before reaching its appropriate frequency place. Under purely mechanical forces, the cochlea cannot develop a strong and sharp TW image.

The mammalian cochlea has evolved a unique mechanism for replacing TW energy lost by viscosity, at least for weak stimuli. The idea of a 'cochlear amplifier' to overcome physical limitations was first proposed by Gold[19]. It was revived following the discovery of OAEs[3,20], but became a credible possibility only after the discovery of hair cell motility by Brownell[21]. Electro-motility (Ashmore, this volume) is the only known functional characteristic of the outer hair cells, which out-number the inner hair cells by 3:1 (Fig. 4A).

Figure 5 illustrates how OHC motility results in TW amplification. In so far as the OHC motile forces exactly oppose the forces of viscous drag, the degrading effect of the drag on the TW 'image' can be regarded as being neutralised. If OHC forces exceed that necessary to overcome viscosity, then excitation will be increased above that delivered by the stimulus, providing the possibility of amplification – as implied in Figure 5B. This process of TW enhancement in the cochlea by stimulated mechanical energy release parallels with what happens to light inside the laser.

Oto-acoustic emissions and the 'imperfect' cochlear amplifier

The cochlear amplifier is physically essential to the high sensitivity of hearing and to the formation of a sharp ~0.25 octave resolution tonotopic 'image' of the acoustic environment along the length of the cochlea. As Figure 5 indicates, OAEs are a by-product of this 'cochlear amplifier'. They arrive in the ear canal as a result of BM disturbances that escape from the cochlear amplifier mechanism and travel away from the sensory cells back to the base of the cochlea. Here the 'up-and-down' motion of the BM exerts a differential oscillating fluid pressure on the oval and round windows causing vibration of the oscicles and ear drum and hence OAEs.

OAEs can only be generated if the cochlear amplifier mechanism is present and to some degree operational. But, paradoxically, the reasons why vibrations are sent back to the base to form OAEs all relate to natural imperfections in this mechanism. What kind of amplifier imperfections result in OAEs?

As illustrated in Figure 5B, if OHC motility is not completely uniformly distributed, a stimulus frequency OAE will be generated. In a travelling wave amplifier, any lack of uniformity in construction or function places an upper limit on the level of stable amplification. By scattering amplified energy back to the base of the cochlea, energy is wasted and appears as stimulus frequency OAEs.

It is not only spatial imperfections that can generate OAEs. If the forces exerted by OHCs on the BM do not exactly follow the stimulus waveform (*i.e.* if the OHC electromotility is 'non-linear'), they will add distortion signals to the forward travelling wave, which are one cause of aural combination tones. As explained in Figure 5, OHC electromotility distortion can also propagate back to the middle ear *via* two competing routes, to cause 'wave' and 'place' fixed 'distortion product' OAEs in the ear canal[22,23]. TEOAEs contain both stimulus frequency and distortion product OAEs according to Yates and Whithnell[24].

Another type of 'imperfection' arises from positive feedback, leading to instability and self-oscillation and is a common property of TW amplification systems. In the cochlea, most energy travels apically and is absorbed, but any energy that escapes basally to reach the base can be partially reflected back, forming a new forward TW. This can re-stimulate the OHC mechanism. Under conditions of high amplification, endless recirculation of the TW leads to sustained oscillation inside the cochlea and to spontaneous OAE of one or more pure tones into the ear canal.

Oto-acoustic emissions as a 'window' on cochlear function

To what extent can the functional status of a cochlea be characterised and quantified using OAEs? OAEs are only a by-product of cochlear function. As we have seen, the factors which govern the escape of energy to produce OAEs relate to 'imperfections' of the cochlear amplifier, *i.e.* non-linearity and irregularities. Also, several different cochlear locations may contribute to a single frequency component of an OAE and these may fortuitously summate or interfere with each other (Fig. 5C). The transmission back to the ear canal also depends on individual middle ear characteristics. The interplay of all these factors cannot yet be accurately modelled, not least because most parameters are unknown. It is not surprising, therefore, that individual healthy ears differ greatly in the level and the spectrum of the OAEs they exhibit. Stimuli of slightly differing frequency or spectral composition can give rise to quite different OAE patterns. Taking an 'average' OAE characteristic over a range of stimuli provides a more meaningful description of cochlear status, but even so the intensity of OAEs alone is a very imperfect index of cochlear status.

The 'frequency' at which an emission can be evoked is more significant. OAEs are frequency-specific responses and tend to emerge only in frequency bands where hearing is near normal. This provides a useful pointer to normally and abnormally functioning parts of a cochlea. But, as Figure 5A–C clearly demonstrates, with OAEs, frequency specificity does not always ensure 'place' specificity, even when pure tone stimuli are used, as with DPOAEs.

Two general rules apply to DPOAE production which are relevant to clinical applications. In any non-linear system, intermodulation distortion is always strongest when the two interacting signals have similar levels at the non-linearity. In the cochlea, the relative intensity and relative frequency of the two stimuli determine where along the organ of Corti this 'physically ideal' condition is met. Referring to Figure 5B, even when the input levels of f1 and f2 are the same, making TW 'f1' and TW 'f2' intensities similar at the base, at the place where TW 'f2' peaks its intensity is much larger than for the TW 'f1'. Making the lower-frequency stimulus relatively more intense than f2 at the input will shift the place of greatest intermodulation towards the f2 peak of the TW and so enhance DP production. Increasing the f1 level too much will be counter-productive. Therefore, for each stimulus level, there is an optimum stimulus intensity ratio for maximum DP production.

DP production does not ensure DP emission, which is governed by the second rule. The extent to which all the elemental OHC DP sources re-inforce each other to produce a strong backwards DP travelling wave (and hence a DPOAE) depends on the spatial distribution of DP phases. This depends on the relative travelling wave velocities of f1 and f2 at the non-linearity. When the ratio f2/f1 is nearly one (*e.g.* 1.05), f1 and f2 TW velocities are very similar at all points. The phase distribution of DP elements then necessarily forms a forward (apical) TW with little DP sent backwards to form a DPOAE. Even so, some DPOAE will escape via the SOAE route, as illustrated in Figure 5C. For large f2/f1 (*e.g.* 1.5), the densely packed phase changes within the f2 envelope generate an undulating DP phase distribution that will be largely self-cancelling and little DP wave will propagate from that region. However, because there is a minus sign in '2f1–f2', for f2 > f1, the spatial phase gradients of TW 'f1' and TW 'f2' counteract each other in 2f1–f2 DP production. Consequently, at some optimum f2/f1 ratio (around 1.2), the relative velocities of TW 'f1' and TW 'f2' are such that the spatial distribution of DP elements actually becomes that of a backward travelling wave over a considerable length of OHCs. Maximum DPOAE is delivered to the ear canal via this 'wave-fixed' mechanism[25]. Interestingly, there is no optimum frequency ratio for the 'alternative' DPOAE 2f2–f1 (see Fig. 5C), which emanates from a place basal to both f1 and f2 peaks over a wide range of f2/f1 ratios. The clinical significance of this DPOAE has not been fully evaluated.

Clinical DPOAE measurements are generally made with both stimulus intensity and frequency ratios optimised for maximum DPOAE 2f1–f2 intensity[26]. As Figure 3 illustrates, many different DPOAEs co-exist and their generation is intimately linked to the operating characteristics of the outer hair cells. It is possible that we will one day be able to reconstruct OHC operating characteristics from DPOAE data.

Spontaneous OAEs (SOAEs) are typically highly stable pure tones of level –10 to 30 dB SPL, which are found in 30–40% of healthy young ears[27,28]. Their presence indicates simply a 'chance' combination of factors. Strong TW amplification must co-exist with irregularities to cause a strong wave to be returned to the base and the proportion reflected back into the cochlea by the middle ear must, after re-amplification and re-emission, be sufficient to sustain a continuous oscillation of the middle ear and along a substantial section of the BM. The round trip travel time also has to be exactly right for this to occur and so can happen only at one precise frequency, just as in the laser. The precise frequency of an SOAE does not imply an origin at a precise place in the cochlea, but only a particular co-incidence of travel time and reflection from an ill-defined region of high OHC activity. But, because of their intrinsic stability and critical dependence on cochlear status, SOAEs are, when present, particularly sensitive indicators of metabolic and physiological changes in the cochlea.

All OAE forms show a high degree of sensitivity to changes in cochlear status. Exposure to noise levels causing temporary threshold shift depresses TEOAEs[29,30] and low stimulus level DPOAEs[31]. Changes in cerebrospinal fluid pressure induced by posture changes affect SOAE frequency and evoked OAE intensity – probably by their influence on cochlear fluid pressure and stapedial position[32]. Drugs known to depress hearing, including aspirin and quinine, also depress OAEs, and loop diuretics known to depress the endocochlear potential also depress OAEs[33,34].

OAEs also exhibit a physical analogue of 'masking' where the perception of one sound is blocked by another (see BJM Moore, this volume). This may indicate that some forms of masking originate preneurally in the cochlea. Tracing the suppression of an OAE response to one tone by adjusting the intensity and frequency of a second suppressor tone allows an OAE suppression-tuning curve to be constructed[35–37]. The sharpness of such curves confirms the close association between OAEs and auditory function, and demonstrates that sharp mechanical tuning is present at the cochlear level.

Perhaps the most interesting suppression effect is the slight depression of OAE level (by 0.5–3 dB) caused by noise or irregular acoustic stimulation applied to the contralateral ear[38,39]. First discovered by Collet *et al* in 1990, this effect has been identified as being largely due to the influence of the medial cochlear efferent system. This terminates directly on the OHC bodies and presumably normally plays a role in the day-to-day maintenance of effective OHC status. The contralateral suppression effect is best seen on TEOAEs evoked by a uniform train of click stimuli of less than 74 dB SPL p.e., but can also be seen on DPOAEs evoked by primaries below 60 dB SPL. The neural mechanism and function remain somewhat obscure. Absence of a contralateral OAE suppression effect can be the result of a brain stem lesion, but Collet has also reported it in certain stages of sleep, and it can be absent in some healthy individuals. It has even been suggested that absence of contralateral OAE suppression may correlate with autism and dyslexia[40–42]. The phenomenon of contralateral OAE suppression is not well understood.

In general, OAE responses carry a large amount of information about the status, activity and environment of OHCs, which we are currently unable to interpret. OAEs tend to be dominated by microscopic details of little relevance to hearing. Nevertheless, OAEs provide the only detailed non-invasive window on the cochlea and by their very presence confirm normal presynaptic cochlear function. Although useful today, if we can learn how to extract definitive data on OHC status from OAE data, then their clinical importance will be greatly enhanced.

Key points for clinical practice

OAEs are already an essential part of the audiological diagnostic test battery[43]. Key points for clinical use are summarised below.

Recording otoacoustic emissions

- Advanced OAE techniques need a sound attenuating booth, but useful OAEs can be made in a quiet office environment. Background room noise levels of 40 dB or below are recommended. A good probe fit helps block out external noise, although this effect is minimal with neonate ears. Short bursts of more intense noise (*e.g.* speaking to the patient, or a cough), which can be detected and rejected by the instrumentation, are less troublesome than continuous or reverberant sounds. Patient movement is also not a problem with OAEs provided it does not result in cable-rub noise. Jaw action, swallowing and vocalisations cause ear canal noises, which can prevent good OAE recordings.

- Patency of the ear canal is essential for successful recordings. Obstruction by wax in older patients, or by fluid or birth debris in neonates, or by collapse of the canal in the latter, prevent OAEs from reaching the ear canal and are major causes of OAE recording failure. Sleep and sedation have minimal effects on OAEs[44].

Types of otoacoustic emissions

- There are two widely used OAE measurements: transient evoked OAEs (TEOAEs) and dual-tone evoked distortion product OAEs (DPOAEs).

DPOAE measurements are better suited to advanced clinical investigation on adult patients, even though DPOAE analysis is complex and interpretation is difficult. The DP technique is more flexible and potentially more powerful than TEOAE analysis, having a wider useful frequency range. Waveform-based TEOAE measurements, as originally used in universal new-born hearing screening programmes, are also useful as a sensitive initial screen prior to full clinical examination. TEOAEs are also more sensitive to cochlear status changes manifested in subtle changes in the TEOAE waveform. DPOAE instruments can be used for screening with an appropriately low stimulus level (*e.g.* 65/55 dB SPL), but DPOAE screening instruments are generally not flexible enough for clinical applications.

Middle ear factors

- OAE detection is affected by conductive losses and OAEs will be absent if there is effusion, glue, otosclerosis or ossicular dislocation. Moderate negative pressure and tympanic perforations not exceeding 30% result in the attenuation of only the lower frequency OAEs. Grommets do not greatly affect OAEs. Absent OAEs can re-appear following effective middle ear treatment or surgery if the residual conductive loss is very small and the cochlea is normal. Large and unusual ear canals and perforations can disturb stimulus delivery by 'ringing' and so prevent successful recording. This does not arise with neonates, but their ear canals are extremely small and this needs to be accommodated in the selection of probe size and stimulation intensity.

Oto-acoustic emissions and the nature of sensory hearing loss

- OAEs come exclusively from outer hair cells which do not themselves activate primary auditory nerve fibres, yet a strong relationship exists between the absence of OAEs and hearing loss. This forces a re-definition of the term 'sensory hearing loss'.

  † **Sensory transmissive loss** can be defined as hearing loss resulting from dysfunction of outer sensory hair cell group. Absence of the 'cochlear amplifier' allows natural damping to remove most stimulus energy from the cochlear travelling wave and lowers the resolution of the cochlear imaging mechanism. Inefficient transmission of excitation to the IHCs causes loss of hearing sensitivity and frequency selectivity. Since there remains a pathway for stimulation to reach the IHCs, profound hearing loss cannot be caused by OHC dysfunction alone. Total OHC failure is estimated to cause no more than 60 dB hearing loss. Loss of OAEs with a normal middle ear indicates sensory transmissive loss.

  † **Sensory transduction loss** can be defined as hearing loss resulting from failure of inner hair cells to respond and activate the synapsed auditory nerves. This could give rise to any degree of hearing loss from mild to profound since the auditory nerves themselves have no sensitivity to sound simulation. Loss of frequency selectivity would not necessarily accompany threshold elevation in a pure sensory transductive loss, and OAEs would be normal.

- It is clear from the high correlation between sensory loss and OAE absence that most sensory losses are of the sensory transmissive type. This makes sense, as the outer hair cell mechanism is both highly specialised and highly vulnerable to degradation by excessive noise, anoxia or ototoxic agents. OHCs selectively amplify weak stimuli which would otherwise fall below the threshold for IHCs to trigger a neural response and as a consequence the symptoms of sensory transmissive loss necessarily include loudness recruitment in addition to threshold elevation and reduced frequency selectivity (see BJM Moore, this volume)[45].

Interpretation of otoacoustic emissions

- The presence of robust evokeable OAEs across the key speech frequency range (1.0–4 kHz) indicates a useful degree of normal function in both the middle ear and cochlea and further indicates that speech and language development will not be greatly impeded by peripheral auditory dysfunction. For clinical purposes, it is useful to record OAE status as a function of frequency, averaged over one-half or one-third octave frequency bands. Higher resolution has little physiological meaning.

- The absence of OAEs without middle ear pathology or acoustic obstruction strongly indicates sensory transmissive hearing loss. Depending on the type and intensity of stimulation, OAEs can reveal threshold elevations as small as 20 dB HL and the frequency 'resolution' of OAEs can be as good as one-half octave. The amount of threshold elevation cannot be predicted with any useful accuracy, but if DPOAEs are present with TEOAEs absent, this suggests mild-to-moderate loss only.

- OAEs are normally very stable with time and are valuable as a sensitive monitor of changes in cochlear (and middle ear) status over time, *e.g.* in relation to sudden hearing loss, Ménière's disease or noise trauma.

- Although OAEs can differ enormously between healthy ears, they are usually quite similar in the left and right ears. Substantial left–right differences may, therefore, indicate pathology.

Differential diagnosis

- OAEs are expected to be present in sensory transductive, neural, central and psychogenic hearing losses. OAEs can be either present or absent with 8th nerve tumours, depending on whether the cochlear blood supply has been compromised. If present, OAEs indicate the possibility of hearing recovery with a conservative surgical approach[43].

- OAEs are preneural responses indicating healthy cochlear status and cannot be used to detect sensory transductive or neural hearing losses. With neonates, the absence of an OAE response in clear dry ears should be treated as a strong risk factor for sensory hearing impairment. However, other risk factors need to be considered before presence of an

OAE is taken as evidence of normal hearing. Hyperbilirubinaemia or any risk of neurological damage requires that an ABR test also be conducted.

- Auditory neuropathy is indicated by the presence of normal OAEs but the absence of normal ABR responses. In such rare cases, the application of hearing aids with high amplification may be counterproductive, so in infants ABR and OAE testing should precede hearing aid selection.

Special applications

- OAEs can be slightly depressed by contralateral noise stimulation if the medial cochlear efferent system is operational. The significance of the absence of this effect is not clearly understood but may help clarify the nature of certain neural pathologies[48].

- The objective nature of OAEs can be useful in the investigation and management of inorganic hearing loss by demonstrating normal cochlear function to the patient.

- Serious tinnitus is almost never associated with OAEs, but rather with their absence (*see* Baguley, this volume). Spontaneous OAEs can sometimes be perceived as tinnitus and occasionally cause unnecessary anxiety. Typically, in such cases, hearing threshold is normal and the tinnitus is mild, tonal and easily maskable by noise. Patients can be re-assured by the objective demonstration of spontaneous OAEs.

References

1 Glattke TJ, Robinette MS. Transient evoked otoacoustic emissions. In: Robinette RM, Glattke T. (eds). *Otoacoustic Emissions – Clinical Applications*, 2nd edn. New York: Thieme, 2002; 95–115

2 Norton SJ, Gorga MP, Widen JE *et al.* Identification of neonatal hearing impairment: evaluation of transient evoked otoacoustic emission, distortion product otoacoustic emission and auditory brain stem response test performance. *Ear Hear* 2000; **21**: 508–28

3 Kemp DT. Stimulated acoustic emissions from within the human auditory system. *J Acoust Soc Am* 1978; **64**: 1386–91

4 Margolis RH. Influence of middle ear disease on otoacoustic emissions. In: Robinette RM, Glattke T. (eds). *Otoacoustic Emissions – Clinical Applications*, 2nd edn. New York: Thieme, 2002; 190–212

5 Yates GK. Human transient otoacoustic emissions recorded with a wideband stimulus and response system, *Assoc Res Otolaryngol* 2000; **22**: 5112

6 Harris FP, Probst R. Reporting click-evoked and distortion-product otoacoustic emission results with respect to the pure tone audiogram. *Ear Hear* 1991; **12**: 399–405

7 Harris FP, Probst R. Otoacoustic emissions and audiometric outcomes. In: Robinette RM, Glattke T. (eds). *Otoacoustic Emissions – Clinical Applications*, 2nd edn. New York: Thieme, 2002; 213–42

8 Prieve BA. Otoacoustic emissions in neonatal screening. In: Robinette RM, Glattke T. (eds). *Otoacoustic Emissions – Clinical Applications*, 2nd edn. New York: Thieme, 2002; 348–74

9 Hall III WH, *Handbook of Otoacoustic Emissions*. San Diego, CA: Singular, 2000

10 Kemp DT. Otoacoustic emissions: distorted echoes of the cochlea's travelling wave. In: Berlin C. (ed) *Otoacoustic Emissions: Basic Science and Clinical Applications*. San Diego, CA: Singular, 1998; 1–60

11 Lonsbury-Martin B, Martin GK, Telischi FF. Otoacoustic emissions in clinical practice. In: Musiek FE, Rintelmann WF. (eds) *Contemporary Perspectives in Hearing Assessment*, 3rd edn. Boston, MA: Allyn and Bacon, 1999; 167–96

12 Gorga MP, Neely ST, Dorn PA. Distortion product otoacoustic emissions in relation to hearing loss. In: Robinette RM, Glattke T. (eds). *Otoacoustic Emissions – Clinical Applications*, 2nd edn. New York: Thieme, 2002; 243–72

13 Boege P, Janssen TH. Pure tone threshold estimation from extrapolated distortion product otoacoustic emission I/O-functions in normal and cochlear hearing loss ears. *J Acoust Soc Am* 2002; **111**: 1810–18

14 Robinette RM, Glattke T. (eds). *Otoacoustic Emissions – Clinical Applications*, 2nd edn. New York: Thieme, 2002

15 O'Mahoney CF, Kemp DT. Distortion product otoacoustic emission delay measurement in human ears. *J Acoust Soc Am* 1995; **97**: 3721–35

16 von Bekey G. *Experiments in Hearing*. New York: McGraw Hill; 1960

17 Johnstone BM, Patuzzi R, Yates GK. Basilar membrane measurements and the travelling wave. *Hear Res* 1986; **22**: 147–53

18 Brass D, Kemp DT. Analyses of Mossbauer mechanical measurements indicate that the cochlea is mechanically active, *J Acoust Soc Am* 1993, **93**: 1502–15

19 Gold T. Hearing II. The physical basis of the action of the cochlea. *Proc R Soc Lond B Biol Sci* 1948; **135**: 492–8

20 Kemp DT. Evidence of mechanical nonlinearity and frequency selective wave amplification in the cochlea. *Arch Otorhinolaryngol* 1979; **224**: 37–45

21 Brownell WE. Observations on a motile response in isolated outer hair cells. In: Webster WR, Aitken L. (eds) *Mechanisms of Hearing*. Clayton, Australia: Monash University Press, 1983; 5–10

22 Knight RD, Kemp DT. Wave and place fixed DPOAE maps of the human ear. *J Acoust Soc Am* 2001; **109**: 1513–25

23 Shera CA, Guinan JJ. Evoked otoacoustic emissions arise from by two fundamentally different mechanisms: a taxonomy for mammalian OAEs. *J Acoust Soc Am* 1999; **105**: 782–98

24 Yates GK, Whithnell RH. Intermodulation distortion in click evoked otoacoustic emissions. *Assoc Res Otolaryngol* 1998; **21**: 17

25 Kemp DT, Knight RD. Virtual DP reflector explains DPOAE wave and place fixed dichotomy. *Assoc Res Otolaryngol* 1999; **22**: 39

26 Harris FP, Lonsbury-Martin BL, Stagner BB, Coats AC, Martin GK. Acoustic distortion products in humans: systematic changes in amplitude as a function of f2/f1 ratio. *J Acoust Soc Am* 1989; **85**: 220–9

27 Penner MJ, Zhang T. Prevalence of spontaneous otoacoustic emissions in adults revisited. *Hear Res* 1997; **103**: 28–34

28 Burns EM, Arehart KH, Campbell SL. Prevalence of spontaneous otoacoustic emissions in neonates. *J Acoust Soc Am* 1992; **91**: 1571–5

29 Lepage EL, Murray NM. Latent cochlear damage in personal stereo users: a study based on click-evoked otoacoustic emissions. *Med J Aust* 1998; **169**: 588–92

30 Kemp DT. Cochlear echoes: implications for noise-induced hearing loss. In: Hamernik RP, Henderson D, Salvi R. (eds) *New Perspectives on Noise-Induced Hearing Loss*. New York: Raven, 1982; 189–207

31 Engdahl B, Kemp DT. The effect of noise exposure on the details of distortion product otoacoustic emissions. *J Acoust Soc Am* 1996; **99**: 1573–87

32 Wilson JP. Evidence for a cochlear origin of acoustic re-emissions threshold fine structure and tonal tinnitus. *Hear Res* 1980; **2**: 233–52

33 Wilson JP, Evans EF. Effects of furosemide, flaxedil, noise and tone over-stimulation on the evoked otoacoustic emissions in the ear canal of gerbil, *Proceedings of the International Union of Physiological Science* 1983; **15**: 100

34 Long GR, Tubis A. Modification of spontaneous and evoked otoacoustic emissions and associated psychoacoustic microstructure by aspirin consumption. *J Acoust Soc Am* 1988; **84**: 1343–53

35 Kummer P, Janssen T, Arnold W. Suppression tuning characteristics of the 2f1–f2 distortion product emission in humans. *J Acoust Soc Am* 1995; **98**: 197–210

36 Harris FP, Glattke T. The use of suppression to determine the characteristics of otoacoustic emissions. *Semin Hear* 1992; **13**: 67–80

37 Brown AM, Kemp DT. Suppressibility of the 2f1–f2 stimulated acoustic emissions in gerbil and man. *Hear Res* 1984; **13**: 29–37

38 Collet L, Kemp DT, Veuillet E, Duclaux R, Moulin A, Morgon A. Effect of contralateral auditory stimuli on active cochlear micro-mechanical properties in human subjects. *Hear Res* 1990; **43**: 251–62

39 Velenovsky DS, Glattke TJ. Contralateral and binaural suppression of otoacoustic emissions. In: Robinette RM, Glattke T. (eds). *Otoacoustic Emissions – Clinical Applications*, 2nd edn. New York: Thieme, 2002; 163–89

40 Perrot X, Micheyl C, Khalfa S, Collet L. Stronger bilateral efferent influences on cochlear biomechanical activity in musicians than in non-musicians. *Neurosci Lett* 1999; **262**: 167–70

41 Veuillet E, Bazin F, Collet L. Objective evidence of peripheral auditory disorders in learning impaired children. *J Audiol Med* 1999; **8**: 18–29

42 Veuillet E, Khalfa S, Collet L. Clinical relevance of medial efferent auditory pathways. *Scand Audiol Suppl* 1999; **51**: 53–62

43 Robinette MS, Cevette MJ, Webb TM. Otoacoustic emissions in differential diagnosis. In: Robinette RM, Glattke T. (eds). *Otoacoustic Emissions – Clinical Applications*, 2nd edn. New York: Thieme, 2002; 297–324

44 Widen JE, O'Grady GM. Evoked otoacoustic emissions in the evaluation of children. In: Robinette RM, Glattke T. (eds). *Otoacoustic Emissions – Clinical Applications*, 2nd edn. New York: Thieme, 2002; 375–415

45 Moore BCJ. *Cochlear Hearing Loss*. London: Whurr; 1998

46 Kemp DT, Ryan S, Bray P. A guide to the effective use of otoacoustic emissions, *Ear Hear* 1990; **11**: 93–105

47 Kemp DT. Exploring cochlear status with otoacoustic emissions. In: Robinette RM, Glattke T. (eds). *Otoacoustic Emissions – Clinical Applications*, 2nd edn. New York: Thieme, 2002; 1–47

48 Collet L, Veuillet E, Bene J, Morgon A. Effects of contralateral white noise on click-evoked emissions in normal and sensorineural ears: Towards an exploration of the medial olivocochlear system. *Audiology* 1992; **31**: 1–7

Index

Vaccination

Scientific Editors: Peter C L Beverley, Leszek Borysiewicz, Adrian V S Hill, Ian G Jones and J G Patrick Sissons

http://www.bmb.oupjournals.org